Cardiopulmonary Bypass: Physiology, Related Complications, and Pharmacology

Edited by

Pierre A. Casthely, MD

Professor of Anesthesiology,
Seton Hall University School of Graduate Medical Education,
South Orange, New Jersey *and* Department of Anesthesiology,
Division of Cardiothoracic Anesthesia,
St. Joseph Hospital and Medical Center, Paterson, New Jersey

and

David Bregman, MD

Professor of Surgery,
Seton Hall University School of Graduate Medical Education,
South Orange, New Jersey *and* Chief, Department of Surgery,
St. Joseph's Hospital and Medical Center,
Paterson, New Jersey

FUTURA

Futura Publishing Company, Inc.

Mount Kisco, NY
1991

Library of Congress Cataloging-in-Publication Data

Cardiopulmonary bypass: physiology, related complications, and pharmacology / edited by Pierre A. Casthely and David Bregman.
p. cm.
Includes bibliographical references and index.
ISBN 8-87993-396-8
1. Cardiopulmonary bypass. I. Casthely, Pierre A. II. Bregman, David.
[DNLM: 1. Cardiopulmonary Bypass—methods. 3. Cardiovascular Agents—pharmacology. WG 168 C2657]
RD598.C37 1991
617.4'12059—dc20
DNLM/DLC
for Library of Congress 91-16171
CIP

Published by
Futura Publishing Company, Inc.
2 Bedford Ridge Road
Mount Kisco, New York 10549

Every effort has been made to ensure that the information in this book is as up to date and accurate as possible at the time of publication. However, due to the constant developments in medicine, neither the author, nor the editor, nor the publisher can accept any legal or any other responsibility for any errors or omissions that may occur.

Printed in the United States of America.

Foreword

Knowledge is of two kinds: we know a subject ourselves, or we know where we can find information upon it.

Samuel Johnson, quoted in Boswell's Life and Samuel Johnson, April 18, 1775.

Information's pretty thin stuff, unless mixed with experience.

Clarence Day, "The Three Tigers". The Crow's Next, 1921.

In the nearly 40 years since the use of cardiopulmonary bypass was initiated, we have challenged the complexities of congenital heart disease and the ravages of valvular and coronary artery disease with more aggressive surgery. Much of that is due to a better understanding of physiology in addition to improved equipment for artificial perfusion and substantial improvements in anesthesia and pharmacology. Indeed, there are now nearly 400,000 procedures performed yearly in the United States alone that require cardiopulmonary bypass support. Coronary artery bypass surgery is one of the most frequent of all surgeries and consumes a large portion of the nation's health financial resources. Although it is clear from the literature that the patient population has changed, overall morbidity and mortality has not increased drastically. Whether we are personally involved in the perioperative patient care for such surgeries, or are in the midst of training for such responsibilities, or are simply curious about this specialized field we often seek authoritative texts such as *Cardiopulmonary Bypass:*

Physiology, Related Complications, and Pharmacology organized by Drs. Casthely and Bregman. This text represents the accumulation and organization of a large body of knowledge. A significant portion of these discussions addresses the multiorgan dysfunctions that may occur with cardiopulmonary bypass. Whether grossly obvious or extremely subtle in nature, these "side effects" of cardiopulmonary bypass point to the direction that future investigative studies must go.

In a multiple author text such as this, we anticipate each subject to be thoroughly researched and to combine the most recent information available prior to submission for publication with the experience gained through patient care by the individual authors. The chapters found here represent that combination of scientific information with practical application.

In addition, one must expect differences between authors in their styles of presentation, some of which may reflect institutional preferences as well as similar material presented from different perspectives. That can be instructional as well, for it affords the reader the opportunity to analyze differences in philosophy as well as concepts.

The knowledge and information presented in this book is very up-to-date and is a solid base on which to add the even more recent scientific discoveries found in the respected journals.

Norman J. Starr, MD
Chairman, Department of
Cardiothoracic Anesthesiology
Cleveland Clinic Foundation
Cleveland, Ohio

Preface

The advent of cardiopulmonary bypass in 1953 and its further and continuous refinements have securely established the specialty of cardiovascular surgery and, in conjunction with improved methods of myocardial preservation, have allowed the safe repair of acquired and complex congenital cardiac defects. During the years, the many variables of the cardiopulmonary bypass system have been altered to the point that most operations are now reproducible with very low morbidity and mortality. Although in its present form the system is quite adequate for most routine surgery, it is far from perfect and the continued quest for alterations to improve the system is an ongoing process. The cardiopulmonary bypass system has also been used as a unique and ingenious method for partial cardiac support in patients undergoing percutaneous transluminal angioplasty. Albeit, certain complications of open heart surgery are part and parcel of the procedure, many new and unique approaches to the concept of organ protection and the treatment of these complications have been developed, refined, and expounded upon in recent years. An area of continued development and exciting success has been in the pharmacological support of the failing heart and in modern anesthetic management in the pre- and postoperative setting.

This book is an effort to bring together the most modern concepts and treatment in the area of cardiopulmonary bypass and its clinical ramifications. The complications engendered during cardiopulmonary bypass are dealt with in detail, as well as the use of both pharmacological support and mechanical circulatory support techniques in the pre- and postoperative period. Finally, aside from routine cardiac surgical procedures, surgery of the thoracic aneurysm and cardiac transplantation are dealt with in detail, including their anesthetic considerations. This book represents the latest information in the developments in cardiac surgery cardiac anesthesia and perfusion technology by a group of experts who collectively represent the leaders in their fields.

We want to thank our families for their complete support during those long working hours required to complete this project. A special thanks goes to Mr. Steven Korn, who has guided us from the beginning with constructive comments and has been very instrumental in the making of this book. We thank his editorial staff, especially Ms. Ann Kerr who has reviewed and corrected the entire manuscript. We would like to thank all the authors from whose work I have borrowed important illustrative material. We also acknowledge the help of Ellen Jackson, Wilma Rivera, Zoraida Rivera and Rose Trottain in the preparation of the manuscript, and Ken Morris for preparing the illustrations for this book. We also gratefully acknowledge the help of our colleagues in cardiac anesthesia, cardiac surgery, and cardiology for their outstanding contributions and their expertly written chapters.

Pierre A. Casthely, MD
David Bregman, MD

Contributors

Karl A. Bocchieri, BS, CCP Long Island Jewish Hospital and Medical Center, New Hyde Park, New York

David Bregman, MD Professor of Surgery, Seton Hall University School of Graduate Medical Education, South Orange, New Jersey *and* Chief, Department of Surgery, St. Joseph's Hospital and Medical Center, Paterson, New Jersey

Pierre A. Casthely, MD Professor of Anesthesiology, Seton Hall University School of Graduate Medical Education, South Orange, New Jersey *and* Department of Anesthesiology, Division of Cardiothoracic Anesthesia, St. Joseph's Hospital and Medical Center, Paterson, New Jersey

Jairo E. Castillo, MD Department of Anesthesiology, Long Island Jewish Hospital and Medical Center, New Hyde Park, New York

B. Chandrasekaran, MD Associate Professor of Medicine, Seton Hall University, Division of Nephrology, St. Joseph's Hospital and Medical Center, Paterson, New Jersey

Ellise Delphin, MD Associate Professor of Clinical Anesthesiology, Columbia University, Columbia Presbyterian Medical Center, New York, New York

John Dluzneski, MD Department of Anesthesiology, Division of Cardiovascular Anesthesiology, Englewood Hospital, Englewood, Florida

Charles M. Fermon, MD Department of Anesthesiology, Long Island Jewish Hospital and Medical Center, New Hyde Park, New York

Phillip Fyman, MD Department of Anesthesiology, Division of Cardiac Anesthesia, Long Island Jewish Hospital and Medical Center, New Hyde Park, New York

Michael J. Given, MD Instructor in Medicine, Seton Hall University School of Graduate Medical Education, South Orange, New Jersey *and* Department of Medicine, Division of Pulmonary Medicine, St. Joseph's Hospital and Medical Center, Paterson, New Jersey

Sheldon Goldstein, MD Assistant Professor of Anesthesiology, Health Science Center, Division of Cardiac Anesthesia, State University of New York, Brooklyn, New York

Alexander W. Gotta, MD Professor of Clinical Anesthesiology, Vice-Chairman for Academic Affairs, Department of Anesthesiology, Health Science Center, State University of New York, Brooklyn, New York

James Harding, MD Department of Anesthesiology, Columbia University, Columbia Presbyterian Medical Center, New York, New York

Roberta Hines, MD Associate Professor of Anesthesiology, Yale University School of Medicine, New Haven, Connecticut

Douglas Jackson, MD Assistant Professor of Anesthesiology, Columbia University, Columbia Presbyterian Hospital, New York, New York

Ayad Jihayel, MD Assistant Professor of Surgery, Seton Hall University School of Graduate Medical Education, *and* Department of Surgery, Division of Cardiothoracic Surgery, St. Joseph's Hospital and Medical Center, Paterson, New Jersey

Andrew Karlin, MD Assistant Professor of Anesthesiology, Health Science Center, State University of New York, Brooklyn, New York, *and* Clinical Director of Anesthesia, Kings County Medical Center, Brooklyn, New York

Michael B. Kesselbrenner, MD Associate Professor of Medicine, Seton Hall University School of Graduate Medical Education, *and* Department of Medicine, Division of Cardiology, St. Joseph's Hospital and Medical Center, Paterson, New Jersey

M. Anees Khan, MD, FACP, FCCP Associate Clinical Professor of Medicine, University of Medicine and Dentistry, Newark, New Jersey, *and* Professor of Medicine, Seton Hall University School of Graduate Medical Center, South Orange, New Jersey, *and* Chief, Pulmonary Division, St. Joseph's Hospital and Medical Center, Paterson, New Jersey

Bruce Kleiman, MD Associate Professor of Anesthesiology & Medicine, Loyola University Medical Center, Maywood, Illinois

Claudia Komer, MD Assistant Professor of Anesthesiology, Seton Hall University School of Graduate Medical Education, South Orange, New Jersey

Soomyung Lee, MD Director of Cardiothoracic Anesthesia, The Jack D. Weiler Hospital of the Albert Einstein College of Medicine, *and* Assistant Professor, Department of Anesthesiology, Albert Einstein College of Medicine/Montefiore Medical Center, Bronx, New York

Youngick Lee, MD Assistant Professor of Surgery, Seton Hall University School of Graduate Medical Education, South Orange, New Jersey *and* Department of Surgery, Division of Cardiothoracic Surgery, St. Joseph's Hospital and Medical Center, Paterson, New Jersey

Charles Marrin, MD Assistant Professor of Surgery, Dartmouth Hitchcock Medical Center, Hanover, New Hampshire

Robert C. Mayer, MD Department of Cardiovascular Anesthesia, Lutheran General Hospital, Park Ridge, Illinois

Gerard McCloskey, MD Assistant Professor of Anesthesiology, Yale University School of Medicine, New Haven, Connecticut

Haroutune Mekhjian, MD Chief, Division of Cardiothoracic Surgery, St. Joseph's Hospital and Medical Center, Paterson, New Jersey

Bennett A. Mitchell, MA, CCP Albert Einstein College of Medicine, School of Perfusion Technology, Bronx, New York

John Niedzinski, CCP St. Joseph's Hospital and Medical Center, Paterson, New Jersey

William C. Nugent, MD Professor of Surgery, Dartmouth School of Medicine, *and* Chairman, Division of Cardiothoracic Surgery, Dartmouth-Hitchcock Medical Center, Hanover, New Hampshire

Jeffrey Sack, MD Clinical Instructor of Medicine, Department of Cardiology, Montefiore Hospital, Pittsburgh, Pennsylvania

George Vretakis, MD Department of Anesthesiology, Long Island Jewish Hospital and Medical Center. New Hyde Park, New York

Thil Yoganathan, MD Professor of Anesthesiology, Seton Hall University School of Graduate Medical Education, South Orange, New Jersey *and* Department of Anesthesiology Division of Cardiothoracic Anesthesia, St. Joseph's Hospital and Medical Center Paterson, New Jersey

This book is dedicated to our mentors:

Herman Turndorf, MD

Norman J. Starr, MD

James R. Malm, MD

Keith Reemtsma, MD

Frederick O. Bowman, Jr, MD

Contents

Chapter 1

Historical Aspects of Cardiopulmonary Surgery

Jairo E. Castillo, MD,
Karl A. Bocchieri, BS, CCP,
Phillip Fyman, MD,
and Charles Fermon, MD

The current practice of cardiopulmonary bypass (CPB) surgery is the outgrowth of many lines of development, all designed to maintain the patient in as a physiologic a state as possible during the operation. In this chapter the principal developments are traced from their origins in the last century to the present.

Transfusion Practices

During the early days of CPB, in the mid-1950s, one of the largest obstacles was the large volumes of blood needed to prime the bypass pump, which made heart surgery cumbersome and dangerous.[1] At first, fresh heparinized blood was used. This presented

From Casthely PA, Bregman D, (eds): *Cardiopulmonary Bypass: Physiology, Related Complications, and Pharmacology.* Mount Kisco, NY, Futura Publishing Company, Inc., © 1991.

a problem, however, as blood had to be drawn from seven or eight donors on the day of surgery, often delaying the beginning of the operation until late afternoon or evening. To avoid this delay, hospitals began collecting blood the day before. Again, heparin was used to store the whole blood because of the concern about the effects of citrated blood on the calcium balance of the myocardium. The need for large volumes of blood for heart surgery created a strain on blood banks and transfusion services throughout the country, as reflected in the parallel increases in demand for blood and blood components and the growth in cardiac surgery.[2] In some institutions, two thirds of the blood resources were used for patients undergoing cardiovascular surgery.[2]

The dangers of large volume blood transfusions that were to assume such importance in the 1980s became apparent early. In 1962, Gadboys, Slonim and Litwak[3] made an important advance in heart surgery with the description of a homologous blood syndrome. Blood from different donors was shown to interact, causing various reactions that led to the sequestration of blood in the periphery. The risk of infectious complications was recognized as early as in the 1930s.[4] Transfusion-associated hepatitis marked by jaundice was reported in 1943.[5]

Because of these problems, other means of priming the bypass pump had to be developed. In the early 1960s, crystalloid priming evolved and was used effectively.[6] This development reduced the requirement for blood and also enabled surgeons to operate on patients of the Jehovah's Witness faith and others to whom blood transfusion is unacceptable. Pumps also evolved with a decrease in the necessary priming volume.

The introduction of plastic tubing and bags in the 1950s helped produce blood component therapy in the 1960s.[7] Prior to that time, blood banks were able to supply only two items: whole blood and plasma. With the development of differential centrifugation, whole blood could be separated into various components: red blood cells (RBC), platelets, and plasma by virtue of their different specific gravities. Contemporary transfusion services can provide 25 or more blood products.[8] The reliance on component therapy has permitted a more efficient use of the blood available for open heart surgery. Specific components can be given as available when needed, and the administration of unnecessary components is avoided. With the advancement in surgical technique and the availability of pumps, the 1970s saw a rapid growth in cardiac surgical procedures. In addition to receiving several units of RBC, most patients also received platelets and fresh frozen plasma prophylactically.[7]

Several factors led to a lowering of the number of homologous blood exposures during open heart surgery in the 1980s. We have to keep in mind that during the decades that cardiac surgery was developed, the medical community knew about, but assigned minimal clinical importance to the many risks of blood transfusions. The most common of these risks has been febrile and urticarial reactions that were associated with only minor morbidity. Serious morbidity and death from transfusion-associated sepsis and viral infections had been so rare that few physicians altered their clinical practices to decrease the risks. In 1984, however the epidemiologic linking of the uniformly lethal acquired immunodeficiency syndrome (AIDS) to transfused blood and blood products led to accelerated and dramatic changes in transfusion practices.[4] Researchers soon developed the technology to detect infectious agents or identify associated markers. Therefore, the wave of public concern came at a time when blood banks were intensifying efforts at providing a generally safe blood supply. Also in the 1980s, it became common practice to accept lower hematocrits in the postoperative period.[9] Moreover, prophylactic fresh frozen plasma and platelets were discontinued in many centers.[10] In recent years, emphasis has been placed on autologous blood transfusions, and the development of intraoperative blood salvage devices has allowed open heart surgery to be performed with minimal blood transfusion. A final development is that more emphasis has been given to understanding and improving oxygen delivery to the tissues.[11] Of course, many factors play a role in oxygen delivery but this research has opened the door to means of maintaining oxygen delivery without directly increasing the red cell mass.

There has been a resurgence of interest in the use of whole blood in open heart surgery.[7] One group of investigators has shown that one unit of whole blood is at least as effective on platelet aggregation as eight to ten units of platelets.[12] Use of single units of whole blood definitely decreases the number of donors to whom a patient is exposed and therefore decreases the risk of transmitting infection.

Thus, blood transfusion during cardiac surgery has gone through many phases of evolution. The extremes of clinical practice ranged from the shotgun approach of recipe transfusion to the more detailed work-up of coagulation deficiencies and targeted therapy. Today, the emphasis is more conservative because of the impending risk of deadly infections transmissible by transfusions.

Anticoagulation During Cardiopulmonary Bypass

Despite years of research since the early heart-lung machines were developed by Dewall, Lillehei, Cooley and others, extracorporeal circulation systems are still being made of materials that stimulate the coagulation process. Thus, one problem faced in the early days of cardiac surgery, dating back to Cradford and associates[13-15] in the 1920s remains. It is clear that sufficient anticoagulation must be established to prevent the formation of both macrothrombi and microthrombi during the pump run, but the means of achieving, maintaining and monitoring an adequate level of anticoagulation is still an area of much debate.

Heparin has been used to inhibit coagulation since the introduction of CPB.[16] This natural substance has been highly satisfactory because it is specific and has few side effects if used properly. Throughout the years, heparin has therefore endured as the most popular anticoagulant, probably because of the absence of a time limit and the fact that it has an antidote.[16]

Loading and maintenance dosages of heparin have been studied extensively by various investigators.[17-21] In the early days of CPB, patients were given a fixed dose based on their weight, height, and age.[19] With time, however, it was found that the heparin response has a large variability and that the amount of heparin required to produce an arbitrary prolongation in the clotting time can vary as much as threefold from patient to patient.[19] This discovery showed that a fixed protocol dose of heparin was too rigid. Low-dosage heparin may not prevent invisible low-grade coagulation and has the disadvantage of depleting coagulation factors with concurrent fibrinolysis.[22-25] By the same token, high dosage heparin has the disadvantage of masking an antithrombin III deficiency, causing platelet dysfunction, and creating a difficult reversal.[26-29]

It was clear that a useful and efficient method of administering individualized dosages was needed.

It was the landmark work of Bull and associates[18,19] that demonstrated that the fixed dose heparin regimen resulted in some patients being inadequately heparinized as well as others overheparinized. Those investigators stressed the importance of maintaining the clotting time at an appropriate level as well as of the appropriate reversal of heparin at the termination of bypass. This work pointed to the establishment of a dose-response relation using the activated clotting time as an endpoint. The dose-response curve allowed a more precise approach to heparin and protamine dosage. Bull and coworkers[18,19] used celite ACT determinations because of their accuracy and simplicity, and made the observation that no clot was apparent in the operative field or was captured in the oxygenator if the manual ACT exceeded 300 seconds. They recommended a minimum value of 480 seconds. Ellison and associates[21] made similar observations using protamine titration and the ACT. Young et al.[25] recommended a 400-second minimum ACT in humans. The studies by Bull and coworkers[18,19] have led to a more precise control of heparinization that has eliminated the development of disseminated intravascular coagulation, hyperheparnimia, and protamine excess.

Reversal of Anticoagulation

In the same fashion that heparin was administered in the early days, protamine was administered in a fixed dose ratio, i.e., 1–1.5 times the initial dose of heparin.[30] However, protamine has not been found to be benign, with substantial hemodynamic changes and a degree of anticoagulant activity appearing when the drug is used in excess.[31]

In 1956, Perkins et al.[32] described a method for protamine titration in the operating room. Later, in 1966, Hawskley and coworkers[30] reported on the effectiveness and accuracy of protamine titration. More recently, Umlas and colleagues[33] described the direct measurement of heparin level by a method that does not depend on clotting (i.e., direct measurement of procoagulant levels). This method allowed for a reasonably accurate calculation of the total body heparin content and thus of a direct protamine dosage.

The Role of Desmopressin Acetate

Despite the rapid success of cardiovascular surgery and the advancement in anticoagulation and reversal, postoperative bleeding has been a persistent concern, with hemorrhagic complications forcing the surgeon to reexplore the chest in many cases.[34] Bick[35] demonstrated that the hemorrhagic tendency accompanying CPB is a complex reflection of many hemostatic defects, such as thrombocytopenia, platelet function abnormality, mild fibrinolysis, unneutralized heparin, and excessive protamine.[36,37]

Desmopressin acetate (DDAVP) is a synthetic vasopressin analog that lacks vasoconstrictor abilities. It first came into use in the mid-1970s for patients with mild hemophilia A or von Willebrand's disease, in whom it was found to shorten the bleeding time by inducing release of factor VIII.[38-41] The drug was also shown to reduce the bleeding time and surgical blood loss in patients with abnormal platelet function and certain thrombopathic states.[42,43] Because platelet dysfunction was thought to be a significant etiologic actor in bleeding after CPB, Salzman et al.[36] studied the use of DDAVP in postbypass patients. Those investigators demonstrated a significant reduction in bleeding and postoperative transfusion requirements. The mechanism of action of DDAVP may be complex, but it seems to involve an elevation in factor VIII concentrations and a subsequent increase in platelet activity.

Myocardial Preservation

Since the beginning of cardiac surgery, special attention has been devoted to developing a proper technique for myocardial preservation. As an example, Melrose et al.[44] in 1955 used chemical potassium citrate cardioplegia to induce cardiac arrest experimentally. A significant drawback was that normal ventricular function could not be restored in some animals despite the normal microscopic appearance of the treated tissue. Potassium citrate cardioplegia was abandoned in the late 1950s when reports described a significant incidence of ventricular fibrillation without adequate ventricular decompression.[45] This response led to fatty degeneration after a short period of ischemia. It thus became evident that myocardial protection was complex and entailed different measures to reduce tissue oxygen consumption and thus to decrease the amount of damage during the ischemic period. Myocardial oxygen demand was decreased by cardiac standstill[46] which was accomplished by aortic crossclamping, continuous electrical fibrillation, or both. Also, cardiac metabolic demands were reduced by lowering the temperature.

In 1957, Gollan and Nelson Gollan[47] reported on the use of systemic hypothermia. A few years earlier, Shumway and associates[48] described selective topical hypothermia for the heart. Maloney and Nelson[49] reviewed the literature prior to 1975 and concluded that the safe ischemic period of 20 minutes at 32°C, could be extended to 30 minutes at 16° to 20°C.[49] The relation between hypothermia, the heart rate, and subendocardial blood flow was described by Swan in the early 1970s.[50]

Because of the increasing demand for repair of major lesions, necessitating longer periods of cardiac arrest, new methods of arrest had to be developed. In 1973, Gay and Ebert[51] substituted potassium chloride for potassium citrate cardioplegia and reduced the potassium concentration. Their cardioplegic solution produced slight myocardial edema, but the normal architecture of the myocytes was maintained.

Adequate myocardial protection required a thorough understanding of the detrimental cellular changes resulting from ischemia and of the mechanisms through which cardioplegia protects; energy conservation during rapid diastolic arrest, slowing of metabolic and degenerative processes through hypothermia, and selective prevention of ischemic changes. Obtaining this knowledge required a special analysis of myocardial ion balances, substrate need, and oxygen balance. It was found that if high-potassium cardioplegia was used to maintain arrest, the heart had a higher incidence of AV dissociation dysrythmias. Reidemeister and coworkers[52] suggested the use of potassium chloride cardioplegia in a solution containing 20 mEq of potassium per liter to produce asystole, with repeated infusions of potassium chloride at 5 mEq per liter being given to maintain arrest. Also, it was found that potassium chloride in a concentration greater than 30 mEq per liter produced intimal damage and increased coronary vascular resistance secondary to a calcium-activated rise in left ventricular tension.[53]

Magnesium also plays an important role in myocardial protection. When magnesium levels are elevated to a cardioplegic concentration; i.e., 15 mEq per liter, the inherent rhythmicity of pacemaker cells and contractility are depressed.[54] Magnesium is important for enzyme activation in reactions that convert ATP to ADP, thereby making energy available. Magnesium also is involved in the production of cyclic AMP.[55] Recent studies suggest that patients with left ventricular hypertrophy may suffer from hypomagnesemia. Pretreatment with oral magnesium salts and the addition of magnesium sulfate to the pump prime may reduce the incidence of dysrrythmias in patients with left ventricular hypertrophy.[56]

Analysis of the principles of ischemic arrest has revealed that control of calcium movement is critical in effective protection of the heart.[57] Calcium movement is involved in contracture and relaxation of the myocardium. In hypoxia, the cell membrane becomes excessively permeable to calcium from the extracellular space, causing an accumulation that leads to a contraction, a response that became known as the "stone heart syndrome." This condition is life-threatening, and therefore, it is imperative to prevent the accumulation of calcium. There is also a condition known as the calcium paradox. In this condition, the heart has been perfused for some time with a solution containing less than 0.05 mmol of calcium per liter and then reperfused with a solution that has a normal calcium concentration. Tissue damage ensues, and contracture occurs. Massive calcium influx to intracellular sites seems to be responsible.[58] In laboratory and clinical research on calcium antagonists and slow calcium channels, these medications were found to have a protective effect on the heart.[57] Hearse and coworkers[59] stressed that calcium channel blockers could act as an insurance policy against regional poor perfusion and poor cooling. It has therefore become the practice to use calcium channel blockers during open heart surgery.[57]

Significant breakthroughs have been made in myocardial preservation in the last 30 years, as shown by the reduction of the early mortality rate of aortocoronary surgery to 1% in first operations. Nevertheless, there are many gaps to be filled.

The History of Pumps and Oxygenators

In the development of CBP, there were two basic functions that had to be addressed: methods to oxygenate the blood and the means to pump the blood through this device and back to the patient. Today many different oxygenators and pumps are available commercially, enabling perfusionists and surgeons to choose the one that best fills their requirements. However, the pioneers of CPB had to build everything they needed. The earliest pumps were adapted from research physiologists methods to study organ function in isolation.[60]

Porter and Bradley were granted a patent on a forerunner of the roller pump in 1855, but this device was not widely used until DeBakey in the United States, and Henry and Jouvelet in France, made some modifications and adapted it for CBP in 1934.[60,61] Many of the early experiments used a pump developed by Dale and Schuster in 1928[62] that caused blood within it to move forward. Another early machine that was used clinically was the sigmamotor pump.[63] This device had occlusive "fingers" that rhythmically compressed the tubing to propel the blood in a forward direction. These pumps produced a pulsatile waveform and were thought at the time to be more physiologic than the roller pump. However, because of their complexity, the difficulty with synchronization at high flow rates, and the extensive hemolysis they caused, the pulsatile device lost favor over time, and the roller pump became the standard. Its advantages include ease of set-up and use. Also in the event of power failure or malfunction (common in early CBP cases), the pump could be cranked by hand, and the roller pump delivered a more even pulse wave that was less traumatic to the blood, causing less hemolysis. As the pumps became more refined, they incorporated auto shut-off systems triggered by high pressure, low level, or gas emboli. These developments all led to ease of use and greater patient safety. The roller pump had become the standard.

In the early 1970s the centrifugal pump was developed as a type of implantable artificial heart. This application was soon abandoned, although the pumps are used as left ventricular assist devices. After further development, some centers began using this device instead of the arterial roller pump. The Biomedicus device

(Medtronic Cardiopulmonary Division, Anaheim, CA, USA) consists of cone-shaped impellers encased in a cone-shaped housing. They are magnetically coupled to a motor in the console. This device uses the principle of a constrained vortex to generate pressure and flow. More recently, another type of centrifugal pump was marketed by Sarns 3M (Sarns, 3M Health Care, Ann Arbor, MI, USA). This Delplim pump has impeller blades that rotate and thus generate flow and pressure within the head. The centrifugal pumps have the advantage of depriming when faced with a large bolus of air, making it difficult to pass gross air to the patient. However, small amounts of air will be broken down into many small emboli, and many would be carried out of the unit, especially at high flow rates.[64] Both manufacturers claim that their units reduce hemolysis and platelet destruction, and there have been numerous studies to prove this. However, some surgeons feel that for the short CPB times of today, it makes no difference to the patient whether a centrifugal pump is used and also that the added cost is prohibitive. Also, these pumps are not without their disadvantages. Because they are nonocclusive, their forward flow is dependent on the internal pressure in the head created by rotation and the peripheral resistance. As the peripheral resistance increases, the flows are independent. A separate flow sensor is used to measure the actual outlet blood flow.

Many different paths were likewise taken to accomplish oxygenation of the blood. For a short period, some surgeons used cross-circulation with a living donor; others used human donor lungs incorporated into the bypass system.[65] Both of these approaches were abandoned early because of their high risk and complexity in a clinical setting. Others turned to mechanical methods, which were adapted and refined to the state we have today.

In 1915, Hooker[66] described an oxygenator in which blood was dropped on a rotating horizontal disc. The centrifugal force spread the blood out to a thin film, and it was then thrown off the disc to the inside of a cylinder, where it fell to the bottom and was collected and transfused. Bayliss and his coworkers[67] modified this device to include more than one disc. This adaptation increased the surface area, enabling perfusion of large subjects.

Also in 1915, Richards and Drinker[68] reported on an oxygenator for isolated organ perfusion.[68] Their device used silk screens over which blood was poured. The blood ran down the screens, which exposed two sides to oxygen, giving twice the efficiency of the solid disc oxygenator. The blood also ran down the screens in a turbulent fashion, which caused mixing and more even oxygenation of the deeper layer of the blood film. These screen and disc oxygenators became widely used in research, and eventually Dewnis, in 1951, reported on his modifications to the apparatus (he replaced the solid disc with rotation screens) and its first use in human patients.

This report was soon followed by the use by Gibbon and coworkers[69] of a stationary vertical screen oxygenator to perform the first successful bypass in man. The developments by Melrose[70] (1953) and Crosss et al.[71] (1956) of the disc oxygenator were to help spread its dominance throughout the United States and the world.

There were many problems with the early pump and oxygenator machines. They were large and cumbersome, with complex assemblies that had to be dismantled, cleaned, sterilized, and reassembled each time a procedure was performed. The early pumps were completely automatic. They sensed venous blood inflow and varied their output in relation to it. They had numerous safety devices to sense pressure, oxygenation, volume, and venous return. Even though these features enabled surgeons to work without total attention to the pump, they increased the complexity of the machine greatly and thus increased the chance for a malfunction. Moreover, these pumps and oxygenators all used electric motors capable of creating sparks during a time when anesthesiologists were still widely using flammable anesthetic gases. To prevent explosions the motors and equipment had to be sealed from the atmosphere, greatly reducing the ability to monitor the equipment.

As cardiac surgery became more common, simpler and more efficient devices were developed. Most tubing was disposable, and soon, oxygenators were to be made that were similarly disposable.

Direct injection of oxygen into the blood was introduced by von Schroder in 1882,[72] and this method had been used in the laboratory as the standard for organ perfusion. The first bubble oxygenator was presented by Clark et al.[73] in 1950. By using a sintered-glass filter in the venous blood path, they directly oxygenated the blood. This method necessitated the development of a way to remove the millions of microbubbles before retransfusing the oxygenated blood. This group developed a method to decrease surface tension by having the blood flow over a foam screen coated with siloxane antifoaming agents.

A device described by De Wall and coworkers in 1956[74] was to pave the way for others. It was the first totally disposable oxygenator. It was followed by devices designed by Hyman in the United States and Rygg and Kyusgaard in Denmark.[75,76] These disposable devices reduced the complexity and the variation between devices.

During this period, the pump itself was becoming less complex, and many centers turned over its control to technicians the surgeons had trained. This step eliminated the need for complex automatic control and simplified the pump greatly.

Many investigators were not in agreement that bubble oxygenators were the last step in the development of methods to oxygenate blood. They held that any introduction of gas directly into blood was damaging, creating emboli-producing bubbles, and so was best avoided. Kolff and Berk[77] reported that cellophane would let oxygen pass across its surface. In 1955, Kolff and Blazer[78] used a coil dialyzer as an oxygenator in animal experiments. Clowes[79] was the most persistent and was able to overcome many early difficulties with membrane oxygenators. In 1958, he reported the clinical use of a 25 m^2 oxygenator in an adult patient.

The main thrust of research in membrane design was to find materials that were inert but provided good gas exchange.[80] The human lung's capillary system is enormous and the smallest capillaries in the lung are much smaller and more numerous than the passages in even the modern oxygenators, one of the many reasons the lungs are so efficient compared with these units. Also, in the lung, the boundary layer between the capillary and the alveolar air sac is very thin and creates almost no resistance to complete diffusion of gases. This boundary layer is much thicker in artificial membranes, which causes the inner path of fast moving blood to be less able to transfer gas than the slower moving blood in contact with the membrane itself. Much of the research in membrane oxygenators has attempted to reduce this boundary layer or to promote mixing of the blood within the layers to equalize diffusion of gases.

Initially silicone elastomers were developed that had high permeability to O_2 and CO_2 and were biologically inert. These materials were used in the 1960s to develop clinical oxygenators.[81-83] Such membranes have since been replaced by microporous polypropylene membranes in the sheet and hollow-fiber type oxygenators.

The latest developments in the these new oxygenators enable them to come very close to the performance of a human lung with low priming volumes, yet they are still relatively inexpensive and compact.

Filtration During Cardiopulmonary Bypass

Gaseous and particulate microemboli passed on during CBP can significantly influence the patient's neurologic status.[84-89] Tissue fragments, bone, fat emboli, and aggregates formed by blood components damaged by suction and air-blood interfaces can be a leading source of microemboli in the CPB circuit.[90-92] It was apparent very early then that some type of filter was needed to remove this material. Work was begun by Swank[93] using a Dacron wool filter in the cardiotomy line to remove contaminants before blood returned to the pump.

In the 1970s Pall Biomedical (Pall Biomedical Products, Glen Cove, NY, USA) developed a polyester mesh screen for use as a filter in both the cardiotomy and the arterial lines. During the same period, Pioneer-Swank developed a Dacron depth filter for the same purpose. Because of its inherently better design and lesser blood trauma, the screen-type filter became more popular. Other filters were offered by other manufactures, most of which use the screen design.

The arterial line filter serves two functions: it removes microbubbles and emboli and it helps prevent massive air emboli. Microemboli are continuously being generated in bubble oxygenators, and the internal defoamers do not eliminate all of them.[94-96] Membrane oxygenators do not have this obvious source of microemboli, but small membrane leaks can force gas into the blood side of the membrane under the right circumstances. With both types of oxygenators, emboli also can occur from blood stagnation in low flow areas, formation of microaggregates because of blood exposure to the foreign surfaces of the oxygenator and tubing, and turbulence in the oxygenator.[97-102] Massive air embolism can be caused by defects in the arterial line and sudden roller pump acceleration.

The mechanism of filter action depends on which type it is. The depth filters contain a medium through which the blood flows.

This large wet surface blocks many particles and thus prevents them from being carried in the fluid stream; they are retained on the internal medium surface by adsorptive forces. The efficiency of particle removal depends on the amount of surface area, the depth versus the width of the medium, the size of filter in relation to the flow rate, and the range of particle sizes. These filters can be easily clogged if many large particles block the initial outer surface. They also can exhibit saturation breakthrough, where in all of the filter's available adsorptive surfaces become coated. Particles of all sizes can then flow through without absorption.

Screen-type filters have pores in a medium that are of a particular size. Filtering of particles happens only on the surface and is directly related to the pore size. Screen filters are made of hydrophilic materials. These fibers are said to be "wetted", and adhesive forces try to hold fluid in direct contact with them. The pores of the membrane have cohesive forces that hold back water. These two forces together let liquid pass through the pores but tend to hold gas back. The pressure required to force microbubbles across a modern screen filter is great and this can be enhanced by using a vent line from the inlet side of the filter to the cardiotomy reservoir. Leaving the purge line open to the operator can decrease the chance of exceeding the pressure at which air will pass through the filter pores (bubble point pressure). Also, keeping the filter as low as possible increases the bubble point pressure.

If enough air is pumped into the filter, the bubble point pressure and air will pass across the membrane, even with the purge line open. However, this point will take longer to appear possibly giving the perfusionist and surgeon time to correct the problem.

Pall Corporation has developed a filter that self-purges. It has a gas permeable membrane on the top side of the surface that allows incoming air to be vented regardless of whether the purge line is open or closed.

Most filters in use today have pores ranging from 20 to 40 μm. The size of the pores is basically determined by the manufacturing design and materials used in filter construction.

A common practice is to flush the filter and the entire CBP circuit with CO_2 prior to priming to displace the air in the circuit. When the priming fluid is added, the CO_2 is more soluble and so is absorbed quickly, providing faster debubbling. Most filter manufacturers recommend retrograde priming and flushing with CO_2.

The high concentration of CO_2 absorbed by the priming fluid can be removed by ventilating the membrane while recirculating the priming solution.[103-105]

Another filter developed for CBP is the pre-bypass filter. These filters, with pore sizes between 5 and 0.2 μm, trap particulate contaminants that can be formed during the production and assembly of the oxygenator and tubing or be present in the primary solutions themselves.[106-108] These filters are used for approximately 15 to 30 minutes of recirculation of the priming fluid and then removed from the circuit before CPB is begun. Because of the small pore size, blood primes cannot be used with them.

Another area where filters are used is in the cardioplegia system. During infusion of cardioplegia solution, there is always a risk of infusing air or particulate emboli.[109] There are specific filters that minimize the chance of this infusion when one is using crystalloid solutions. With the increasing popularity of blood-containing cardioplegia systems, manufacturers are sure to address this important topic.

A filter that is almost automatically placed in CBP circuits is a gas line filter. These filters prevent bacterial and particulate contamination from the compressed gas source. These filters were more important when a bubble oxygenator was used, as gas is injected directly into the blood path. With membrane oxygenator systems, the direct blood-gas interface is eliminated, so contamination becomes less of a concern. Thus, such filters probably are not needed, but for an added measure of safety, most perfusionists still use them in all circuits.

Today, there is no reason not to incorporate adequate filtration into the CBP circuit. The numerous studies cited all point to a reduction of embolic complications when proper filters and techniques are used. The cost of modern filters is reasonable compared with the total cost of CBP circuit, yet they have one of the most important functions. Many studies have shown decreases in morbidity and mortality rates when using adequate filtration,[110,111] and a majority of centers use them routinely for all CBP cases.

Filters made of polyester mesh do not increase hemolysis or aggregation of platelets.[112] However, because of the difficulty in assessing the subtle neurologic changes that occur in patients before and after CBP, it is not yet possible to determine which filter and what construction and materials are most beneficial.[113] With increasing sensitivity of the methods used to assess brain function and injury, these questions will be answered.

REFERENCES

1. Cooley D. Recollections of early development and later trends in cardiac surgery. *J Thorac Cardiovasc Surg* 98:817-822, 1989.
2. Milam J. Blood transfusion in heart surgery. *Surg Clin North Am* 63:1127-1147, 1983.
3. Gadboys HL, Slonim R, Litwak RS. Homologous blood syndrome I: preliminary observations on its relationship to clinical cardiopulmonary bypass. *Ann Surg* 156:793, 1962.
4. Warner WA, Faust RJ. Risks of transfusion. *Anesthesiol Clin North Am* 8:501-517, 1990.
5. Beeson PB. Jaundice occurring one to four months after transfusion of blood or plasma: Report of seven cases. *J Am Med Assoc* 121:1332-1334, 1943.
6. Cooley DA, Beall AC, Grondin P. Open heart operations with disposable oxygenators, 5 percent dextrose prime, and normothermia. *Surgery* 52:713, 1962.
7. Steghling L. Trends in transfusion therapy. *Anesthesiol Clin North Am* 8:519-531, 1990.
8. Blajchman MA. Transfusion medicine—the coming age of a new specialty. *Transfusion Med Rev* 1:1, 1987.
9. Cosgrove D, Loop F, Lytle B, et al. Determinants of blood utilization during myocardial revascularization. *Ann Thorac Surg* 14:380, 1985.
10. Simon TL, Ak BF, Murphy W. Controlled trial of routine administration of platelet concentrates in CPB. *Ann Thorac Surg* 37:359, 1984.
11. Tuman KJ. Tissue oxygen delivery: the physiology of anemia. *Anesthesiol Clin North Am* 8:451-469, 1990.
12. Lavee J, Martinowitz U, Mohr R. The effect of transfusion of fresh whole blood versus platelet concentrates after cardiac operations. *J Thorac Cardiovasc Surg* 97:204, 1989.
13. Cradfoord C. Two cases of obstructive pulmonary embolism successfully operated upon. *Acta Chir Scand* 64:172, 1928.
14. Cradfoord C, Nylin G. Congenital coarctation of the aorta and its surgical treatment. *J Thorac Surg* 14:347, 1945.
15. Cradfoord C, Senning A. Artificial circulation. Extrait du Vive Congres de la Societe Internacionale de Chirurgie Paris. Sept 23-29, 1951.
16. Ellison N, Jobes D. Hemostasis during cardiopulmonary bypass. In: Tinker JH, ed. *Cardiopulmonary Bypass: Current Concepts and Controversies. A Society for Cardiovascular Anesthesiologists Monograph.* Philadelphia, PA: WB Saunders; 1989:99-10.
17. Young JA. Coagulation abnormalities with cardiopulmonary bypass. In: Utley JR. ed. *Pathophysiology and Techniques of Cardiopulmonary Bypass I.* Baltimore, MD: Williams & Wilkins; 1982:88-105.

18. Bull BS, Korpman RA, Huse WM, et al. Heparin therapy during extracorporeal circulation: I. *J Thorac Cardiovasc Surg* 69:674, 1975.
19. Bull BS, Huse WM, Brauer FS, et al. Heparin therapy during extracorporeal circulation: II. *J Thoracic Cardiovasc Surg* 69:685, 1975.
20. Verska JJ. Control of heparinization by activated clotting time during bypass with improved postoperative hemostasis. *Ann Thorac Surg* 24:170, 1977.
21. Ellison N, Edmunds HL, Colman RW. Platelet aggregation following heparin and protamine administration. *Anesthesiology* 48:65-68, 1978.
22. Nilson IM, Sweddeberg J. Coagulation studies in cardiac surgery with extracorporeal circulation using a bubble oxygenator. *Acta Chir Scand* 117:47, 1959.
23. Tsuji HK, Redinton JB, Kay JH, et al. The study of fibrinolytic and coagulation factors during open heart surgery. *Ann NY Acad Sci* 146:763, 1968.
24. Kalter RD, Saul CM, Wetstein L, et al. Cardiopulmonary bypass-associated hemostatic abnormalities. *J Thorac Cardiovas Surg* 77:427, 1979.
25. Young JA, Kisker CT, Doty DB. Adequate anticoagulation during cardiopulmonary bypass determined by activated clotting time and the appearance of fibrin monomer. *Ann Thorac Surg* 26:321, 1978.
26. Zucker MB. Effect of heparin on platelet function. *Thromb Diath Haemorrh* 33:63-65, 1974.
27. Barrer MJ, Ellison N. Platelet function. *Anesthesiology* 46:202-211, 1977.
28. O'Brien JR. Heparin and platelets. *Curr Ther Res* 18:79-90, 1975.
29. Tinker J, Roberts SL. Management of cardiopulmonary bypass. In: Kaplan JA, ed. *Cardiac Anesthesia.* 2nd Ed. Philadelphia, PA: WB Saunders; 1987:895-920.
30. Hawskley M. De-heparinisation of blood after cardiopulmonary bypass. *Lancet* I:563-565, 1966.
31. Ellison N, Osminsky AJ, Wollman H. Is protamine a clinically important anticoagulant? *Anesthesiology* 35:621, 1971.
32. Perkins HA, Osborn JJ, Hurt R, et al. Neutralization of heparin in vivo with protamine. Simple method of estimating required dose. *J Lab Clin Med* 48:223-226, 1956.
33. Umlas J, Gauvin G, Taff R. Heparin monitoring and neutralization during cardiopulmonary bypass using a rapid plasma separator and a fluorometric assay. *Ann Thorac Surg* 37:301-303, 1984.
34. Bachman F, McKenna R, Cole RE, et al. The hemostatic mechanism after open heart surgery. I: Studies on plasma coagulation factors and fibrinolysis in 512 patients after extracorporeal circulation. *J Thorac Cardiovasc Surg* 70:76-85, 1975.
35. Bick RL. Hemostasis defects associated with cardiac surgery, prosthetic devices and other extracorporeal circuits. *Semin Thromb Hemost* 11:249-280, 1985.

36. Saltzman EW, Weinstein RM, Wientraub JA, et al. Treatment with desmopressin acetate to reduce blood loss after cardiac surgery. *N Engl J Med* 314:1402-1406, 1986.
37. Yehuda T, Aledort L, Puszkin E, et al. Functional changes in platelets during extracorporeal circulation. *Ann Thorac Surg* 19:639-647, 1975.
38. Mannucci PM, Canciani MT, Rota L, et al. Response of factor VIII/von Willebrand factor to DDAVP in healthy subjects and patients with haemophilia A or von Willebrand's disease. *Br J Haematol* 47:283-293, 1981.
39. Mannucci PM, Ruggeri ZM, Pareti FI, et al. 1-Deamino-8-D-arginine vasopressin: a new pharmacological approach to the management of haemophilia and von Willebrand's disease. *Lancet* 1:869-872, 1977.
40. Ruggeri PM, Mannuci PM, Lombardi R, et al. Multimetric composition of factor VIII/von Willebrand factor following administration of DDAVP: implications for pathophysiology and therapy of von Willebrand's disease subtypes. *Blood* 59:1272-1278, 1982.
41. Gader AMA, daCosta J, Cash JD. A new vasopressin analogue and fibrinolysis. *Lancet* ii:1417-1418, 1978.
42. Mannucci PM, Remmuzzi G, Pusineri F, et al. Deamino-D-8-arginine vasopressin shortens the bleeding time in uremia. *N Engl J Med* 308:8-12, 1983.
43. Kobrinsky NL, Israels ED, Gerard GM, et al. Shortening of bleeding time by 1-deamino-8-D-arginine vasopressin in various bleeding disorders. *Lancet* 1:1145-1148, 1984.
44. Melrose DG, Dreyer B, Bentail HH, et al. Elective cardiac arrest. *Lancet* 269:21, 1955.
45. Helmsworth JA, Kaplan S, Clark LC, et al. Myocardial injury associated with asystole induced with potassium citrate. *Ann Surg* 149:200, 1959.
46. Buckberg GD, Hottonerott CE. Ventricular fibrillation: its effect on myocardial flow, distribution, and performance. *Ann Thorac Surg* 20:76, 1975.
47. Gollan F, Nelson IA. Anoxic tolerance of beating and resting heart during perfusion at various temperatures. *Proc Soc Exp Biol Med* 95:485, 1957.
48. Shumway NE, Lower RR, Stofer RC. Selective hypothermia of the heart in anoxic cardiac arrest. *Surg Gynecol Obstet* 109:750, 1959.
49. Maloney JV, Nelson RL. Myocardial preservation during cardio pulmonary bypass: an overview. *J Thorac Cardiovasc Surg* 70:1040, 1975.
50. Swan H. Clinical hypothermia: a lady with a past and some promise for the future. *Surgery* 73:736, 1973.
51. Gay WA, Ebert PA. Functional, metabolic and morphologic effects of potassium induced cardioplegia. *Surgery* 74:284, 1973.
52. Reidemeister JC, Heberer G, Bretschneider HJ. Induced cardiac arrest by sodium and calcium depletion and application of procaine. *Int Surg* 47:535, 1967.

53. Kirsch V, Rodewald G, Kalmar P. Induced ischemic arrest in clinical experience with cardioplegia in open heart surgery. *J Thorac Cardiovasc Surg* 77:803-815, 1979.
54. Skaredoff MN, Roaf E, Datta S. Hypermagnesaemia and anaesthetic management. *Can Anaesth Soc J* 29:35, 1982.
55. Lehr D, Chau R, Irene S. Possible role of magnesium loss in the pathogenesis of myocardial fiber necrosis. *Rec Adv Stud Cardiac Struct Metab* 6:95, 1975.
56. Krasner BS, Girdwood R, Smith H. The effect of slow releasing oral magnesium chloride on the QT internal of the electrocardiogram during open heart surgery. *Can Anaesth Soc J* 28:329, 1981.
57. Jan W, de Jong JW. Cardioplegia and calcium antagonists: a review. *Ann of Thorac Surg* 42:495-593, 1986.
58. Fox KAA, Bergmann SR, Sobel BE. Pathophysiology of myocardial reperfusion. *Ann Rev Med* 36:125, 1985.
59. Calcium antagonists and cardioplegia in cardiac surgery. Abstract and discussion at the International Symposium on Cardioprotection: Quo Vadis? *Eur Heart J* 4(Suppl C):7-91, 1983.
60. Miller BJ. The development of heart lung machines. *Surg Gynecol Obstet* 154:403-414, 1982.
61. De Bakey ME. Simple continuous flow blood transfusion instrument. *N Orleans Med Surg J* 87:386, 1934.
62. Dale HH, Shuster EHJ. Double perfusion pump. *J Physiol* 64:356, 1928.
63. De Wall RA, et al. A simple expendable artificial oxygenator for open heart surgery. *Surg Clin North Am* 36:25-34, 1956.
64. Khoury GF, Mann ME, Porot MJ et al. Air embolism associated with veno-venous bypass during orthotopic liver transplantation. *Anesthesiology* 67:848, 1987.
65. Lillehei CW, Varco R. The results of direct vision closure of ventricular septal defects in eight patients by means of controlled cross circulation. *Surg Gynecol Obstet* 447-466, 1955.
66. Hooker DR. The perfusion of the mammalian medulla: the effect of calcium and potassium on the respiratory and cardiac center. *Am J Physiol* 38:200, 1915.
67. Rayliss LE, Fee AR, Ogden EA. A method of oxygenating blood. *J Physiol* 66:443, 1928.
68. Richards AN, Drinker CK. An apparatus for the perfusion of isolated organs. *J Pharmacol Exp Ther* 7:476, 1915.
69. Gibbon JM Jr, Miller BJ, Dobel A. The repair of interventricular septal defects under direct vision with the assistance of a pump oxygenator. *J Thorac Surg* 28:235, 1954.
70. Melrose DG. A Heart-lung machine for use in man. *J Physiol* 127:51-53, 1955.
71. Cross FS, et al. Evaluation of a rotation disc type reservoir oxygenator. Proc Soc Exp Biol Med 93:210-214, 1956.
72. Von Schroder W. Uber die Bildungsstatte des Harnstoffs. *Arch Path Pharm* 15:364-402, 1882.

73. Clark LC, et al. The oxygenation of blood by gas dispersion. Science, 111:85, 1950.
74. De Wall RA, et al. A simple, expendable artificial oxygenator for open heart surgery. *Surg Clin North Am* 36:1025-1034, 1956.
75. Hyman ES. Simple disposable, autoclavable plastic unit to substitute for heart and lungs. *Trans Am Soc Artif Intern Organs* 2:1, 1956.
76. Rygg IH. Discussion of oxygenators. In: Thomas C, Allen JG, eds. *Extracorporeal Circulation.* Springfield, IL: 1958:108.
77. Kolff WJ, Berk MT Jr. Artificial kidney: a dialyser with a great area. *Acta Med Scand* 117:121, 1944.
78. Kolff WJ, Blazer RR. Artificial coil lung. *Trans Am Soc Artif Intern Organs* 1:39, 1955.
79. Clowes GHA Jr. Experimental procedures for entry into the left heart to expose mitral valve. Ann Surg 134:957-968, 1951.
80. Clowes GHA Jr, Hopkins AL, Neville WE, et al. An artificial lung dependent on diffusion of oxygen and carbon dioxide through plastic membranes. *J Thorac Surg* 32:630, 1956.
81. Bramson ML, Osborn JJ, Main FB, et al. A new disposable membrane oxygenator with internal heat exchanger. *J Thorac Cardiovasc Surg* 50:391, 1965.
82. Kolobow T, Bowman RL. Construction and evaluation of alveolar membrane artificial heart lung. *Trans Am Soc Artif Intern Organs* 9:238, 1963.
83. Lande AJ, Fillmore SJ, Subramanian VA et al. 24 hour veno-arterial perfusion of awake dogs with a simple membrane oxygenator. *Trans Am Soc Artif Intern Organs* 15:181, 1969.
84. Alldyce DB, Yoshida SH, Ashmore PG, et al. The importance of microembolism in the pathogenesis of organ disfunction caused by prolonged use of the pump oxygenator. *J Thorac Cardiovasc Surg* 52:706, 1956.
85. Branthwaite MA. Detection of neurological damage during open-heart surgery. *Thorax* 28:464-472, 1973.
86. Clark RE, Dietz DR, Miller JG, et al. Continuous detection of microemboli during cardiopulmonary bypass in animal and man. *Circulation* 54:III74-III78, 1975.
87. Geruin AS, Oervin AS, McNeer JF, et al. Ultrapore hemofiltration during extracorporeal circulation. *J Thorac Cardiovasc Surg* 67:237-243, 1974.
88. Hill JD, Aguilar MJ, Baraneo A, et al. Neuropathological manifestations of cardiac surgery. *Ann Thorac Surg* 7:409, 1969.
89. Kritikou PE, Branthwaite MA. Significance of changes in cerebral electrical activity at onset of cardiopulmonary bypass. *Thorax* 32:534-538, 1977.
90. Dutton RC, Edmunds LH. Measurement of emboli in extracorporeal perfusion systems. *J Thorac Cardiovasc Surg* 65:523, 1973.
91. Solen KA, Whiffer JD, Lightfoot EN, et al. The effect of shear specific surface and hemolysis. *J Biomed Mater Res* 12:381-399, 1978.

92. Wright G, Sanderson JM. Cellular aggregation and trauma in cardiotomy suction systems. *Thorax* 34:621, 1979.
93. Swank RL. Alteration of blood on storage: measurement of adhesiveness of "aging" platelets and leukocytes and their removal by filtration. *N Engl J Med* 265:728-733, 1961.
94. Kessler J, Patterson RH. Production of microemboli by various blood oxygenators. *Ann Thorac Surg* 9:221-224, 1970.
95. Mollison DR, Streczyn MV. In depth evaluation of arterial line filtration of air emboli in bubble and membrane oxygenators. *Am Soc Extracorp Tech Proc* 99, 1976.
96. Patterson RH, Kesster J. Microemboli during cardiopulmonary bypass detected by ultrasound. *Surg Gynecol Obstet* 129:505-510, 1969.
97. Chenoweth DE, Cooper SW, Hugli PE et al. Complement activation during cardiopulmonary bypass: evidence for generation of C3a and C5a anaphylatoxins. *N Engl J Med* 304:497, 1981.
98. De Leval MR, Hill PD, Mielkec CH Jr, et al. Blood platelets and extracorporeal circulation. *J Thorac Cardiovasc Surg* 69:144, 1975.
99. Dutton RC, Edmunds DH, Hutchinson JC, et al. Platelet aggregate emboli produced in patients during cardiopulmonary bypass with membrane and bubble oxygenators and blood filter. *J Thorac Cardiovasc Surg* 67:258, 1974.
100. Jones HM, Mattews N, Vaughn RS, et al. Cardiopulmonary bypass and complement activation: involvement of classical and alternative pathways. *Anaesthesia* 37:629, 1982.
101. Loop FD, Szabo J, Rowlinson RD, et al. Events related to microembolism during extracorporeal perfusion in man: effectiveness of in-line filtration recorded by ultrasound. *Ann Thorac Surg* 21:412, 1976.
102. Page US, Bigelow JC, Carter CR, et al. Emboli (debris) produced by bubble oxygenators: removal by filtration. *Ann Thorac Surg* 18:164, 1974.
103. Kurusz M, Shaffer CW, Christman EW, et al. Runaway pump head: new cause of gas embolism during cardiopulmonary bypass. *J Thorac Cardiovasc Surg* 77:792, 1979.
104. Mills NL, Ochsner JL. Massive air embolism during cardiopulmonary bypass. *J Thorac Cardiovasc Surg* 80:708, 1980.
105. Stoney WS, Alford WC, Burns GR, et al. Air embolism and other accidents using pump oxygenators. *Ann Thorac Surg* 29:336, 1980.
106. Ashmore PG, Sulter V, Ambrose B, et al. The incidence and effects of particulate aggregation and microembolism in pump-oxygenator systems. *J Thorac Cardiovas Surg* 55:691, 1968.
107. Reed CC, Romangnoli A, Taylor PE, et al. Particulate matter in bubble oxygenators. *J Thorac Cardiovasc Surg* 68:971, 1974.
108. Pastoriza-Pinol JV, McMillan J, Smith BF, et al. An analysis of microembolic particles originating in the extracorporeal circuit before bypass. *J Extracorp Technol* 11:211, 1979.
109. Mortensen JD, Yates WG, Schoenberg AA, et al. Cardiopulmonary bypass systems: a study of safety and performance TR5534-010. Bureau of Medical Devices of the US food and Drug Administration,

University of Utah Research Institute Salt Lake City, Utah, 84108, April 1981.
110. Hill JD, Aguilar MJ, Baranco A, et al. Neuropathological manifestation of cardiac surgery. *Ann Thorac Surg* 7:409, 1969.
111. Aberg T. Effect of open heart surgery on intellectual function. *Scand J. Thorac Surg* 1(Suppl. 15):63, 1974.
112. Guidoin R, Laperche V, Martin L, et al. Disposable filters for microaggregate removal from extracorporeal circulation. *J Thorac Cardiovasc Surg* 71:502, 1976.
113. Willner AE, Caramonte L, Garvey JW, et al. The relationship between arterial filtration during open heart surgery and mental abstraction ability. *Proc Am Acad Cardiovasc Perf* 4:56, 1983.

Chapter 2

The Anatomy of Cardiopulmonary Bypass

Pierre A. Casthely, MD

The essential goals of cardiopulmonary bypass (CPB) are to maintain adequate circulation and respiration by diverting blood flow to an extracorporeal circuit that functionally replaces the heart and lung to facilitate surgery of the heart and great vessels.

Normal circulation is as follows: deoxygenated blood returns to the heart via the superior vena cava (SVC) and inferior vena cava (IVC) into the right atrium. From the right atrium, it goes to the right ventricle, then is pumped via the pulmonary arteries into the lungs. There, the blood is oxygenated and carbon dioxide is removed as it passes through the alveolar capillary network. After oxygenation, the blood is returned to the left atrium by way of the four pulmonary veins, then passes into the left ventricle, and is pumped back into the systemic circulation. Tissues remove oxygen from hemoglobin and release carbon dioxide as the blood passes through the body's capillary system. The blood is then returned to the venous system, and the cycle is repeated over and over.

Adequate knowledge of the basic cardiopulmonary bypass circuit will make it easier to understand the functions of other extra-

From Casthely PA, Bregman D, (eds): *Cardiopulmonary Bypass: Physiology, Related Complications, and Pharmacology.* Mount Kisco, NY, Futura Publishing Company, Inc., © 1991.

corporeal circuits such as hemodialysis, femoral-femoral cardiopulmonary support (CPS), or extracorporeal membrane oxygenation (ECMO). The essential components of the CPB machine remain the same despite different machine designs (Fig. 1). The artificial circuit is composed of venous cannula, venous line tubing, venous and cardiotomy reservoirs, arterial and suction pumps, arterial cannula, arterial line tubing, arterial filter, a flow

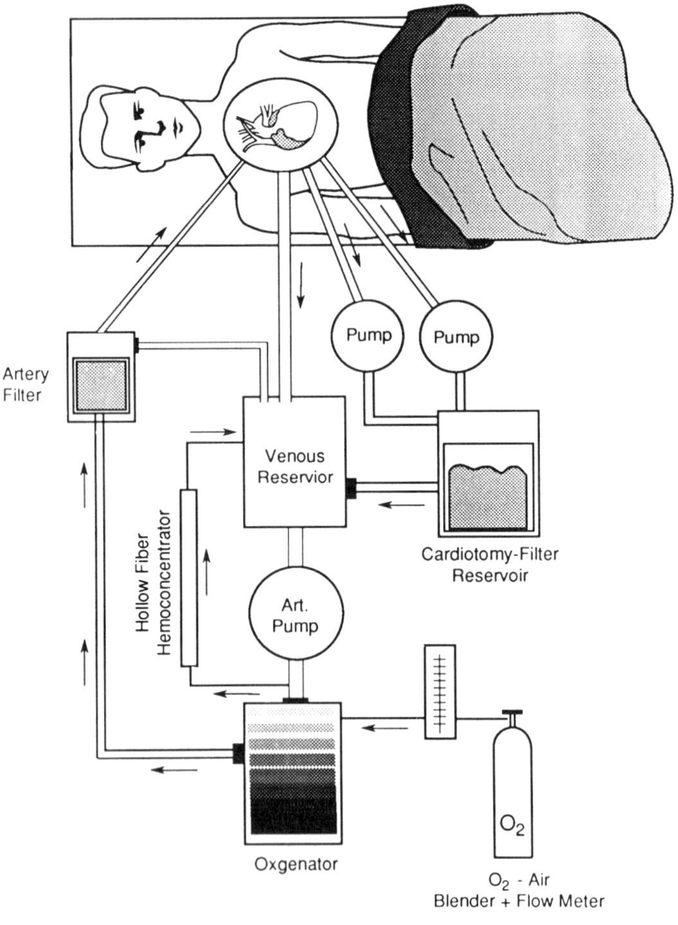

Figure 1. Essential components of the cardiopulmonary bypass circuit.

meter, an oxygenator, and hemoconcentrator. Venous blood is drained from the patient by gravity via the cannulae inserted in the right atrium, vena cava, or femoral veins into a reservoir.

Two types of venous cannulae and cannulation sites are commonly used (Table I). The first is the single right atrial cannula with multiple drainage holes that is inserted via the right atrial appendage into the IVC. This cannula provides superb venous drainage and right ventricular decompression. However, jugular venous hypertension may occur, especially when the surgeon rotates the heart to expose the circumflex coronary artery. Alternatively, individual SVC and IVC cannulae may be inserted. Tourniquets are tightened around them to prevent vena cava blood from entering the right heart. However, the right heart may become distended by blood from the coronary sinus unless the right atrium has been opened. Jugular venous hypertension can still occur if the SVC cannula is malpositioned (e.g., in the innominate vein) (Table I). A pump returns arterialized blood to the patient via an arterial cannula inserted in either the aorta or femoral artery. The circuit includes a blood reservoir to absorb fluctuations in venous return and a heat exchanger which permits either warming or cooling of the blood and thereby the patient. A microfilter and a bubble trap are also inserted into the arterial line to provide protection against air or debris that may be present in the circuit. Additional roller pumps power the cardiotomy suction and the left ventricular vent. The former retrieves blood from the surgical field; the latter prevents distention of the left ventricle during fibrillation or aortic cross clamping. Blood from the suction systems passes through a filter before being returned to the oxygenator.

Table I
Comparison of Venous Cannulation Sites

	Single	*Double*
Positioning for adequate drainage for all types of procedures	Difficult	Easy
Right heart exclusion	Incomplete	Complete
Technical difficulty	Easy	Difficult
Coronary sinus return	Included	Excluded
Myocardial preservation	Suboptimal	Best

The roller pump, in most modern heart-lung machines, can deliver either pulsatile or nonpulsatile flow. Although many experiments and clinical trials indicate that pulsatile flow is advantageous,[1-3] particularly for prolonged cardiopulmonary bypass, others demonstrate no benefit.[4,5] These experimental inconsistencies can be attributed to differences in the amount of extra energy imparted to the blood by various techniques of pulsation. Advantages ascribed to pulsatile flow during CPB are shown in Table II. The most consistently demonstrable benefits of pulsation include decreased systemic vascular resistance, increased systemic oxygen consumption, decreased "stress hormone" production,[6,7] and improved urine output. Pulsation may improve cerebral circulation.[2] Recent data suggest decreased cerebral oxygen consumption during nonpulsatile flow in humans. In experimental animals, pulsation has been shown to improve cerebral blood flow in ischemic brain regions.[2]

Table II
Advantages of Pulsatile Flow

Increased urine volume
Less metabolic acidosis
Decreased "stress hormone"
Decreased peripheral vascular resistance
Increased oxygen consumption
Improved myocardial perfusion

Cannulae and Tubing

Cannulae and tubing are simple conduits for moving blood through the components of the extracorporeal circuit. Venous tubing is a large volume, low-pressure funnel. Both arterial and venous are meant to channel the flowing blood with a minimal degree of turbulence.

Tubing is manufactured for extracorporeal circuits in virtually any combination of length, size, thickness, and flexibility. The tubing should be stiff enough to limit any tendency to kink or collapse, yet it should remain flexible enough to be handled easily. A partially kinked or collapsed tube represents an obstruction to flow and is a source of turbulence.

Plastic or metal tubes are used to connect cannulae to the extracorporeal circuit. The connections must be smooth and leak-proof to prevent turbulence that may result in hemolysis, possible platelet adhesion and clot formation.

Pumps

The deoxygenated blood leaves the patient via the venous cannula and is subsequently driven through the circuit by a pump. Roller pumps and centrifugal pumps are the two types of pumps most commonly used.

Roller pumps are simple in concept and are the most commonly used. They consist of an electric motor that controls, and the roller head. The pump mechanism itself never comes in direct contact with the blood. Tubing is inserted between the pump head wall and the rollers. The roller pump causes blood to flow by compressing plastic tubing between the roller and the horseshoe-shaped backing plate. Each pump usually has two roller heads placed 180° apart to maintain continuous roller head contact with the tubing. Typical occlusion of roller pump tubing as shown in Figure 2 will prevent destruction of formed blood elements. The quantity of blood moved is determined by the diameter of the tubing and the circumference of the pump head volume displacement. The larger the diameter of the tubing and the longer the length, the larger the volume of blood pushed with each revolution of the motor. The disadvantages of the roller pump are that they can pump air as easily as blood and they will overpressure the circuit if obstruction to flow occurs. They are also traumatic to the red blood cells and can produce spallation of the tubing.

Those pumps with computerized speed controls can be made to rotate in a manner that will produce a pulsating flow. This can be achieved by having the pump rotate at a high speed for several revolutions, and low speed for several more. Repeated many times, this sequence causes the blood to be ejected from the pump in a manner that is very much like the pumping action of the heart.

Centrifugal pumps are the other pumps in common use in extracorporeal circuits. Currently, there are only two manufactur-

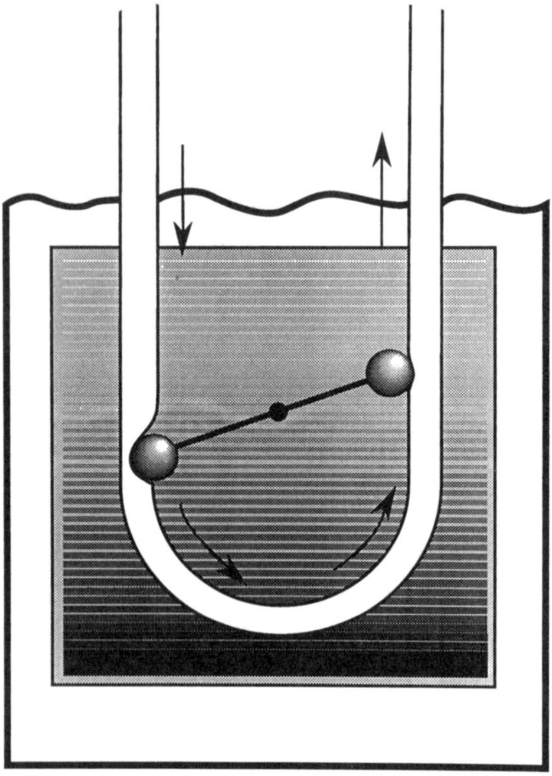

Figure 2. Demonstration of occlusion of roller pump tubing.

ers of centrifugal pumps: the Biopump (Biomedicus, Eden Prairie, MN, USA) and the Sarns/Centrimed pump (Sarns, 3M Health Care, Ann Arbor, MI, USA). The Vortex biopump consists of a series of rotor cones mounted in a clear plastic housing that spin at high speed causing circular motion of the blood. The rotation of the spinning pump imparts its energy to the blood through friction, driving it out of the circuit. The cones spin by means of a magnetic connection to a drive shaft. Blood enters along the central axis of the pump and exits the pump at the periphery.

Flow is dependent upon the pressure change created by the spinning cones in the pump. The flow rate is usually affected by the size of the cannula, length and diameter of the tubing, restrictions in the tubing, and changes in the patient's peripheral vascular resistance. If there is an obstruction or resistance to the blood flow, the flow will decrease or stop. Such decreases in flow can be, in part, compensated by increasing the pump speed. A flow meter is mandatory when using a centrifugal pump and should be inserted in the arterial line in order to accurately determine the actual flow rate. Centrifugal pumps cannot function if they become filled with air because they rely on the centrifugal force to generate pressure. However, if small bubbles are accidentally present in the blood, centrifugal pumps can easily pump them into the blood stream.

Reservoirs

During the course of a cardiac surgical procedure, considerable amounts of blood may need to be shifted from the patient's circulation into a reservoir in order to empty the heart and lungs.

Our typical circuit has two reservoirs. The first, the venous reservoir, is a receiving chamber for the deoxygenated blood that has just left the patient's venous system. The second is the cardiotomy reservoir, which receives blood that has been removed from the surgical field by the suction system. A filter is incorporated in each reservoir. In the cardiotomy reservoir, the filter is designed to remove any debris (tissue, fat, suture material, etc.) that is sucked into the circuit along with the blood by the coronary suction. Blood that leaves the venous reservoirs should also be free of bubbles before returning to the circulation. Nonsurgical procedures, such as ECMO, dialysis, and CPS may not require or use reservoirs in their circuits.

Oxygenators

Oxygenators are designed to produce an environment similar to the alveolar capillary membrane in order to oxygenate the blood and remove carbon dioxide. However, in designing any oxygenator, it is important to separate ventilation (carbon dioxide elimination) from oxygenation in order to control them independently.

They are all designed to optimize gas transport and should have the capability of delivering 300 mL/min of oxygen into the venous blood to produce 95% to 100% saturation at a flow rate varying from 50 mL to 80 mL/kg/min in the adult and remove 250 mL/min of carbon dioxide.

There are two types of oxygenators in common use: (1) bubble, and (2) membrane. In bubble oxygenators, oxygen is bubbled through venous blood, which flows into the oxygenation chamber with a direct blood-gas interface. They all have three main compartments: an oxygenation section, a defoamer, and a reservoir. Venous blood that enters the oxygenator is directed over a source of flowing oxygen that causes the blood to foam. As the blood passes through the oxygenating chamber, the gas exchange takes place at the surface of the bubbles. Oxygenation and carbon dioxide removal are determined by the size and number of bubbles. The number of bubbles is proportional to the rate of gas flow. Small bubbles create more surface area for blood to gas exposure, thereby improving oxygenation. Bubbles of oxygen that are too small will result in inadequate carbon dioxide removal because they are absorbed very quickly.

An elaborate defoaming mechanism is required to prevent bubbles from embolizing the patient. This is accomplished by passing the bubbles through a sponge impregnated with a defoaming agent. Because it requires time, a large portion of actual gas exchange occurs while the blood is passing through the defoamer. In time, the antifoam agent is washed away or consumed, thereby limiting the usefulness of bubble oxygenators to a few hours. From the defoamer, the blood passes into a reservoir and is then pumped into the circulation.

Bubble oxygenators have their limitations. They tend to cause hemolysis and disrupt the clotting mechanisms. Direct gas contact causes denaturation of the proteins that is considerably worse than the damage to the red cells.

The membrane oxygenators mimic more closely the natural pulmonary capillary by interposing a thin membrane between the blood and gas (oxygen-air mixture). Current membrane oxygenators have a large surface area (2-4 m^2) that is either fanfolded, coiled, or shaped into capillary tubes. The blood passes through the oxygenator as a thin film, minimizing the diffusion distance for gases in the blood, therefore optimizing the net gas exchange. The membrane materials commonly used are sheets of polypropylene, Teflon, silicone rubber. The sheets of silicone rubbers are nonporous; the polypropylene sheets have pores that are physical connections between the gas and blood space.

Nonporous membrane oxygenators are manufactured by coiling silicone rubber sheets in a cylindrical fashion. The membrane separates the blood from the gas. Gas transfer through the membrane depends on the diffusion distance of the gas in blood, the driving pressure of either gas in the membrane, and the permeability of the membrane. Those membranes must be more permeable to carbon dioxide than to oxygen because of the lower driving pressure of carbon dioxide.

Hollow fiber (microporous) membranes were manufactured to mimic the capillary bed by packing together in a parallel or spiral fashion microporous fibers. The blood may either flow through the capillaries surrounded by gas, or the gas may flow through the capillaries surrounded by blood. The membrane oxygenators, in which the blood passes through the capillaries, may produce plugging of the hollow fibers leading to decreased gas transfer. That is the reason why they are not suitable for long-term ECMO. The oxygenator of choice for ECMO is the coiled silicone membrane of the Sci-Med Oxygenator (SciMed Life Systems, Inc., Minneapolis, MN, USA).

A comparison between the bubble and membrane oxygenators is illustrated in Table III. When compared to membrane oxygenators, bubble oxygenators cause significantly more damage to red blood cells, platelets, and formed elements and also significantly increases postoperative blood loss.[8-11] Gaseous microemboli are detectable in the systemic circulation during perfusion with bubble, but not with membrane oxygenators.[10]

Table III
Comparison of Oxygenators

	Bubble	*Membrane*
Method of oxygenation	Direct contact of gas and blood	O_2-CO_2 transfer through membrane
Antifoam compound	Necessary	Unnecessary
Microembolism	Likely	Rarely

Membrane oxygenators are more expensive than bubble oxygenators. However, the membrane's ability to process blood in a gentle, more physiological manner has allowed their users to justify their preference in spite of the added expense.

Hemoconcentrators

A close relative of hollow fiber oxygenators are hollow fiber ultrafilters. Hemoconcentrators have an important role in the CPB circuit that resembles the function of the kidney in the body. As the fluid is removed, the dilution of the blood components is reversed, and the hematocrit is increased. The microporous construction is too small to let plasma proteins pass, but large enough to allow the passage of water and electrolytes. The higher the pressure difference across the membrane, the greater the rate of filtration. Unfortunately, this is where the similarity to the kidneys ends. Ultrafilters do not have the selectivity of the kidneys, thus filtered electrolytes are not reabsorbed. In comparison with diuretics, ultrafilters are readily controllable and excessive losses of potassium can be avoided.

Heat Exchangers

A great deal of heat is lost by the blood as it travels the circuit. Without a method to warm the blood, the patient would become hypothermic in a very short time. Most extracorporeal circuits include a heat exchanger between the venous reservoir and the oxygenator. In fact, it is common for the heat exchanger to be incorporated inside the venous reservoir. Blood flowing over or through the heat exchanger is warmed or cooled by exchange with warmer or cooler water flowing on the other side of a heat conductive surface. Application of extracorporeal techniques in the resuscitation of accidental hypothermia victims was made possible because of the presence of heat exchangers in the circuit.[12]

Filters

In an extracorporeal circuit, filters are very important to prevent air and microparticular emboli from entering the circulation. Two types of filters are used during cardiopulmonary bypass: depth filters and screen filters. Depth filters are composed of fibers of Dacron and are very seldom used nowadays. They filter by absorption on their large surface areas and act as a barrier to any particle larger than the pore in the filter material. Screen filters are made of a woven mesh of polyester materials. Some screen fibers remove debris by attracting particles that carry an electric charge opposite to that of the filter material. Intact blood components have a negative environment. They are, therefore, repelled by each other and by normal vessel walls that also have a negative charge. Damaged tissue, including blood cells and proteins, lose their negative charge and are then attracted by the filter. Arterial filters are the most important ones in the extracorporeal circuit because they not only filtrate particulate matter, but act as a last barrier against the introduction of microemboli into the circulation.

Controls

The perfusionist controls the extracorporeal process. He or she is proficient in interpreting and using the stream of information from the blood gas and chemistry laboratories. They are the interface between the CPB machine and all the information provided by the arterial pressure and temperature monitors and blood coagulation monitors to safely manage the patient during the extracorporeal bypass. They anticipate and meet the physiologic needs of the patient before they become apparent. Over the years, techniques and equipment have been developed with the goal to increase the safety of the process. Many safety devices have been added to the CPB circuit. They include devices to detect and prevent air embolism such as low-level alarm, air bubble detector, arterial line filter or bubble trap, one-way vent valve, and purge lines. Devices to monitor blood oxygenation, ventilation, and acid-base status on CPB have progressed from becoming intermittent to continuous, making possible the rapid detection of changes in the patient's perfusion status. Devices to monitor the coagulation status during CPB have progressed from the whole blood clotting time to the activated clotting time (ACT) and the use of sonoclot and thromboelastography. In the years to come, developments in this field will continue to make safety the number one priority, even as new devices are being developed such as heparin-coated CPB circuits that would obviate the need for patient heparinization. For example, computers will be used to enhance date acquisition and processing to a greater degree than is done at the present.

There will be more reliable blood gas and blood chemistry probes appearing as integral parts of the oxygenator. The control network will be improved with the use of probes implanted in the patient's core tissues giving instant, continuous physiological feedback. (muscle oxygen tension) Use of extracorporeal devices outside of the cardiac surgical suite have been increasing. The use of blood salvagers in orthopedic surgery is a direct outgrowth of extracorporeal techniques, and CPS is also being used in cardiac catheterization laboratories for patients too sick to tolerate balloon angioplasty safely without some mechanical help for their weak and failing hearts.[13]

REFERENCES

1. Williams GF, Seifen AB, Lawson NW, et al. Pulsatile perfusion versus conventional high flow non-pulsatile perfusion for rapid core cooling and rewarming of infants for circulatory arrest in cardiac operation. *J Thorac Cardiovasc Surg* 78:667-677, 1979.
2. Andersen K, Waaben J, Husum B, et al. Non-pulsatile cardiopulmonary bypass disrupts the flow metabolism couple in the brain. *J Thorac Cardiovasc Surg* 90:570-579, 1985.
3. Habal SM, Weiss MB, Spotnitz HM, et al. Effects of pulsatile and non-pulsatile coronary perfusion on performance of the canine left ventricle. *J Thorac Cardiovasc Surg* 72:742-745, 1976.
4. Frater RWM, Wakayama S, Oka V, et al. Pulsatile cardiopulmonary bypass: failure to influence hemodynamics or hormones. *Circulation* 62(Suppl):19-25, 1980.
5. Kono K, Philbin DM, Coggins CH, et al. Adrenocortical hormone levels during cardiopulmonary bypass with and without pulsatile flow. *J Thorac Cardiovasc Surg* 85:129-133, 1983.
6. Taylor KM, Wright GS, Reid JM, et al. Comparative studies of pulsatile and non-pulsatile flow during cardiopulmonary bypass. III. Response

of anterior pituitary gland to thyrotropic releasing hormone. *J Thorac Cardiovasc Surg* 75:579-584, 1978.
7. Sink JD, Chitwood WR, Hill RC, et al. Comparison of non-pulsatile and pulsatile extracorporeal circulation on renal cortical blood flow. *Ann Thorac Surg* 29:57-62, 1980.
8. Clark RE, Beauchamp RA, Magrath RA, et al. Comparison of bubble and membrane oxygenators in short and long perfusions. *J Thorac Cardiovasc Surg* 78:655-666, 1979.
9. Van Oevern W, Kazachkine MD, Descamps-Latscha B, et al. Deleterious effects of cardiopulmonary bypass. A prospective study of bubble versus membrane oxygenation. *J Thorac Cardiovasc Surg* 89:888-899, 1985.
10. Blauth CL, Arnold JV, Schulenbed WE, et al. Cerebral microembolism during cardiopulmonary bypass. *J Thorac Cadiovasc Surg* 95:668-676, 1988.
11. Boonstra PW, Van Imhoff GW, Eysman L, et al. Reduced platelet activation and improved hemostasis after controlled cardiotomy suction. *J Thorac Cardiovasc Surg* 89:900-906, 1985.
12. Laub GW, Banaszak D, Kupferschmid J, et al. Percutaneous cardiopulmonary bypass for the treatment of hypothermia circulatory collapse. *Ann Thorac Surg* 47:608-611, 1989.
13. Riley JB, Litzie K, Overlie P, et al. Supported angioplasty: a new contribution for extracorporeal circulaion technology. *J Extracorporeal Technol* 20(4):134-137; 1988.

Chapter 3

Physiologic Changes of Cardiopulmonary Bypass

Claudia Komer, MD

Since Gibbon first utilized cardiopulmonary bypass in the repair of an atrial septal defect in 1953,[1] technical advances in the design of the extracorporeal circuit as well as the quality of biosynthetic components have been made. The introduction of hemodilution and hypothermic techniques have improved oxygen delivery and organ preservation. These factors, along with better understanding of the physiologic alterations associated with cardiopulmonary bypass (CPB), have greatly contributed to the sharp reduction in bypass related morbidity and mortality over the past three decades.

Specific changes occur to varying degrees in all patients who undergo cardiac surgery with cardiopulmonary support. Although most patients convalesce uneventfully, others may develop sequelae such as pulmonary, renal, and neural dysfunction, coagulopathy, and increased susceptibility to infection are sequelae. This chapter will discuss the physiologic alterations imposed by extracorporeal circulation as well as address current controversies in CPB management.

From Casthely PA, Bregman D, (eds): *Cardiopulmonary Bypass: Physiology, Related Complications, and Pharmacology.* Mount Kisco, NY, Futura Publishing Company, Inc., © 1991.

Oxygenation

The primary purpose of extracorporeal circulation (ECC) is to perfuse vital organs and maintain function by ensuring adequate oxygen transport. Through the use of an oxygenator in the extracorporeal circuit, desaturated hemoglobin is oxygenated and dispersed into the circulation. The oxygen within the hemoglobin matrix will diffuse down a concentration gradient from the plasma, across the capillary wall, and ultimately through the cell membrane to the target system of the cell. It is the oxygen tension of the red blood cell being greater than 100 mm Hg and that of the mitochondria being 1-2 mm Hg, that maintains a gradient facilitating transfer at the cellular level. Oxygenation is influenced not only by cellular supply and demand, but also by the cells' ability to effectively extract and utilize the oxygen delivered.[2]

It is the oxygenator within the extracorporeal circuit that allows efficient gas exchange. Two basic types of gas exchange devices are used today. A direct gas interface oxygenator in which oxygen is bubbled directly through blood allowing oxygen transfer and carbon dioxide removal. Prior to entering the arterial cannula, the blood is defoamed through a filtering chamber. With this type of oxygenator, oxygenation depends on the matching of gas flow to blood flow.[3] Direct blood gas contact permits extremely efficient oxygenation, even in patients with unusually high oxygen requirements. This bubble oxygenator, however, has been associated with greater blood trauma especially platelet destruction,[4] as well as the potential for dispersal of gaseous microemboli.[5] The bubble oxygenator is limited in its use to under 6 hours.

The other type of commonly used oxygenator requires a gas porous membrane that separates the circulating blood from the oxygen/carbon dioxide mixture. Membrane oxygenation is efficient for several days and is associated with significantly less trauma to blood components.[6] As long as flow through either type of oxygenator is maintained according to the manufacturer's specifications, blood will be fully saturated and O_2 will be delivered to the tissues both as oxygen dissolved in plasma and saturated hemoglobin.

The actual flow of oxygenated prime through a tissue is a function of afferent arteriolar tone and therefore directly influenced by vasoactive agents, changes in locally occurring hormone levels, local tissue temperature, and metabolic activity. Vasoconstriction is associated with increased shunting through larger arteriovenous channels and may result in poor oxygenation while apparently maintaining adequate tissue flow. In addition, vasoconstriction may impair flow of the hypothermic perfusate through the microcirculation. This will result in failure to achieve the desired temperature reduction and thus tissue oxygenation will be further compromised by poor flow and normal cellular activity. Cellular oxygenation is also influenced by factors affecting the oxyhemoglobin dissociation curve, namely $PaCO_2$, intracellular pH, temperature, and 2,3-diphosphoglutamate (2,3-DPG). These factors are further influenced by blood viscosity, colloid osmotic pressure, complement activation, and the liberation of oxygen free radicals.

Oxyhemoglobin Dissociation Curve

The oxyhemoglobin dissociation curve relates O_2 content to the partial presure of oxygen in the blood. Its sigmoidal shape allows hemoglobin to remain highly saturated at a pO_2 value of 100 mm Hg, and to release large amounts of oxygen with a small drop in pO_2. The position of the oxyhemoglobin dissociation (OxyHb) curve is best described by the PO_2 tension at which hemoglobin is 50% saturated (p50). The normal P50 is 26.7 mm Hg. A P50 value greater than 27 mm Hg describes a right shifted OxyHb curve, meaning that at any given PO_2, hemoglobin has a low affinity for O_2 and is therefore less saturated than normal. This may allow lower than normal tissue perfusion to produce the normal amount of O_2 unloading. A decrease in P50 value is reflective of an increase in hemoglobin oxygen affinity.

Many conditions encountered during CPB affect the slope and position of the oxyhemoglobin dissociation curve, including changes in pH, temperature, pCO_2, and 2,3-DPG.[7-9] These variables will affect oxygen delivery over the same range of pO_2 values.

A change in pH from 7.4 to 7.2 results in a shift of the curve by approximately 15% to the right (Fig. 1). On the other hand, an increase in pH from 7.4 to 7.6 would shift it to the left, reducing O_2 availability at the tissue level.[10]

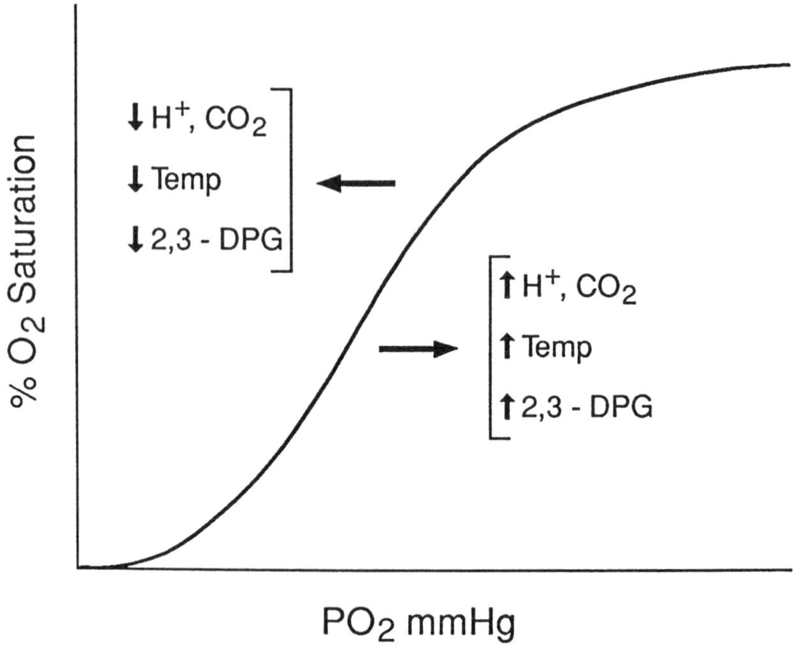

Figure 1. Oxygen hemoglobin dissociation curve.

Hypothermia decreases O_2 availability by increasing oxygen hemoglobin affinity, with a shift of the curve to the left. During rewarming however, this relationship reverses with increased O_2 availability.

An increase in CO_2 tension and decrease in red blood cell 2,3-DPG content also shift the curve to the right, resulting in decreased hemoglobin affinity for oxygen and subsequent increase in O_2 availability for transfer to the cell.

The organic phosphate 2,3-DPG is required for blood to maintain a normal O_2 hemoglobin dissociation relationship. Reduced 2,3-DPG, as in aged blood, results in decreased O_2 delivery over a normal arterial-venous pO_2 range and shifts the curve to the left.

Moores et al.[11] studied the significance of 2,3-DPG content using a right heart bypass model in swine. Animals receiving blood depleted in 2,3-DPG (decreased P50), clearly demonstrated depressed cardiac performance. Conversely, Valeri et al.[12] reported that patients transfused with 2,3-DPG enriched blood demonstrated an increased cardiac index immediately following CPB.

Monitoring Oxygenation

The adequacy of oxygenation during CPB may be assessed by serial measurements of arterial blood gases. The arterial oxygen tension will indicate the efficiency of the oxygenator and reveal the environment of O_2 perfusing the tissues. With tissue hypoxia there will be a fall in pH and secondary reduction in bicarbonate due to anerobic metabolism. Therefore, these values will provide additional evidence of inadequate tissue oxygenation.

Various in-line oximetric systems have become available for the monitoring of pH, PCO_2, and O_2 saturation, that provide continuous information regarding the patient's state of oxygenation.

Perfusion

Widespread controversy regarding adequate perfusion pressure and systemic flow has existed since the earliest days of extracorporeal circulation (ECC). Presently, various protocols are in use throughout the country for the maintainence of pressure and flow during CPB.

Initially, Kirklin et al.[13] (1955) postulated that flows during CPB parallel that of the resting adult. Utilizing dye dilution, cardiac output of multiple adults was assessed and it was concluded that systemic flows be calculated at 60 cc/kg/min or 2.4 L/min/m^2.

As our understanding of myocardial preservation has evolved, and techniques such as hypothermia and aortic occlusion with cold ischemic cardioplegic introduced, the potential value of reduced arterial pressure and flow has been recognized. Advantages of low pressure and flow include a reduction in blood trauma from the pump oxygenator system, improved surgical exposure, a decrease in noncoronary collateral flow, and more effective isolation of the heart from systemic perfusate during aortic occlusion thereby enhancing myocardial protection.[14] This contributes significantly toward preservation of myocardial hypothermia. High arterial blood pressure during CPB possibly increases risk of cerebral hemorrhage in anticoagulated patients, and, in addition, pump tubing disconnections are more likely.[15]

To assess optimal flow and pressure, the association between cerebral blood flow, hypothermia, and oxygen consumption were studied. Early work of Kety and Schmidt[16] in 1945 indicated that cerebral blood flow should decrease linearly as cerebral perfusion pressure is decreased below 50 mm Hg during CPB. Subsequently, in 1979, Selkoe and Meyes[17] demonstrated in monkeys that a mean arterial pressure as low as 25 mmm Hg was tolerated without cerebral ischemia. In fact, mean arterial pressures (MAP) of 35-40 mm Hg were sustained for up to 3 hours without evidence of neurologic or cardiovascular sequelae. Kollka and Hilberman[18] reported that the duration of MAP less than 50 mm Hg was not predictive of outcome. Recent studies have clearly shown no correlation between arterial hypotension during CPB and postbypass neurologic dysfunction. Govier et al.[19] demonstrated that cerebral blood flow was relatively constant down to a MAP of 30 mm Hg, in patients normotensive preoperatively.

Kollka and Hilberman reported that the use of the "Stanford technique of low flow/low pressure CPB", resulted in an overall incidence of cerebral dysfunction of less than 3%, in 450 patients.[18] Ellis et al.[20] performed a similar study, and reported a comparably low incidence of neurologic complications.

To further evaluate the safety of low flow, Hickey and Hoar[21] investigated total body oxygen consumption ($\dot{V}O_2$) as an indicator of adequacy of perfusion. Induced hypothermia to 25°C reduced $\dot{V}O_2$ by 50%. Cardiopulmonary bypass flow rate reduction from 2.1 to 1.2 L/min/m^2, while allowing arterial pressure to decrease, did not alter $\dot{V}O_2$. They concluded this as evidence for the adequacy of low flows.[21] In 1982, Fox et al.[22] measured $\dot{V}O_2$ during profound hypothermia and randomly altered flow rates from 0.25 to 2.0 L/min/m^2 as opposed to gradually reducing flows as Hickey and Hoar did. They reported that $\dot{V}O_2$ did decline in relation to reductions in CPB flow, but suggested that 1.2 L/min/m^2 might be the lower limit with respect to adequacy of tissue oxygenation.

Most recently, Govier et al.[19] measured cerebral blood flow (CBF) with 133 Xenon washout at pump flows of 1.6 L/min/m^2. Cerebral blood flow was measured at whatever MAP resulted, and ranged from 30-110 mm Hg. They found no correlation between CBF and perfusion pressure until a MAP of 30 mm Hg (at 28°C). They concluded that the lower limit of cerebral autoregulation is extended down to 30 mm Hg during hypothermic CPB at 1.6 L/mim/m^2.

Rubeyka et al.[23] assessed cerebral function using somatosensory cortical evoked potentials (SSEP) and cerebral metabolism measuring cortical adenosine triphosphate (ATP) concentrations while decreasing flow from 2.0-1.5 L/mim/m^2 during nonpulsatile CPB. Cortical ATP concentrations decreased significantly as flow decreased, but SSEPs remained unchanged at flows of 1.0/min/m^2 (MAP 40 mm Hg), at 20-25°C. Increased latency of SSEPs was apparent at flows of 0.5 L/min/m^2 (MAP 25 mm Hg).[23]

These data suggest that during hypothermic CPB 20-25°C, flow rate rather than perfusion pressure per se influences cerebral function, and during low flow CPB a minimum flow of 1-1.2 L/min/m^2 is required to maintain oxygen delivery.[24]

Kirklin et al.[25] devised a normogram based on the results of several animal studies relating oxygen consumption to pump flow rates at various temperatures (Fig. 2). The small *x* on each curve represent clinically used flow rates. A greater than 2.2-2.4 L/min/m^2 flow rate at normothermia does not result in greater tissue O_2 consumption, and only exposes blood to greater damage from high shear stress.

Monitoring Pressure and Perfusion

Arterial Blood Pressure

The adequacy of arterial pressure during CPB should be assessed from an indwelling arterial catheter. Although the ideal blood pressure during bypass is not known, as discussed above, a MAP of less than 30 mm Hg is below the critical closing pressure of some vascular beds, and the risk of hypoperfusion exists.

Hypotension during CPB may result from a low systemic vascular resistance (SVR), a low flow rate, or mechanical problems involving cannulation and or the CPB circuit. A decrease in SVR

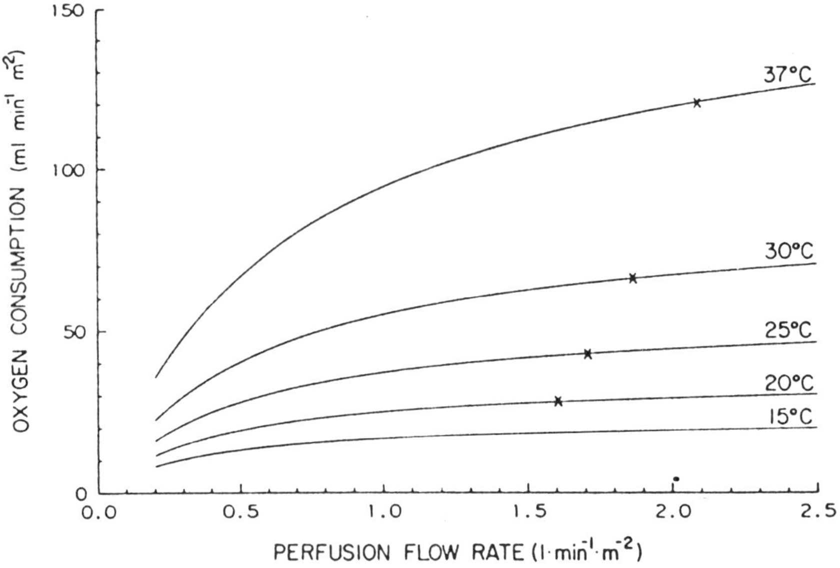

Figure 2. Normogram of an equation expressing the relationship of oxygen consumption (VO_2) to perfusion flow rate (Q) and temperature (T). The small *x*'s represent perfusion flow rate used clinically at these temperatures. (With permission from J.W. Kirklin and B.G. Barratt-Boyes. Hypothermia, circulatory, and cardiopulmonary bypass. In: J.W. Kirklin, B.G. Barratt-Boyes, eds. *Cardiac Surgery.* New York, NY: Churchill Livingstone; 1986:35.

secondary to hemodilution and reduced blood viscosity commonly occurs at the onset of CPB. Anesthetic agents and vasodilators also decrease SVR. In addition, hyperthermia and metabolic factors may be factors. Mechanical factors such as kinked cannula, decreased venous return, or inaccurately calculated flow rate may result in arterial hypotension. Cannulation complications including aortic dissection, and inadvertent innominate artery cannulation may also result in inadequate arterial pressure.[26]

On the other hand, an elevated arterial pressure commonly reflects an increased SVR, which may be secondary to catecholamine release, hypothermia, inadequate anesthesia, the use of vasoconstricting agents such as neosynephrine, as well as metabolic factors. High perfusion flow rates may also increase mean pressure. In addition, technical considerations such as innominate arterial cannulation with right radial pressure monitoring may be reflected as an unexplainably elevated arterial pressure during bypass.

Mixed Venous Oxygen Content

The Fick equation relates cardiac output (Q) to oxygen consumption ($\dot{V}O_2$) and the difference between the mixed arterial venous oxygen content (CaO_2-CvO_2).

Therefore,

$$CvO_2 = CaO_2 - \dot{V}O_2 / \dot{Q}.$$

During CPB, CvO_2 is represented by PvO_2, the partial pressure of oxygen in mixed venous blood. Under normal physiologic conditions, oxygen consumption and arterial oxygen content (CaO_2) are relatively constant and are independent of perfusion, so based on the Fick equation, venous oxygen content should be a useful index of perfusion.

Kirklin and Kirklin[27] reported that a PvO_2 of 30 mm Hg or more is consistent with normal convalescence. However, PvO_2 in itself may be a deceptive measurement in that an abnormally high value could represent either excess cardiac output, or hypoperfusion with microvascular shunting. Swan et al.[28] reported a strong relationship between venous oxygen tension and lactic acid levels. Use of mixed venous oxygen tension monitoring with the goal of maintaining PvO_2 level above 35 mm Hg, correlated with insignificant lactic acid levels. Significant lactic acidemia during hypothermic CPB will not occur even if PvO_2 occasionally falls below 30 mm Hg.

Oxygen Consumption

Actual measurement of $\dot{V}O_2$ considers both cardiac output and CvO_2, and thus provides an even better index of perfusion. A normal

$\dot{V}O_2$ for any given temperature usually indicates at least adequate tissue perfusion. The difficulty arises in determining what is a normal $\dot{V}O_2$ for a given patient at a given temperature. Fox et al.[22] suggested that a measured $\dot{V}O_2$ of 85% of maximal predicted value for a given temperature will ensure adequate tissue perfusion and oxygen delivery.

However, accurate determination of $\dot{V}O_2$ is obtained only if the actual arterial and venous oxygen content are measured. Serial measurements are necessary to assess the efficiency of tissue oxygenation and perfusion.

Lactate Levels

If tissue hypoperfusion exists, serum lactate levels should in fact rise secondary to increased anerobic metabolism. Various conditions will affect this relationship. For example, intravascular shunting may result in an accumulation of lactic acid that is not released into the circulation until more optimal blood flow is restored. Thus serum lactate levels have not proven to be useful in the regular monitoring of tissue perfusion due to their variable nature.[15]

Hypothermia

Varying degrees of hypothermia are introduced in the majority of cardiac surgical procedures performed. The primary reason for utilizing this technique is to reduce O_2 consumption and high-energy phosphate utilization during CPB. It has been shown that within the range of 0°C to 42°C, O_2 consumption will fall 50% for each 10°C decrease in temperature.[29] As the rate of temperature falls, the rate of O_2 consumption in general decreases more rapidly than supply (cellular), and local stores are consumed more slowly. Hypothermia thereby exerts a protective effect on the cells from anoxia.[30]

Moderate hypothermia affords the option of cross clamping the aorta, eliminating coronary perfusion and providing a dry field at 32°C. This can be carried out safely for 20-30 minute intervals, and if necessary extended further with cardioplegic techniques. Another major advantage in using hypothermic techniques is the safety factor it affords the surgeon. In the event of a CPB catastrophe, the entire circuit can be turned off for periods of 10 minutes at 30°C to 45 minutes at 16-25°C (Table I).[25]

Hypothermia is associated with an increase in blood viscosity that may cause sludging of red blood cells in the microcirculation, adversely affecting flow.[31] Because of this, all patients are hemodiluted to hematocrits of 20%-25% during CPB. Although O_2 carrying capacity is decreased with hemodilution, O_2 delivery and microcirculatory flow is improved, secondary to the concomitant decrease in viscosity.

As temperature decreases, the binding affinity between oxygen and hemoglobin is increased, thus less efficient release of O_2 from hemoglobin occurs at the tissue level. Utley et al.[32] assessed the effect of hypothermia on organ blood flow. They demonstrated that hypothermia is associated with a decrease in cerebral blood flow and O_2 delivery, and has a protective effect on the brain from edema.

Hypothermia is associated with a decrease in blood flow to all regions of the kidney, decreasing glomerular filtration rate and osmolar clearance. Overall however, hypothermia does not alter total body water balance.[33]

With regard to myocardial function, hypothermia is commonly used to protect the myocardium from ischemic damage. In fact, during aortic clamping the myocardium is often maintained at temperatures of 10-12°c. This reduces basal energy utilization, and may have a protective effect on intracellular membranes possi-

Table I

Temperature (°C)	*O_2 Consumption (%)*	*Circulatory Arrest (min)*
37	100	4–5
29	50	8–10
22	25	16–20
16	12	32–40
10	6	64–80

(Adapted from Meijne: Archivum Chirurgicum Neerlandicum, 25:227, 1973)

bly reducing oxygen mediated reperfusion injury. Hypothermia does have its disadvantages. Immersion hypothermia of the myocardium is associated with subendocardial hemmorhage and myocardial damage, suggesting vascular effects.[34] In addition, it may impair the sodium-potassium transmembrane pump and result in increased myocardial cellular edema. Furthermore, hypothermia has been shown to reduce myocardial diastolic compliance.[35]

Monitoring Temperature

Both central and peripheral temperature should be monitored during CPB. A nasopharyngeal probe is frequently used as central while a toe probe is used as a peripheral monitor. Recent studies have found a good correlation between blood temperature and bladder temperature which has resulted now in the frequent use of bladder probes.[36] However, the bladder probe will be affected by urine flow. Rectal temperature monitoring does not reflect central temperature.

Both absolute core as well as the core-peripheral gradient is important in assessing the adequacy of cooling and rewarming. A progressive increase in temperature gradient suggests increasing vasoconstriction, and rewarming can be facilitated by the use of vasodilators.

Termination from CPB should never be considered unless central temperature is stable and at least 37°C, and the peripheral temperature at least 32°C. Recooling of the body can occur with its adverse sequelae unless CPB rewarming time has been sufficient. Heating humidified gases, as well as the use of the heating blanket has been controversial with regards to their value in preventing a postbypass temperature reduction.[37,38] The use of pulsatile perfusion however has been reported to improve rewarming.[39,40] Blood temperature in the arterial line, and coolant temperature should be continuously monitored as well during CPB.

Acid Base Management During Hypothermia

The subject of appropriate acid-base management during hypothermic CPB remains controversial. Two specific forms of management may be used: (1) pH-stat: the clinical objective of this technique is to maintain a pH of 7.4 at the patients core temperature. This requires the addition of exogenous CO_2 to the pump oxygenator to maintain a temperature corrected $PaCO_2$ at 35-40 mm Hg. Until recently, pH-stat was the most common method of management; (2) α-stat: the nontemperature corrected pH is kept at 7.4 and the $PaCO_2$ is kept at 40 mm Hg (measured at 37°C), so the actual pH varies with body temperature (Table II).

The pH-stat method has been used since the early work of Severinghaus in which he detailed normograms for temperature changes in arterial blood gases.[41,42] A temperature corrected pH of 7.4 was thought to be "normal" and thus more physiologic. This set the precedent for the use of normal corrected values of arterial pH and $PaCO_2$ during the first two decades of hypothermic CPB. In addition, with an inherently greater $PaCO_2$, and as $PaCO_2$ is a potent vasodilator, it was thought that cerebral blood flow would be enhanced.

Subsequent research has suggested that the α-stat method may be a more physiologic approach to acid-base management. To evaluate these two methods of management, it is necessary to understand the alterations in acid-base homeostasis as a function of temperature. If a sample of blood is held in an airtight syringe, (constant CO_2), it is known that there will be an inversely proportional change in pH of $-$ 0.0147° per °C temperature change. As temperature decreases, CO_2 becomes more soluble and $PaCO_2$ falls. Plasma bicarbonate concentration and total CO_2 do not change. These same changes are seen in arterial blood during hypothermic bypass. If the arterial blood sample is warmed to 37°C, in a blood gas analyzer, it would read the same uncorrected values of 7.40 and 40 mm Hg as total CO_2 stores are unchanged.[43]

On a biochemical level, it is known that acid-base regulatory systems provide a constant ratio of hydrogen and hydroxide (H/OH) ions. Therefore the appropriate pH for a given temperature is that which maintains neutrality (i.e., constant H/OH ratio). This is often referred to as the neutral pH of water.[44-46] During hypothermia, the dissociation of water is proportionately decreased, and intracellular pH rises. A buffering mechanism first identified by Reeves[47] ensures that a constant H^+ ion gradient is maintained across the cell membrane and that intracellular pH is kept at a neutral state. This protein buffer is the imidazole group of the

Table II
Different Hypothermic Acid-Base Regulatory Strategies

Strategy	*Aim*	*Total CO_2 Content*	*pH and Paco Maintenance*	*Intracellular State*	*Alpha-Imidazole and Buffering*	*Enzyme Structure and Function*	*Cerebral Blood Flow and Coupling*
pH-stat	Constant pH	Increases	Normal corrected values	Acidotic (excess H^+)	Excess (+) charge Buffering decreased	Altered and activity decreased	Flow close to normothermic ? Flow and metabolism uncoupled
Alpha-stat	Constant OH^-/H^+	Constant	Normal uncorrected values	Neutral (H^+ = OH^-)	Constant net charge Buffering constant	Normal and activity maximal	Flow decreases (appropriate) ? Flow and metabolism coupled

(Adapted with permission from Hickey PR, Hansen DD. Temperature and blood gases: the clinical dilemma of acid-base management for hypothermic cardiopulmonary bypass. In: tinker JH, ed. *Cardiopulmonary Bypass: Current Concepts and Controversies.* Philadelphia, PA: W.B. Saunders; 1989:16.)

amino acid histadine. As temperature drops, this imidazole buffer changes its dissociation constant in parallel with the neutral pH of water (pN). Because of this parallelism, intracellular pH increases along the same slope as blood pH when temperature falls as long as total CO_2 stores remain unchanged. The degree of buffer dissociation is expressed as α. Constancy of α at all temperatures preserves optimal transmembrane H gradient, and electrochemical neutrality. Electrochemical neutrality maintains normal protein structure and function as well as other as other aspects of intracellular homeostasis. The essence of α-stat management is what has just been described, i.e., the fraction of unprotonated imidazole groups remains constant, total CO_2 remains constant, and pH changes as temperature changes.

Subsequently, it has been found that the optimal pH of most enzyme systems, including that of the cytochrome c system, sodium/potassium ATPases, enzymes involved in glycolysis, fatty acid synthesis, and aerobic as well as anerobic metabolism vary with temperature to maintain a neutral intracellular pH. Thus these enzyme systems function in a manner consistent with α-stat management.[48]

White's review[44] of comparative physiology shows that in all organisms, most functioning tissues maintain their pH at or close to the α-stat requirements as tissue temperatures change. When the organism as a whole must function, blood pH also follows α-stat acid-base balance.

Studies on cerebral blood flow and acid-base balance have demonstrated that with α-stat management, cerebral blood flow correlates with cerebral oxygen consumption during hypothermia, and is independant of cerebral perfusion pressure over 20 to 100 mm Hg. This confirms intact autoregulation. On the contrary, with pH-stat management, cerebral oxygen consumption and cerebral blood flow vary independently.[49] Cerebral blood flow changes significantly with perfusion pressure. pH-stat is associated with increased cerebral blood flow secondary to the potent vasodilatory property of CO_2. This is potentially deleterious, paradoxically increasing regional ischemia by diverting blood away from maximally dilated, collateral-dependent regions. CO_2 induced vasodilatation can also reduce driving pressure, jeopardizing areas supplied by critically stenosed vessels.[50] In addition, excessively high cerebral flows may increase amount of air and microaggregates delivered into the microcirculation.[51]

The effects of acid-base management on myocardial function have also been studied. McConnell and associates[52] evaluated function in the canine heart during CPB at 28°C, and made comparisons at a pH of 7.4 and 7.7. Under the α-stat regime (pH 7.7 corrected) they reported significant elevations in coronary blood flow, left ventricular oxygen consumption, and lactate utilization by comparison to the pH-stat regimen (pH 7.4 corrected). Swan et al.[53] also reported a maintenance of left ventricular function after CPB with α-stat regimen as opposed to when pH-stat was used. Poole-Wilson and Langer[54] evaluated the performance of hypothermic perfused papillary muscle and found the pH of well-oxygenated perfusate to the alkaline side of pH 7.4, resulted in preservation of greater contractility. They later observed that acidosis, induced by increasing perfusate PCO_2 was associated with a rapid fall in myocardial tension development as well as alteration in calcium transport.[54]

Swain et al.[55] reported the effect of acid-base regulation on cardiac electrophysiology and noted that during hypothermia, electrical stability of the heart was increased using α-stat. Conversely, Gillen[56] reported a decrease in ventricular fibrillatory threshold in dogs using the pH-stat regimen.

In summary, the α-stat method of acid-base management during hypothermic bypass clearly has theoretical merit, however additional clinical studies need to be performed to ascertain the significance of this merit.

Hemodilution

In the face of increased risks of hepatitis and AIDS, as well as greater awareness of the adverse responses to homologous blood transfusions, it has become common practice in the United States to use a nonhemic CPB prime solution.

Hemodilution to a hematocrit of 20%-25% is most often used for adult surgical cases and is associated with diminished O_2 carrying capacity and a fall in blood viscosity and vasodilation, counteracting the deleterious effects of hypothermia. In experimental studies, hemodilution increases blood flow to the myocardium, outer cortex of the kidney, cerebral cortex, spleen, and intestine. Thus the diminished O_2 carrying capacity of hemodilution is compensated by increased flow to ensure normal oxygen delivery.[57]

The lower limit of hematocrit necessary to support organ function in not clearly known. Some investigators have warned against hemodilution to hematocrits lower than 20% in open heart operations.[58,59] Buckley and coworkers, and Laver and Buckley described operations in which the hematocrit was decreased below 10% under severe hypothermia without signs of tissue hypoxia, or pulmonary edema.[60,61] In the work of Lilleaasen and Stokke,[62] the average hematocrit during perfusion was 18% in patients having extreme hemodilution. No attempt was made to lower body temperature that was stable between 34°C to 35°C. They reported no adverse sequelae.

Moores[63] demonstrated preservation of left ventricular function in swine when hematocrit was reduced to 15%. Kleinman and others[64] demonstrated that, in dogs, a decrease in hematocrit to 20% resulted in maldistribution on subendocardial blood flow between regions of the left ventricle with normal and those with collateral flow. In dogs with normal coronaries and adequate myocardial perfusion during acute normovolemic anemia, at a hemoglobin level of less than 5 mg/dL, subendocardial ischemia clearly developed as a result of a decrease in the ratio of endocardial to epicardial blood flow .

Nimikowski demonstrated that during CPB with hemodilution, although the PaO_2 was consistently greater than 300 mm Hg, the mean tissue PO_2 fell to as low as 14 mm Hg, suggesting redistribution of blood flow, and probably poorly perfused subcutaneous tissue.[65]

Hemodilution was shown by Utley to be the main cause of fluid retention during CPB, when compared to the effect of hypothermia or the pump oxygenator. Hemodilution decreases plasma colloid oncotic pressure which correlates with a fall in plasma proteins, particularly the albumin fraction.[33] This may ultimately lead to increased fluid requirements and tissue edema. Webber found that the colloidal oncotic pressure and albumin levels remained at 80% of normal even during the week following surgery.[66]

The safety of hemodilution has been well established. The improvement in blood coagulation, lung function, renal, and myocardial function is probably related to the absence of homologous blood in the priming solution. However, certain considerations must be kept in mind. First of all, if hemoglobin concentration is reduced by 50%, blood flow must be able to double if O_2 transport is to remain unchanged. Such a marked rise in flow is not feasible during CPB, thus the importance of always combining hemodilution with hypothermia. Secondly, the limits of hemodilution cannot be accurately predicted, such that in a patient having stenosis of critical arteries feeding various organs, the ability to increase flow as the concentration of hemoglobin declines decreases.

The most vulnerable periods for myocardial metabolism during extreme hemodilution are during the first few minutes of CPB, the time of aortic cross clamping, the phase of recirculation as the heart is fibrillating, and the time of rewarming when the heart is regaining its original rhythm, periods when optimal O_2 delivery are crucial.

Foreign Surface Activation

Interaction between the cellular and humoral components of blood with the foreign surfaces of the extracorporeal circuit has been well described.[67] The deleterious effects of this interaction include protein denaturation, activation of various enzyme systems, depletion or activation of clotting factors, platelet aggregation, lipid peroxidation, and activation of the complement cascade.[68,69] These pathophysiological effects are implicated in the varied postoperative sequelae associated with CPB that include impairment of alveolar gas exchange, renal insufficiency, coagulopathy, cerebral dysfunction,[70] and often a vague "systemic toxicity reaction".[71]

Upon initial contact of the blood with the foreign components of the extracorporeal circuit, plasma proteins adsorb to the surface and denaturation occurs. This primary event appears to dictate all subsequent events. Denatured proteins may adhere to the red blood cell membranes and increase red cell adhesiveness, aggregate formation, and impairment of the microcirculation. Contact with foreign surfaces also results in the denaturation of lipoproteins, with the release of free lipid globules into the circulation. These lipid emboli may ultimately cause vascular occlusion. In addition, protein denaturation is a strong activator of the complement, kallikrein/kinin cascade, as well as the coagulation and fibrinolytic cascade systems.[72-74]

Complement Activation

The human complement system is composed of more than 20 plasma proteins, which are an integral part of the humoral immune system.[75] They act in a concerted fashion to promote host defense mechanisms.

Almost immediately after the onset of CPB, exposure of blood to the nonendothelial surfaces initiates activation of the coagulation cascade and fibrinolytic system. This in turn activates the complement cascade.[76]

Complement may be converted from its inactive to active form via the classical or alternate pathway. In general, antibody dependant activation of complement proceeds via the classical pathway, whereas foreign materials such as the biosynthetic components used in the extracorporeal circuit tend to promote activation via the alternate pathway. The alternate and classical pathway converge to promote the enzymatic activation of C3, which in turn initiates a sequence of events that comprises the final common pathway. C5 is activated in this common pathway (Fig. 3).

C3a and C5a are potent inflammatory mediators known as anaphylatoxins. These anaphylatoxins are smooth muscle spasmogens and result in tissue changes including vasoconstriction, increased vascular permeability, induction of histamine release, and modulation of host immune responses.[77]

Chenoweth et al.[76] demonstrated that complement anaphylatoxin C3a is released within minutes after the onset of CPB and production continued in a time dependant manner (Fig. 4). The rate of formation of C3a however, is slowed during the hypothermic phase of CPB and enhanced during rewarming, implying some sort of protective benefit of hypothermia.

Overall levels of C3a were directly dependent on the duration of CPB. A prospective clinical study at the University of Alabama found that cardiac dysfunction in the first 24 hours postsurgery was significantly related to C3a levels 3 hours after CPB, prolonged

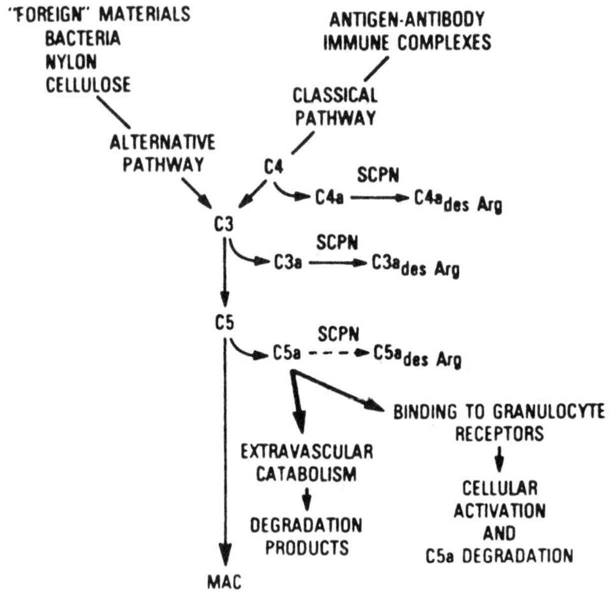

Figure 3. (Reproduced with permission from Chenoweth De. Complement activation during cardiopulmonary bypass. In: Utley J, ed. *Pathophysiology of Cardiopulmonary Bypass*. Williams and Wilkins; 1983:51.)

duration of CPB, and younger age at operation. Postoperative pulmonary dysfunction was related to the same factors.[71]

C5a is unique in that it is rapidly bound to circulating neutrophils that are sequestered in the pulmonary circulation. The C5a stimulated cell release superoxides, lysosomal enzymes and proteases. The protease elastase level was measured by Antonsen and found to be elevated 10-30 times above normal during CPB. A rise of this magnitude implies extensive degranulation or destruction of neutrophils circulating in the course of CPB.[78]

Microaggregates of these injured leukocytes form and when filtered lodge in the alveolar microcirculation. In addition O_2 free radicals are generated that contribute to lipid peroxidation and damage to the alveolar capillary membrane, resulting in alterations in permeability and accumulation of extravascular water.

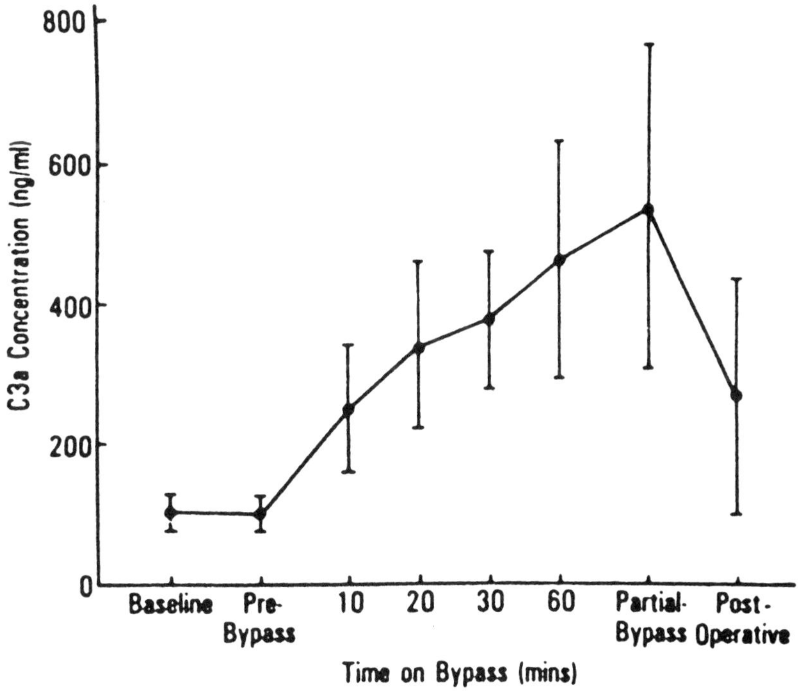

Figure 4. Pasma levels of $C3_a$ in patients undergoing cardiopulmonary bypass. (Reproduced with permission from Chenoweth DE, et al. Complement activation during cardiopulmonary bypass: evidence for generation of $C3_a$ and $C5_a$ anaphylatoxins. *N Engl J Med* 304:497, 1981).

Activation is now known to be promoted by both bubble and membrane oxygenators.[79,80] In particular, the nylon fiber often used is one of the most potent sources of complement activation. Nylon is capable of producing 15-20 times more C3a than the process of oxygenation. Biopolymers also play a significant role in the formation of complement derived inflammatory mediators.[71,80]

It was the hypothesis that protease enzyme release may be implicated in pulmonary membrane damage and whole body inflammation that led to an investigation of the value of antiproteases in an attempt to attenuate the complement response. Van Oeveren et al.[81] infused aprotinin, a protease inhibitor in patients undergoing CPB. Aprotinin had little effect on complement activation; however, it did inhibit the production of fibrin degradation products and the decrease in platelet numbers.

Recent investigation has targeted in on what can reduce anaphylatoxin formation. Reigal et al.[82] demonstrated inhibition of granulocyte activation with nifedipine infusion during CPB. Oral administration of calcium channel blockers also have a similar effect.[82] Methylprednisolone at doses of 30 mg/kg administered prior to CPB has been shown to be associated with reduced anaphylatoxins levels.[80]

Complement activation is universal in all patients undergoing CPB. Activation is increased at the extremes of age, and in particular with CPB runs of greater than 120 minutes.[71,80] Although it is difficult to imply complement activation is a direct cause of specific subsystem organ dysfunction, in a cause-effect manner, it seems reasonable that reducing complement activation could reduce tissue injury. Investigation is continuing in this area, with particular emphasis on the development of biomaterials for use in oxygenation and in the extracorporeal circuit. Improvements in circuit design and components could certainly improve outcome for the open heart surgical patient.

Pulsatile Perfusion

Since the introduction of various pulsatile perfusion systems, there has been ongoing controversy regarding the importance of pulsatile flow, and its inherent physiologic advantage. Initial laboratory studies of pulsatile versus nonpulsatile perfusion were performed by Weslowski and associates.[83] These studies showed no pronounced differences between the two forms of perfusion. It was Wesolowski's work that made nonpulsatile perfusion the "gold standard" for CPB. Subsequently, in 1966, Shepard suggested a value to pulsatile flow. He stated that the product of pulsatile flow depended not on a pressure gradient but on an energy gradient; this energy may be utilized by the tissues.[84]

More recently, intra-aortic balloon pulsation technique, advances in pump technology, and organ preservation studies have rekindled interest in pulsatile perfusion. Reports however, have only bred further controversy. Advantages found in many studies are in contrast with the lack of benefits observed in other studies. Difficulty exists in evaluating the results ot these studies, due to differences in the various forms of pulsation used, and lack of quantification of the critical aspects of pulsatile flow. In the literature there is no standardization of pulsatile components, or definition of what represents effective pulsatile force. In addition, numerous variables including vascular impedance and the hydraulic energy involved alter the effectiveness of flow.

Pulsatile perfusion during CPB has been associated with various hemodynamic and metabolic advantages. It is well known that during conventional nonpulsatile CPB, peripheral vascular resistance (PVR) increases. Shepard and Kirklin, Dunn, and Trinkle and their coworkers all reported significantly reduced PVR during pulsatile perfusion at comparable flow rates.[85-87] In contrast, two recent studies have shown no difference in PVR between patients having pulsatile and those having nonpulsatile CPB.[88,89] Thus although the majority of animal and human studies show a lower PVR with pulsatile CPB, a few studies fail to show this decrease in PVR. No consistent pattern of pumps, flow, temperatures or other variables explain the differences in the reported findings.

It appears that in changing from pulsatile to nonpulsatile flow there is a marked increase in frequency of carotid sinus baroreceptor discharge. This mechanism may induce reflex vasoconstriction in the peripheral circulation either by direct neural reflexes or by stimulating the release of various hormonal vasoconstrictors. Studies by Angell James and deVurgh Daly showed that this increased baroreceptor afferent activity inhibited vasomoter discharge and decreased PVR.[90]

Giron and colleagues[91] showed that depulsation of the entire systemic arterial circuit increased PVR, but when pulsation in the aortic arch and carotid sinus was maintained without pulsation in the rest of the arterial tree, PVR did not increase supporting an autonomic vasomotor mechanism as a cause of change in PVR. Most probably, it is a combination of vasomotor reflexes, hormones and the physical effects of pulsatile flow that act together to lower PVR during pulsatile perfusion.[91]

Nonpulsatile perfusion has been associated with the presence of microcirculatory shunting and widespread capillary collapse. This results in reduced O_2 consumption and tissue acidosis. In addition, nonpulsatile perfusion has been associated with reduction in lymph flow and increased interstitial fluid.

Parsons and McMaster's classic studies in 1938 provided evidence of the importance of pulsatile flow in the microcirculation.[92,93] Ogata and associates observed that capillary flow in the omentum virtually ceased in nonpulsatile CPB, while normal capillary flow was maintained during pulsatile CPB. No change in omental volume was seen during pulsatile bypass, but a progressive rise was observed during nonpulsatile perfusion suggesting stagnation of lymph and formation of edema. Ogata et al.[94] observed higher O_2 consumption, pH and buffer base levels with pulsatile CPB in dogs at flow rates of 60 and 75 mL/kg/min. At a higher flow rate of 100 mL/kg/min, no difference was seen. Geha and associates[95] also reported lower lactate levels in animals having pulsatile CPB. Dunn and associates[86] noted higher oxygen consumption, pH, and bicarbonate levels with pulsatile CPB.

In most clinical and experimental studies, pulsatile flow has been shown to preserve the microcirculation, improve tissue metabolism and inhibit edema formation. Integrity of the vascular compartment appears to be better maintained with pulsatile perfusion. Transfusion volumes and fluid replacement volumes are significantly less than those required with nonpulsatile flow.[95]

Reported changes in hormonal responses occur with pulsatile perfusion. Philbin et al.[96] noted an increase in epinephrine and norepinephrine levels during pulsatile and nonpulsatile bypass. A significantly higher level of these catecholamines was seen in the nonpulsatile group.

In studies of plasma renin activity, Landymore and colleagues[97] found significantly lower activity after CPB in patients having pulsatile CPB. Watkins and colleagues[98] reported similar results. They also reported significantly lower plasma angiotensin II levels. Frater et al.[89] reported no difference in renin levels in patients pretreated with propanolol, a known inhibitor of renin release.

Plasma vasopressin levels have been reported to increase during nonpulsatile CPB, Philbin and associates[99,100] found this increase attenuated by pulsatile CPB. Increased levels of vasopressin seen during nonpulsatile CPB might contribute to the increased PVR and hypertension seen after nonpulsatile perfusion. Plasma cortisol levels have been found to decrease during nonpulsatile perfusion. Taylor et al.[101] found this response reversed in patients at normothermia with pulsatile CPB.

In addition, prostaglandins have been reported to be affected by pulsatile flow. Watkins and associates[102] found that the elevation of thromboxane, a potent vasoconstrictor and platelet aggregator was much less with pulsatile perfusion, while the increase in prostacyclin, a potent vasodilator and antithrombotic agent was significantly greater with pulsatile perfusion.

The effect of pulsatile flow on organ function has similarly shown mixed results. Studies have uniformly demonstrated improved renal metabolism with pulsatile perfusion.[103] Parquet showed decreased acidosis, incresed O_2 consumption along with improved function, while German and coworkers reported that pulsatile perfusion produced lower renal vein lactate levels and higher pH levels than did nonpulsatile perfusion. They also reported greater renal oxygen consumption and better cortical and medullary tissue oxygen levels with pulsatile CPB, especially after 2 hours.[104] Jacob and colleagues[105] found significantly greater urine output and creatine clearance during pulsatile bypass in dogs. Bregman et al.[106] also reported greater urine volume with pulsatile perfusion. Clinical studies, however, in patients have shown varied results.

In general, studies suggest that pulsatile perfusion better preserves renal function, maintains more normal renal metabolism, preserves outer cortical flow, and prevents ischemic changes, especially during longer periods of perfusion. Myocardial function studies during pulsatile perfusion have also yielded mixed results. Moores and colleagues[107] found no significant change in myocardial oxygen consumption or lactate extraction with pulsatile perfusion in beating or fibrillating hearts with pulsatile flow. Grover and associates[108] demonstrated no difference in myocardial oxygen consumption, coronary sinus lactate level, myocardial lactate levels, or myocardial adenosine triphosphate levels with pulsatile bypass in beating or fibrillating dog hearts.

Maddoux and colleagues[109] reported that left ventricular ejection in patients undergoing coronary bypass grafting with nonpulsatile perfusion declined markedly by the first postoperative day. With pulsatile bypass, ejection fraction increased considerably by the first postoperative day. These patients also had a lower rate of intraoperative infarction. Also Bregman et al.[106] reported a lower incidence of perioperative myocardial infarction when pulsatile perfusion was used. Levine and coworkers,[110] however, failed to find any significant difference in ejection fraction or CPK isoenzymes in the postoperative period between those receiving pulsatile versus nonpulsatile perfusion.

Habal and associates[111] found a marked decrease in left ventricular compliance with nonpulsatile perfusion in the fibrillating heart compared with the maintenance of left ventricular compliance found with pulsatile perfusion.

Thus, many studies have suggested pulsatile CPB improves subendocardial coronary flow and myocardial metabolism at least in the fibrillating heart. However, almost the same number of studies have failed to support these results.

Limited studies have been performed to assess the effects of pulsatile perfusion on pulmonary function. No difference in oxygenation was found. However, a marked increase in pulmonary vascular resistance occurred with nonpulsatile flow. The data regarding the effects of pulsatile perfusion on postoperative pulmonary function are is so inconsistent that it is really not possible to draw any conclusions from them.

Few studies have been performed to assess the effects of pulsatile perfusion on the brain. Sanderson and colleagues[112] noted acute histological changes in the brain following both pulsatile and nonpulsatile bypass. The incidence of discrete focal lesions attributed to microbubbles was the same for both groups. Although higher cerebrospinal fluid oxygen tensions and lower jugular venous lactate levels have been reported with pulsatile flow, no definite evidence exists for improved cerebral metabolism with pulsatile bypass.[113] Further research in this area is needed.

In summary, pulsatile flow is polymorphic in its physical properties and therefore different from those of nonpulsatile flow. Numerous pump systems, as well as variations in the form of pulsatile flow, introduce many factors that alter the effectiveness of pulsatile perfusion. Further studies should be directed toward defining what constitutes effective pulsatile flow and what is most effective in perfusing tissue under specific physiological conditions.

The Effect of Cardiopulmonary Bypass on Organ Function

Endocrine Function

During CPB, there is altered hormone production, secretion, and degradation. In addition, organ perfusion as well as distrbution of blood flow is changed which will affect the hormone triggered response.

During CPB, the lungs are excluded from the perfusion circuit and no longer participate in hormonal secretion and degradation. Systemic heparinization alters tissue release of hormones, cellular affinities, and globulin binding affinities. Moderate to profound hypothermia effects the rate of enzymatic proccesses involved in hormone synthesis and degradation. In addition, hemodilution decreases serum concentration of proteins including hormones.

Catecholamine secretion is dependant on CPB stress, choice of anesthetic, the patient's volume status and body temperature. During CPB and aortic cross clamp, circulating levels of epinephrine and norepinephrine increase significantly (Fig. 5). In fact, epinephrine is increased tenfold over prebypass levels and norepinephrine fourfold over prebypass levels.[97,114] The decrease in blood pressure that occurs with initiation of CPB is probably related to the decrease in concentration of circulating catecholamines secondary to hemodilution. Within minutes after this, catecholamine levels increase and result in peripheral vasoconstriction. It is thought that this increase may be a reflex mediated response triggered by the drop in blood pressure at the onset of CPB. In addition, catecholamine release may also be triggered via reflexes initiated by baroreceptors and chemoreceptors in the heart and lung when these organs are excluded from the circulation. As the lung is the major site of norepinepherine inactivation, the lack of degradation may contribute to the increased levels seen during CPB. Following the reinstitution of pulmonary blood flow, catecholamine inactivation resumes.

Vasopressin or antidiuretic hormone (ADH) is an important determinant of sodium and water homeostasis and peripheral vascular resistance. General anesthesia and surgical stress are known

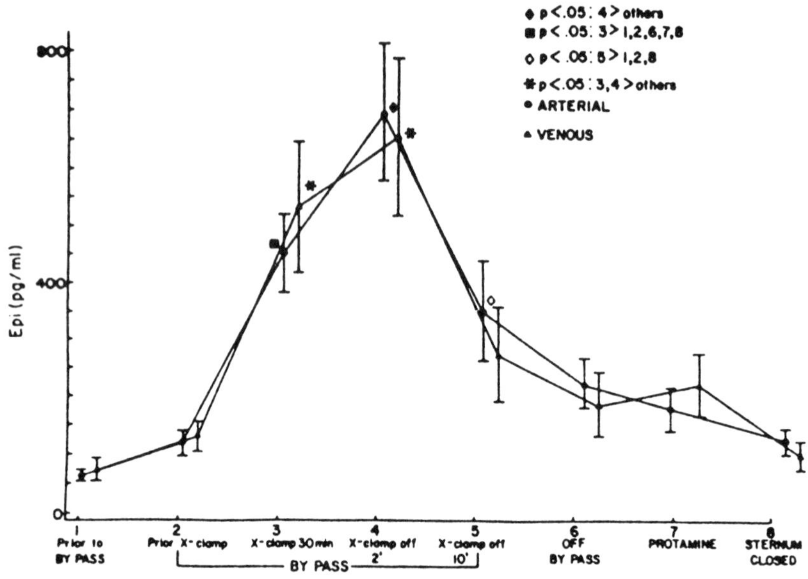

Figure 5. Mean plasma levels of epinephrine (Epi) during cardiac surgery. (Reproduced with permission from Reves, et al. Neuronal and adrenomedullary catecholamine release in response to cardiopulmonary bypass in man. *Circulation* 66:49-55, 1982.)

to moderately increase vasopressin levels. However, increases up to 20 times basal levels often occur with CPB, and these elevations usually persist into the postoperative period.[99,115] Stimuli for vasopressin release include volume receptors, left atrial stretch receptors, as well as pain and light anesthesia.[116] Specifically, large volume changes associated with CPB may play a major role. For example, the decrease in blood volume at the onset of CPB as well as the decrease in left atrial pressure which occurs with left ventricular venting may simulate volume depletion and be a stimulus for vasopressin release.

During CPB, vasopressin and catecholamines potentiate each other's vasoconstricting effects and may lead to intense peripheral vasoconstriction. This is one reason why vasodilating agents have been advocated during CPB to improve peripheral perfusion. In addition, vasopressin causes a paradoxical renal response during

CPB when levels are high, resulting in a profound sodium and water diuresis.

Atrial natriuretic factor (ANF) is a hormonal peptide released from the cardiac atria that regulates vascular volume by increasing sodium excretion and decreasing vasomotor tone and catecholamine synthesis. Normally, ANF release is directly related to atrial filling pressure. Dewar et al.[117] reported that there is a paradoxical rise of ANF during CPB. However, there was no correlation between atrial filling pressure and ANF. The ANF response to pulmonary capillary wedge pressure began to normalize 24 hours after the operation. The significance of this hormone in the pathophysiology of CPB is still unclear.

Cortisol is another hormone known to participate in the stress response and undergo changes associated with CPB. Taylor et al.[101,118] reported that during CPB the cortisol response differs markedly from the typical response to surgical stress, with a fall in levels at the onset of CPB. Oka et al.[119] reported similar results. Uozome et al.[120] demonstrated that these low levels were probably caused by hemodilution.

Hyperglycemia usually occurs during CPB, with peak values being observed during hypothermia. This value begins to decline during rewarming, and approaches normal within 12 hours. Factors associated with this response include; (1) increased glycogenolysis secondary to elevated epinephrine levels during CPB, (2) an abnormal pancreatic insulin response that is probably a function of hypothermia, (3) impaired glucose transport and utilization, and (4) the binding of endogenous insulin to the oxygenator tubing that which occurs during CPB.[121,122]

Due to derangements in glucose transfer during CPB, lipid metabolism becomes dominant with free fatty acids serving as a substrate for energy production. Free fatty acids are elevated two to four times basal levels with bypass, and do not return to normal until the first postoperative day.[123]

Cerebral Function

Cerebral dysfunction is one of the most dreaded complications of CPB. Clinical studies to ascertain the effects of CPB on cerebral blood flow and cerebral metabolism have reported somewhat conflicting results. Variables such as the method of acid-base management, mean arterial pressure, flow rate, and type of perfusion, and their effect on the cerebral circulation remain controversial.

Normally, CBF is independent of cerebral perfusion pressure (CPP) over a range of 50-150 mm Hg, with the primary determinant of flow being cerebral metabolic rate. This phenomenon of autoregulation provides for a stable internal environment of the brain and maintains homeostasic function. Outside of this range of autoregulation, CBF is directly related to CPP.

Several studies indicate preserved autoregulation, while others question it. The implications of this information are significant as it may clearly alter our intraoperative management during CPB. Govier et al.[19] performed the first CBF measurements in humans during hypothermic nonpulsatile CPB, using α-stat acid-base management. They demonstrated that CBF correlated with nasopharyngeal temperature and $PaCO_2$, but was independent of MAP, and therefore concluded that flow metabolism was intact. Because MAP ranged from 30-110 mm Hg, Govier et al.[19] further concluded that during hypothermic CPB the limit of autoregulation is as low as 30 mm Hg. Tanaka et al.[124] reported the presence of autoregulation in the canine cerebral circulation during nonpulsatile CPB at 20°C, stating that as long as the perfusion pressure in the vessels leading to the brain is 40 mm Hg or greater, cerebral metabolic activity remains essentially normal. Murkin et al.[49] subsequently reported that autoregulation appears to be intact over a range of perfusion pressures from 20-100 mm Hg during hypothermic, nonpulsatile bypass.

In studies correlating blood pressure with neurologic outcome, Sotamiemi[125] found no correlation between brain damage and hypotension, even in aged patients. Ellis et al.[126] reported no correlation between psychological dysfunction postbypass and perfusion pressure, flow rate (30 cc/kg/min) and length of time each was reduced, during moderate hypothermia (28°C).[126]

Fedderson et al.[127] studied patients during moderate hypothermic nonpulsatile CPB, using α-stat management. Patients either received placebo or prostacyclin during bypass. Mean atrial pressures averaged 30 mm Hg in the prostacyclin group, and when measured, CBF was reduced by approximately 10 mL/100 gm/min suggesting that at 30 mm Hg pressure autoregulation was not present. The cerebral hypoperfusion in the prostacyclin group however did not impair oxygen delivery as CMRO2 was identical in both groups. The prostacyclin patients compensated for lower CBF with increased O_2 extraction. Somatosensory evoked potentials (SSEP) were unchanged in the prostacyclin group.[127]

As previously discussed in this chapter, acid-base management has been found to profoundly influence CBF, as CO_2 is a potent cerebral vasodilator. Murkin et al.[49] measured Xenon[133] clearance and effluent cerebral venous blood sampling to determine the effects of maintaining temperature-corrected or noncorrected $PaCO_2$, on the regulation of cerebral blood flow and flow/metabolism coupling. The authors found that cerebral oxygen consumption was markedly reduced in both groups at low temperature. With the addition of CO_2 (temperature correction), CBF was significantly increased, beyond that of metabolic demand. When CO_2 was not added (nontemperature correction), CBF decreased, correlating with the drop in $CMRO_2$. In addition, in the latter group CBF was found to be independent of MAP, implying the presence of autoregulation, and clearly dependent on cerebral metabolism and oxygen consumption. Johnsson et al.[128] performed serial blood flow measurements similarly using Xenon[133] to evaluate autoregulation before, during and after bypass. They confirmed that when CO_2 was not added to the oxygenator during CPB, cerebral blood flow remained unchanged compared with prebypass levels, without evidence of byperemia or impairment of autoregulation.

The clinical implications of these studies are important because a global increase in CBF due to elevation of $PaCO_2$, and associated cerebral vasodilatation may critically reduce perfusion pressure and jeopardize areas of the brain dependent on flow through stenosed vessels. In addition, it has been suggested that cerebral hyperperfusion may potentially deliver more gaseous and particulate microemboli into the cerebral circulation. Cerebral blood flow is also affected by anesthetic agents. In general, the intravenous agents commonly used such as narcotics and benzodiazepines decrease CBF, as long as $PaCO_2$ is controlled, and depress $CMRO_2$, maintaining flow/metabolism coupling. Whether inhalational anesthetic agents abolish flow/metabolism coupling during CPB has yet to be determined.

Microembolization that is reported to occur to varying degrees in all patients undergoing CPB, is a well-documented cause of postoperative cerebral dysfunction.[129] These emboli are gaseous, or particulate consisting of platelet, fibrin, leukocyte, and protein microaggregates.[130,131] Air emboli are seen more commonly in open chamber procedures.[132] Oxygen microemboli may result during extracorporeal oxygenation. Gaseous microemboli may form if too great a temperature differential is established between the blood and heat exchanger, especially during attempts at rapid rewarming. Solid microemboli may be introduced via stored bank blood, and particulate matter such as plastic fragments may be released from the CPB circuit itself.

Membrane oxygenators appear to produce fewer cerebral arterial microbubbles than the bubble oxygenator.[133] Sotaniemi[134] noted that the use of the membrane oxygenator was associated with a lower incidence of neurologic dysfunction than the bubble oxygenator. Arterial inflow filters in the CPB circuit have reduced the number of microemboli, and possibly decrease the frequency and extent of cerebral injury.

Although our knowledge of cerebral physiology during CPB is increasing, we still are not clear on the mechanisms of cerebral injury associated with CPB and thus appropriate preventive measures.

Pulmonary Function

Gibbon[135] reported in 1959, that postoperative pulmonary dysfunction contributed more than any other complication to the morbidity of cardiac surgery with extracorporeal circulation. In the 1960s, a frequently fatal complication known to follow prolonged CPB was identified as the "postperfusion syndrome". It is manifest clinically as generalized weakness, anorexia, fever, respiratory insufficiency, hypoventilation, dyspnea, and sometimes cyanosis. Pulmonary function is disturbed as revealed by definite impairment of blood gas diffusion, including hypercapnea and hypoxemia. Microscopically, diffuse atelectasis, severe congestion with perivascular and intra-alveolar hemorrhage are present.[136] With improved technology and surgical methodology, this once frequent complication is rarely seen today.

Extracorporeal circulation (ECC) alters pulmonary function in nearly all patients undergoing cardiac operations. Chenoweth[76] described pulmonary injury as a consequence of complement activation secondary to foreign surface interaction. As discussed previously, complement anaphylatoxins result in leukosequestration in the pulmonary circulation, and lysozomal enzyme release. In addition, generation of oxygen free radicals further contributes to alveolar capillary injury and leads to increasing microvascular permeability, interstitial hemorrhage, and miliary atelectasis. Bando et al.[137] studied the effects of leukocyte depletion via a filter on free radical mediated lung injury after CPB. They reported that pulmonary function post-CPB was better preserved in the leukocyte depleted group, and specifically there was less O_2 free radical activity, pulmonary edema, and vasoconstriction.

Interestingly, it has also been reported that hemodilution reduces alveolar capillary damage and associated increased pulmonary capillary permeability. Specifically, Rabelo et al.[138] reported that adherence of neutrophils to the pulmonary capillary endothelium during CPB, with subsequent alveolar cell damage is markedly diminished with hemodilution.

Despite the decrease serum colloid oncotic pressure, dilute prime does not result in pulmonary edema as there is also a drop in the colloidal osmotic pressure of the proteins in the interstitial fluid and a compensatory increase in pulmonary lymph flow. This system can compensate for low colloidal osmotic pressure of plasma proteins if integrity of the pulmonary capillary membrane is preserved. Therefore, controlled pulmonary capillary hydrostatic pressure is critical to the prevention of postoperative pulmonary edema. Even transient rises in pulmonary capillary pressure can cause disruption of the endothelial cell junctions. Therefore during CPB effective left ventricular venting is essential to prevent this increase in pulmonary pressure. Monitoring pulmonary artery pressure with a pulmonary artery catheter is important. In addition, postoperative control of pulmonary artery pressure with appropriate fluid management and vasodilators is essential.

Injury to the lung can also occur during CPB secondary to air and blood component microemboli. This leads to damage in the underperfused areas and an increase in pulmonary capillary pressure and filtration in the perfused areas.[139]

All patients undergoing open heart surgery with ECC are at high risk for alveolar collapse and consequent intrapulmonary shunting. This is secondary to the increase in capillary permeability, pulmonary capillary pressure, and fall in lung volume due to decreased lung compliance and altered chest wall mechanics. Pennock et al.[140] compared static inflation, deflation, and ventilation during CPB and found all three modes of ventilation associated with decreased lung compliance and markedly reduced functional residual capacity. In principle, probably the best form of ventilation during CPB would be to use air while maintaining lung volume at pre-CPB functional residual capacity level. Certainly, if the cause of lung damage is in fact due to complement activation, and superoxide generation then theoretically high concentrations of oxygen will in fact increase injury.

Much research is in progress to further define the mechanisms of pulmonary injury. Specific factors critical to the development of respiratory insufficiency that have been identified include a CPB pump time of greater than 120-150 minutes, the amount of leukosequestration in the alveolar vasculature, and the normality of the lung prior to surgery.[71] Ratliff et al.[141] clearly demonstrated that a healthy lung is much more resistant to the trauma of CPB than a previously injured lung.

Hematologic Function

The coagulation system is profoundly affected by the foreign surfaces of the extracorporeal circuit, hemodilution, hypothermia, and use of the cardiotomy suction systems.

Platelet Dysfunction and Thrombocytopenia

Alteration in platelet function and number is the most commonly observed hematologic dysfunction seen during CPB. Normally, platelets adhere to both foreign surfaces and to each other by the process of aggregation. Aggregation is activated by chemical substances including adenosine diphosphate (ADP), seratonin, arachadonic acid, and thromboxane A_2. Once activated, platelets undergo both structural and biochemical change and release thromboxane A_2 as well as additional seratonin and ADP. Thromboxane

A_2, a powerful vasoconstrictor and platelet activator promotes further platelet aggregation.

Within minutes following the onset of CPB, plasma proteins also adhere to the synthetic surfaces. Fibrinogen is one of the plasma proteins which rapidly binds to the surfaces, and is then denatured. This denatured fibrinogen in turn stimulates platelet adhesion via platelet fibrinogen receptors and triggers platelet activation and degranulation with the liberation of activator substances which leads to further platelet to platelet adhesion as well as platelet to foreign surface adhesion. New platelets that enter the circulation after the first few minutes of CPB do not adhere to the surfaces since the absorbed fibrinogen is covered with platelets and platelet membrane fragments.[142]

The membrane of the oxygenator provides a very large surface for interaction, and the rapid reduction in circulating platelets seen is due to this large activating surface. With the bubble oxygenator direct platelet injury is superimposed on that which accrues from the foreign surface interaction. The blood-gas interfaces denature proteins, and mechanical obstruction of platelets occurs at this interface. There is a gradual progressive decline in platelets due to destruction.[143] There is evidence suggesting that the larger platelets are more vulnerable to destruction due to their size leaving the older, less functional ones in the circulation.[144]

Platelet aggregates have been demonstrated in the arterial return line, and as peripheral emboli in the brain and other organs. In view of the consequences of platelet aggregation, research has been directed toward the use of platelet inhibitors such as prostacyclin and dipyridamole.[145] Precoating surfaces with albumin has been found to reduce platelet adhesion.[146]

Hypothermia is also associated with platelet dysfunction. In vitro platelet aggregation is abolished below 33°C,[147] while sequestration of platelets occurs below 25°C, primarily to the liver with return into the circulation during rewarming.[148] Platelet count also decreases during CPB due to dilution by the priming solution, blood loss, adhesion to the circuit, as well as fragmentation, and destruction. The platelet count usually decreases by 25%-60% from baseline values. In addition, the cardiotomy suction exposes platelets to blood-air and blood-tissue interfaces, where activation, injury and destruction occur.

Coagulation Factors

A reduction of coagulation factors, fibrinogen, and plasminogen occurs with CPB. This reduction parallels the decrease in hematocrit suggesting that hemodilution is the cause. The range of decrease reported has been variable and may reflect different protocols of pump prime and flow rates. Factor V decreases to lower levels than that predicted by hemodilution alone, the reason being unknown.

The reduction in coagulation factors seen is usually not great enough to result in a bleeding diathesis. Ecxessive red blood cell transfusion coupled with hemodilution however may further reduce these factors.

In addition, variable levels of primary fibrinolytic activity occur during CPB, rarely associated with hypofibrinogenemia or elevated fibrin split products postoperatively and usually are not clinically significant.[149]

Red Blood Cells

Hemodilution upon initiation of CPB results in an immediate 30%-50% reduction in hematocrit. Sheering stress from cardiotomy suction systems, and trauma associated with blood-gas interfaces contribute to red cell damage and immediate hemolysis. This hemolysis is associated with a release of ADP that contributes to platelet activation. In addition it has been shown that CPB is associated with the development of an anemia and shortened red blood cell life span. Possibly the red blood cell losses exceed the human regenerative capacity[150]

In summary, alteration in coagulation function with CPB is unavoidable, and contributes to the morbidity of the cardiac surgical patient. However, with improved bypass circuit components, better oxygenators, use of hemodilution and hypothermia, and low flow rates, hematologic problems have become less severe. In addition, meticulous surgical technique, controlled cardiotomy suction, the use of the membrane oxygenator for bypass runs greater than 2 hours, adequate rewarming, and appropriate heparin reversal will minimize these undesirable effects. Continued research regarding more optimal biosynthetics, as well as pharmacological strategies to minimize the foreign surface interaction is necessary.

Renal Function

The effect of CPB on kidney function is secondary to the type of flow, hemodilution, hypothermia, extracorporeal oxygenation, and the associated hormonal response.

Hemodilution has a known protective effect on the kidney during CPB. In association with a lower plasma oncotic pressure, hemodilution maintains the glomerular filtration rate (GFR) at lower perfusion pressures resulting in an increase in urine output, and decrease in creatinine and sodium clearance during CPB.[151] The diminished urine osmolarity with hemodilution has been demonstrated to protect renal tubular integrity.[152] In addition, hemodilution produces less hemolysis than a blood prime.

Hypothermia decreases both inner and outer renal cortical blood flow in about equal proportions. It also decreases GFR, and osmolar clearance while elevating filtration fraction and potassium excretion. The decreased viscosity associated with hemodilution opposes the vasoconstriction of hypothermia to maintain satisfactory levels of renal perfusion.[153,154]

Utley et al.[33] reported the use of the pump oxygenator to result in diminished outer cortical flow, possibly due to the cortical delivery of microemboli. The rate of production of microemboli appears to be greater in bubble oxygenators than disc oxygenators. Additional factors such as the stimulation of the renin-angiotensin-aldosterone axis in early bypass and the use of various pharmacologic agents contribute to the increased renal vascular resistance seen with CPB.

Unquestionably CPB is associated with altered renal function. The duration of CPB, and aortic cross clamp as well as the entire operation correlates with risk of postoperative renal dysfunction. Decreased renal blood flow and urine output becomes marked with prolonged CPB. Negative free water clearance and creatinine clearance are less in patients who have perfusion for greater than 60 minutes. Although the depression of renal plasma flow, GFR and sodium excretion are reported less at higher pressure and flow rates than at low flow rates, Abel et al.[154] were not able to show any correlation between perfusion pressure, flow rates, or presence of hemoglobinemia with postoperative renal dysfunction. Hemolysis that is known to occur during CPB may precipitate in the renal tubules, impair function and lead to acute necrosis. Pulsatile perfusion has reportedly been associated with lower renin-angiotensin levels, greater urine output and creatine clearance than nonpulsatile flow.[99]

Although renal function is clearly altered by CPB, the incidence of renal failure postoperatively is probably more related to preoperative renal function and postoperative perfusion than the actual exposure to the bypass circuit and the asociated pharmacologic manipulations.

Monitoring Renal Function

Urine output is the simplest measure of renal function during CPB. Both quality and quantity of urine output are good indicators of adequacy of renal perfusion. However, varying perfusion pressures, hypothermia, and mannitol in the pump prime may all effect urine output and make it an inaccurate indicator of perfusion.

Oliguria during CPB should be aggressively evaluated. A kinked or obstructed foley catheter should be first ruled out. Then causes of impaired renal perfusion sought. Inadequate perfusion flow rate, arterial hypotension, nonpulsatile perfusion, renal vasoconstriction secondary to pharmacologic agents, and elevated inferior vena cava pressure all may impair renal blood flow. This can be worsened by elevated circulating catecholamine levels and vasopressin that occur during CPB.

Conclusion

An attempt was made to provide the reader with an overview regarding the physiologic considerations of CPB. Although our knowledge of perfusion is advancing at a rapid pace, continued research regarding the components of the extracorporeal circuit, and clinical studies further defining the mechanisms of organ dysfunction and appropriate measures of intervention are necessary. Many controversies over appropriate management will continue until well-directed clinical studies are performed.

REFERENCES

1. Gibbon JH. Application of a mechanical heart and lung apparatus to cardiac surgery. *Minn Med* 37:171, 1954.
2. Simpson JC. Oxygenation—general review in cardiopulmonary bypass, In: Taylor KM, ed. *Principles of Cardiopulmonary Bypass.* Baltimore, MD: Williams and Wilkins; 1986:149-159.
3. Galletti PM, Richardson PD, Snider MT, et al. A standardized method for defining the overall gas transfer performance of artificial lungs. *Trans Am Soc Artif Int Org* 18:398-392, 1972.
4. Edmunds LH Jr, Ellison N, Colman R. Platelet function during cardiac operations: comparison of membrane and bubble oxygenators. *J Thorac Cardiovasc Surg* 80:805-812, 1982.
5. van Oeveren W, Kazatchkine MD, Descamps-Latscha B, et al. A prospective study of bubble versus membrane oxygenation. *J Thorac Cardiovasc Surg* 89:888-899, 1985.
6. Teoh KH, Christakis GT, Weisel RD, et al. Blood conservation with membrane oxygenators and dypyridamole. *Ann Thorac Surg* 44:40-47, 1987.
7. German B, Wyman J Jr. The titration curves of oxygenated and reduced hemoglobin. *J Biol Chem* 117:553, 1937.
8. Astrup P, Engel K, Severinghaus JW, et al. The influence of temperature and pH on the dissociation curve of oxygenated human blood. *Scand J Clin Lab Invest* 17:515, 1965.
9. Severinghaus JW. Respiration and hypothermia. *Ann NY Acad Sci* 80:384, 1959.
10. Guyton A. Transport of oxygen and carbon dioxide in blood and body fluids. In: Guyton A. *Textbook of Medical Physiology* Philadelphia, PA.: W.B. Saunders Co; 1976:549.
11. Moores WY. Oxygen delivery during cardiopulmonary bypass. In: Utlry J, ed. *Pathophysiology of Cardiopulmonary Bypass I.* Baltimore, MD: Williams and Wilkins; 1983:1-11.
12. Valeri CR, Dennis RC, Hedhtman HB, et al. Transfusion of 2,3-DPG enriched red blood cells to improve cardiac function. *Ann Thorac Surg* 26:17, 1978.
13. Kirklin JW, Dushane JW, Patrick RJ, et al. Intracardiac surgery with the aid of a mechanical pump oxygenator system: report of eight cases. *Proc Mayo Clinic* 30:301, 1955.

14. Conti VR, Bertranou EG, Blackstone EM, et al. Cold cardioplegia versus hypothermia for myocardial protection. *J Thorac Cardiovasc Surg* 76:577-589, 1978.
15. Hild P. Pathophysiology of cardiopulmonary bypass. In: Hensley JA, Martin DE, eds. *The Practice of Cardiac Anesthesia*. Boston, MA: Little, Brown and Co.; 1990:605-623.
16. Kety SS, Schmidt CF. The determination of cerebral blood flow in man by use of nitrous oxide in low concentration. *Am J Physiol* 38:143-53, 1945.
17. Selkoe DJ, Myers RE. Neurologic and cardiovascular effects of hypotension in the monkey. *Stroke* 10:147, 1979.
18. Kollka R, Hilberman M. Neurologic dysfunction following cardiac operations with low-flow, low-pressure cardiopulmonary bypass. *J Thorac Cardiovasc Surg* 79:432-437, 1980.
19. Govier AV, Reves JG, McKay RD, et al. Factors and their influences on regional cerebral blood flow during nonpulsatile cardiopulmonary bypass. *Ann Thorac Surg* 38:559-600, 1984.
20. Ellis RJ, Wisniewski A, Potts R, et al. Reduction of flow rate and arterial pressure at moderate hypothermia does not result in cerebral dysfunction. *J Thorac Cardiovasc Surg* 79:173-180, 1980.
21. Hickey RF, Hoar PF. Whole body oxygen consumption during low-flow hypothermic cardiopulmonary bypass. *J Thorac Cardiovasc Surg* 86:903-906, 1983.
22. Fox LS, Blackstone MD, Kirklin JW, et al. The relationship of whole body oxygen consumption to perfusion flow rate during hypothermic cardiopulmonary bypass. *J Thorac Cardiovas Surg* 83:239-248, 1982.
23. Rubeyka IM, Coles JG, Wilson GJ, et al. The effect of low-flow cardiopulmonary bypass on cerebral function: an experimental and clinical study. *Ann Thorac Surg* 43:391, 1987.
24. Thompson IR. The influence of cardiopulmonary bypass on cerebral physiology and function. In: Tinker JH, ed. *Cardiopulmonary Bypass: Current Concepts and Controversies*. Philadelphia, PA: WB Saunders; 1989:21-37.
25. Kirklin JW, Barratt-Boyes BG. Hypothermia, circulatory arrest and cardiopulmonary bypass. In: Kirklin JW, Barratt-Boyes BG, eds. *Cardiac Surgery*. New York, NY: Churchill Livingstone; 1988:35.
26. High KM, Williams DR, Kurusz M. Cardiopulmonary bypass circuits and design. In: Hensley FA Jr, Martin DE, eds. *The Practice of Cardiac Anesthesia*. Boston, MA: Little, Brown, and Co.; 1990:584-601.
27. Kirklin JK, Kirklin JW. Management of the cardiovascular system after cardiac surgery. *Ann Thorac Surg* 32:311-19, 1981.
28. Swan H, Sanchez M, Tyndall M, et al. Quality of control of perfusion: monitoring venous blood oxygen tension to prevent hypoxic acidosis. *J Thorac Cardiovasc Surg* 99:868-872, 1990.
29. Fuhram GJ, Fuhram FA. Oxygen consumption of animals and tissues as a function of temperature. *J Gen Physiol* 42:215, 1959.
30. Penrod KE. Oxygen consumption and cooling rates in immersion hyopothermia in the dog. *Am J Physiol* 157:436, 1949.

31. Eisenman B, Spencer FC. Effect of hypothermia on the flow characteristics of blood. *Surgery* 52:532, 1961.
32. Karim F, Reza H. Effect of induced hypothermia and rewarming on renal hemodynamics in anesthetized dogs. *Life Sci* 9:1153, 1970.
33. Utley JR, Wachtel C, Cain RB, et al. Effects of hypothermia, hemodilution, and pump oxygenation on organ water content, blood flow and oxygen delivery and renal function. *Ann Thorac Surg* 31:121, 1981.
34. Sarajas HSS. Myocardial damage induced by immersion hypothermia. *Am J Cardiol* 13:355, 1964.
35. Remensnyder JP, Austen WG. Diastolic pressure-volume relationships of the left ventricle during hypothermia. *J Thorac Cardiovasc Surg* 49:339, 1965.
36. Lilly JK, Boland JP, Zekam S. Urinary bladder temperature monitoring: a new index of core body temperature. *Crit Care Med* 8:742-744, 1980.
37. Caldwell C, Crawford R, Sinclair I. Hypothermia after cardiopulmonary bypass in man. *Anesthesiology* 55:86-87, 1981.
38. Ralley FE, Ramsay JG, Wynand JE, et al. Effect of heated humidified gases on temperature drop after cardiopulmonary bypass. *Anesth Analg* 63:1106-1110, 1984.
39. Williams DG, Siefen AB, Lawson NW, et al. Pulsatile perfusion versus conventional high-flow nonpulsatile perfusion for rapid core cooling and rewarming of infants for circulatory arrest in cardiac operations. *J Thorac Cardiovasc Surg* 78:667-677, 1978.
40. Gravelee GP. Delayed warming during cardiopulmonary bypass. In: Reves JG, Hall RD, eds. *Common Problems in Cardiac Anesthesia*. Chicago, IL: Year Book Medical Publishers, 1987:66-74.
41. Severinghaus JW. Respiration and hypothermia. *Ann New York Acad Sci* 80:384-394, 1959.
42. Severinghaus JW. Blood gas calculation. *J Appl Physiol* 21:1108-1116, 1966.
43. Rosenthal TB. The effect of temperature on the pH of blood and plasma in vitro. *J Biol Chem* 173:25-34, 1948.
44. White FN. A comparative physiological approach to hypothermia. *J Thorac Cardiovasc Surg* 82:821-828, 1981.
45. Rahn H, Reeves RB, Howell BJ. Hydrogen ion regulation, temperature, and evolution. *Am Rev Resp Dis* 112:165-172, 1975.
46. Swan H. The hydroxyl-hydrogen ion concentration ratio during hypothermia. *Surg Gynecol Obstet* 155:897-912, 1982.
47. Reeves RB. An imidazole alpha stat hypothesis for vertebrate acid-base regulation: Tissue carbon dioxide content and body temperature in bullfrog. *Resp Physiol* 14:219-236, 1972.
48. Somero GN, White FN. Enzymatic consequences under alpha stat regulation. In: Rahn H, Prakash O, eds. *Acid-Base Regulation and Body Temperature*. Boston, MA: Martinus Nijhoff; 1985:55-80.
49. Murkin JM, Farrar JK, Tweed WA, et al. Cerebral autoregulation and flow/metabolism coupling during cardiopulmonary bypass: the influence of $PaCO_2$. *Anesth Analg* 66:825-832, 1987.

50. Boysen G, Ladegaard-Pederson HJ, Henriksen H, et al. The effects of $PaCO_2$ on regional cerebral blood flow and internal carotid pressure during carotid clamping. *Anesthesiology* 35:286-300, 1971.
51. Hickey PR, Hansen DD. Temperature and blood gases: the clinical dilemma of acid-base management for hypothermic cardiopulmonary bypass. In: Tinker JH, ed. *Cardiopulmonary Bypass: Current Concepts and Controversies*. Philadelphia, PA: W.B. Saunders; 1989:1-20.
52. McConnell DH, White FN, Nelson RL, et al. Importance of alkalosis in maintenance of "ideal" blood pH during hypothermia. *Surg Forum* 26:263-265, 1975.
53. Swan H. The importance of acid-base management for cardiac and cerebral preservation during open heart operations. *Surg Gynecol Obstet* 158:391-414, 1984.
54. Poole-Wilson PA, Langer GA. Effect of pH on ionic exchange in rat and rabbit myocardium. *Am J Physiol* 229:570, 1975.
55. Swain JA, White FN, Peter RM. The effect of pH on hypothermic ventricular fibrillation thresholds. *J Thorac Cardiovasc Surg* 87:445-451, 1984.
56. Gillen JP, Vogel MFX, Holterman RK, et al. Ventricular fibrillation during orotracheal intubation of hypothermic dogs. *Ann Emerg Med* 15:412-416, 1986.
57. Utley JR, Stephens DB. Fluid balance during cardiopulmonary bypass. In: Utley J, ed. *Pathophysiology of Cardiopulmonary Bypass I.* Baltimore, MD: Williams and Wilkins; 1983:23-36.
58. Kawashima Y, Yamatomoto Z, Manabe H. Safe limits of hemodilution in cardiopulmonary bypass. *Surgery* 76:391, 1974.
59. Utley JR, Todd EP, Wachtel CC, et al. Effect of hypothermia, hemodilution, and pump oxygenation on organ water content and blood flow. *Surg Forum* 27:217, 1976.
60. Buckley MJ, Austen WB, Goldblatt A, et al. Severe hemodilution and autotransfusion for surgery of congenital heart disease. *Surg Forum* 22:160, 1971.
61. Laver MB, Buckley MJ. Extreme hemodilution in the surgical patient. In: Messmer K, Schmid-Schonbein E, eds. *Hemodilution: Theoretical Basis and Clinical Application*. Basel: Karger; 1972:215.
62. Lilleaason P, Stokke O. Moderate and extreme hemodilution in open heart surgery: fluid balance and acid-base studies. *Ann Thorac Surg* 25:127, 1978.
63. Moores WY. Oxygen delivery during cardiopulmonary bypass. In: Utley JR, ed. *Pathophysiology of Cardiopulmonary Bypass I.* Baltimore, MD: Williams and Wilkins; 1983:1-11.
64. Kleinman LH, Yarbrough JW, Symmonds JB, et al. Pressure-flow characteristics of the coronary collateral circulation during cardiopulmonary bypass: effects of hemodilution. *J Thorac Cardiovasc Surg* 75:17, 1978.

65. Nimikowski J, Laaksonen V, Meretoja O, et al. Oxygen transport to tissue under normovolemic moderate and extreme hemodilution during coronary bypass operation. *Ann Thorac Surg* 31:134-143, 1981.
66. Webber CE, Garnett ES. The relationship between colloid osmotic pressure and plasma proteins during and after cardiopulmonary bypass. *J Thorac Cardiovasc Surg* 65:234, 1973.
67. Westaby S. Aspects of biocompatibility in cardiopulmonary bypass. CRC Crit Rev Biocompat 3:193-234, 1987.
68. Lee WH Jr, Krumbhaar D, Fonkalsrud EW, et al. Denaturation of plasma proteins as a cause of morbidity and death after intracardiac operations. *Surgery* 50:29-39, 1961.
69. Kalter RD, Saul CM, Wetstein L, et al. Cardiopulmonary bypass associated hemostatic abnormalities. *J Thorac Cardiovasc Surg* 77:427-435, 1979.
70. Chenoweth DE. Complement activation during cardiopulmonary bypass. In: Utley J, ed. *Pathophysiology of Cardiopulmonary Bypass*. Baltimore, MD: Williams and Wilkins; 1983:49-60.
71. Kirklin JK, Westaby S, Blackstone EH, et al. Complement and damaging effects of cardiopulmonary bypass. *J Thorac Cardiovasc Surg* 86:845-857, 1983.
72. Feijen J. Thrombogenesis caused by blood foreign surface interaction. In: Kenedit RM, Courtney JM, Gaylor IDS, et al. eds. *Artificial Organs*. Baltimore, MD: University Park Press; 1977:235-245.
73. Ellison N, Behar M, MacVaugh H III, et al. Bradykinin, plasma protein fraction, and hypotension. *Ann Thorac Surg* 29:15, 1980.
74. Bachman F, McKenna R, Cole ER, et al. The hemostatic mechanism after open heart surgery. I. Studies on plasma coagulation factors and fibrinolysis in 512 patients after extracorporeal circulation. *J Thorac Cardiovasc Surg* 70:76, 1975.
75. Muller-Eberhard HJ. Complement. *Ann Rev Biochem* 44:697, 1975.
76. Chenoweth DE, Cooper SW, Hugli TE, et al. Complement activation during cardiopulmonary bypass: evidence for generation of C3a and C5a anaphylatoxins. *N Engl J Med* 304:497-503, 1981.
77. Hugli TE, Muller-Eberhard HJ. Anaphylatoxins: C3a and C5a. *Immunology* 28:1067, 1975.
78. Antonsen S, Brandshund I, Clemensen S, et al. Neutrophil enzyme and complement activation during cardiopulmonary bypass. *Scand J Thorac Cardiovasc Surg* 21:47-52, 1987.
79. Kirklin JK, Blackstone EH, Kirklin JW. Cardiopulmonary bypass: studies on its damaging effects. *Blood Purif* 5:168-175, 1987.
80. Cavarocchi NC, Pluth JR, Schaff HV, et al. Complement activation during cardiopulmonary bypass. *J Thorac Cardiovasc Surg* 91:252-258, 1986.
81. van Oeveren W, Janse NJG, Bidstrup BP, et al. Effects of aprotinin on hemostatic mechanisms during cardiopulmonary bypass. *Ann Thorac Surg* 44:640-645, 1987.

82. Reigel WE, Spillner G, Schlosser V, et al. Plasma levels of main granulocyte components during cardiopulmonary bypass. *J Thorac Cardiovasc Surg* 6:1014-1019, 1988.
83. Wesolowski SA, Sauvage LR, Pinc RD: Extracorporeal circulation: the role of the pulse in maintenance of the systemic circulation during heart-lung bypass. *Surgery* 37:663, 1955.
84. Shepard RB, Simpson DC, Sharp JF. Energy equivalent pressure. *Arch Surg* 193:730, 1966.
85. Shepard RB, Kirklin JB. Relation of pulsatile flow to oxygen consumption and other variables during cardiopulmonary bypass. *J Thorac Cardiovasc Surg* 58:694, 1969.
86. Dunn J, Kirsh MM, Harness J, et al. Hemodynamic, metabolic, and hematologic effects of pulsatile cardiopulmonary bypass. *J Thorac Cardiovasc Surg* 68:138, 1974.
87. Trinkle JK, Helton NE, Bryant LR, et al. Pulsatile cardiopulmonary bypass: clinical evaluation. *Surgery* 68:1074, 1970.
88. Singh RKK, Barratt-Boyes BG, Harris EA. Does pulsatile flow improve perfusion during hypothermic cardiopulmonary bypass? *J Thorac Cardiovasc Surg* 79:827, 1980.
89. Frater RWM, Wakagama S, Oka Y, et al. Pulsatile cardiopulmonary bypass: failure to influence hemodynamics or hormones. *Circulation* 62(Suppl 1):19, 1980.
90. Angell James JE, de Burgh Daly M. Effects of graded pulsatile pressures on the reflex vasomotor responses elicited by changes of mean pressure in the perfused carotid sinus-aortic arch regions of the dog. *J Physiol (Lond)* 214:51, 1971.
91. Giron F, Birtwell WC, Soroff HS, et al. Hemodynamic effects of pulsatile and non-pulsatile flow. *Arch Surg* 93:802, 1966.
92. McMaster PD, Parsons RJ. Effect of pulse on spread of substances through tissues. *J Exp Med* 68:377, 1938.
93. Parsons RJ, McMaster PD. Effect of pulse upon formation and flow of lymph. *J Exp Med* 68: 353, 1938.
94. Ogata T, Ida Y, Nonoyama A, et al. A comparative study of the effectiveness of pulsatile and non-pulsatile flow in extracorporeal circulation. *Arch Jpn Clin* 29:59, 1960.
95. Geha AS, Salaymeh MT, Tomio A, et al. Effect of pulsatile cardiopulmonary bypass on cerebral metabolism. *J Surg Res* 12:381, 1972.
96. Hickey PR, Buckley MJ, Philbin DM. Pulsatile and non-pulsatile cardiopulmonary bypass: a review of a counter productive controversy. *Ann Thorac Surg* 36:6, 1983.
97. Landymore RW, Murphy DA, Kinley CE, et al. Does pulsatile flow influence the incidence of post operative hypertension? *Ann Thorac Surg* 28:26, 1979.
98. Watkins L Jr, Lucas SK, Gardner TJ, et al. Angiotensin II levels during cardiopulmonary bypass: a comparison of pulsatile and non-pulsatile flow. *Surg Forum* 29:229, 1978.
99. Philbin DM, Levine FH, Emerson CW, et al. Plasma vasopressin levels and urinary sodium excretion during cardiopulmonary bypass in

patients with valvular disease:effect of pulsatile flow. *J Thorac Cardiovasc Surg* 78:779, 1979.
100. Philbin DM, Levine FH, Kono K, et al. Alteration of the stress response to cardiopulmonary bypass by the addition of pulsatile flow. *Circulation* 64:808, 1981.
101. Taylor KM, Wright GS, Reid JM, et al. Comparative studies of pulsatile and nonpulsatile flow during cardiopulmonary bypass II: the effects on renal secretion of cortisol. *J Thorac Cardiovasc Surg* 75:574, 1978.
102. Watkins WD, Moss J, Lappas DG, et al. Vasoactive mediators and human cardiopulmonary bypass (abstract). *Anesthesiology* 51:597, 1979.
103. Pacquet KJ. Hemodynamic studies on normothermic perfusion of the isolated pig kidney with pulsatile and nonpulsatile flow. *J Thorac Cardiovasc Surg (Torino)* 1:45, 1969.
104. German JC, Chalmers GS, Mukherjee D, et al. Comparison of nonpulsatile and pulsatile extracorporeal circulation on renal tissue perfusion. *Chest* 61:65, 1972.
105. Jacobs LA, Klopp EH, Seamone W, et al. Improved organ function during cardiac bypass with a roller pump modified to deliver pulsatile flow. *J Thorac Cardiovasc Surg* 58:703, 1969.
106. Bregman D, Bowman FO, Parodi EN, et al. An improved method of myocardial protection with pulsation during CPB. *Circulation* 56: 157, 1977.
107. Moores WY, Hannon JP, Crum J, et al. Coronary flow distribution and dynamics during continuous and pulsatile extracorporeal circulation in the pig. *Ann Thorac Surg* 24:582, 1977.
108. Grover FL, Fewel JG, Vines J, et al. Effects of aortic balloon pumping during cardiopulmonary bypass on myocardial perfusion, metabolism and contractility. *Chest* 75:73, 1979.
109. Maddoux G, Papas G, Jenkins M, et al. Effect of pulsatile and nonpulsatile flow during CPB on left ventricular ejection fraction early after aortocoronary bypass surgery. *Am J Cardiol* 37:1000, 1976.
110. Levine FH, Grotte GJ, Falon JT, et al. Effects of pulsatile and nonpulsatile reperfusion on the postischemic myocardium (abstract). *Am J Cardiol* 45:394, 1980.
111. Habal SM, Weiss MB, Spotnitz HM, et al. Effects of pulsatile and nonpulsatile coronary perfusion on performance of the canine left ventricle. *J Thorac Cardiovasc Surg* 72:742, 1976.
112. Sanderson JM, Wright G, Sims FW. Brain damage in dogs immediately following pulsatile and nonpulsatile blood flow in the extracorporeal circulation. *Thorax* 27:275, 1972.
113. Geha S, Malt SH, Nara Y, et al. Effect of cardiopulmonary bypass on cerebral metabolism. *J Thorac Cardiovasc Surg* 61:200, 1971.
114. Hirvonen J, Huttunen P, Nuutinen L. Catecholamines and free fatty acids in plasma of patients undergoing cardiac operations with hypothermia and bypass. *J Clin Pathol* 31:949, 1978.

115. Wu W, Zubuzek VK, Bellevue C. Vasopressin release during cardiac operation. *J Thorac Cardiovasc Surg* 79:83, 1980.
116. Shore L. Vasopressin: its bioassay and the physiological control of its release. *Am J Med* 42:701, 1967.
117. Dewar ML, Walsh G, Chiu RC, et al. Atrial natriuetic factor: response to cardiac operation. *J Thorac Cardiovasc Surg* 96(2):266-270, 1988.
118. Taylor KM, Jones JV, Walker MS, et al. The cortisol response during heart-lung bypass. *Circulation* 54:20, 1976.
119. Oka Y, Wakayama S, Oyama T, et al. Cortisol and antiuretic hormone responses to stress in the cardiac surgical patients. *Can Anaesth Soc J* 28(4): 334-337, 1981.
120. Uozone T, Manabe H, Kawashima Y, et al. Plasma cortisol corticosterone and non-protein bound cortisol in the evtracorporeal circulation. *Acta Endocrinol* 69:517, 1972.
121. Mills NL, Beaudet RL, Isom OW, et al. Hyperglycemia during cardiopulmonary bypass. *Ann Surg* 177:203, 1973.
122. Swain JA. Endocrine responses to cardiopulmonary bypass. In: Utley J, ed. *Pathophysiology of Cardiopulmonary Bypass I.* Baltimore, MD: Williams and Wilkins; 1983:24-33.
123. Moffitt EA, Rosevear JW, Molnar GD, et al. Myocardial metabolism in open-heart surgery. Correlation with insulin response. *J Thorac Cardiovasc Surg* 59:691, 1970.
124. Tanaka J, Shiki K, Asou T, et al. Cerebral autoregulation during hypothermic nonpulsatile cardiopulmonary bypass with selective perfusion in dogs. *J Thorac Cardiovasc Surg* 95:124-132, 1988.
125. Sotaniemi KA, Jaolasmaa A, Hokkanen ET. Neuropsychologic outcome after open heart surgery. *Arch Neurol* 38:2, 1981.
126. Ellis RJ, Wisniewski A, Potts R, et al. Reduction of flow rate and arterial pressure at moderate hypothermia does not result in cerebral dysfunction. *J Thorac Cardiovasc Surg* 79:173, 1980.
127. Feddersen K, Aren C, Nilsson NJ, et al. Cerebral blood flow and metabolism during cardiopulmonary bypass with special reference to effects of hypotension induced by prostacyclin. *Ann Thorac Surg* 41:395, 1986.
128. Johnsson P, Messeter K, Ryding E, et al. Cerebral blood flow and autoregulation during hypothermic cardiopulmonary bypass. *Ann Thorac Surg* 43:386-390, 1987.
129. Muraoka R, Yokoya M, Aoshima M, et al. Subclinical changes in brain morphology following cardiac operations as reflected by computed tomographic scans of the brain. *J Thorac Cardiovasc Surg* 81:364-369, 1981.
130. Fish KJ. Microembolization: etiology and prevention. In: Hilberman M, ed. *Brain Injury and Protection During Heart Surgery.* Martinus Nijhoff; 1987:67-83.
131. Shaw PJ. Neurological complications of cardiovascular surgery: procedures involving the heart and thoracic aorta. CNS sequelae of open heart surgery. *Anesthesiol Clin* 24:159-200, 1986.

132. Rodigas PC, Meyer FJ, Haasler GB, et al. Intraoperative 2- dimensional echocardiography: ejection of microbubbles from the left ventricle after cardiac surgery. *Am J Cardiol* 50:1130-1132, 1982.
133. Ellis RJ. Cerebral dysfunction following cardiopulmonary bypass. In: Utley J, ed. *Pathophysiology of Cardiopulmonary Bypass I.* Baltimore, MD: Williams and Wilkins; 1983:4-76.
134. Sotaniemi KA. Brain damage and neurolgical outcome after open-heart surgery. *J Neurol Neurosurg Psychiatry* 43:127, 1980.
135. Gibbon JH Jr. The Lewis A. Conner Memorial Lecture: Maintenance of cardiorespiratory functions by extracoporeal circulation. *Circulation* 19:646-656, 1959.
136. Baer DM, Osborn JJ. The post perfusion pulmonary congestion syndrome. *Am J Clin Pathol* 34:442-445, 1960.
137. Bando K, Pillai R, Cameron DE, et al. Leukocyte depletion ameliorates free radical-mediated lung injury after cardiopulmonary bypass. *J Thorac Cardiovasc Surg* 99:873-877, 1990.
138. Rabelo RC, Oliveira SA, Tannaka H, et al. The influence of the nature of the prime on postperfusion pulmonary changes. *J Thorac Cardiovasc Surg* 66:782, 1973.
139. Peters RM. Effects of cardiopulmonary bypass on lung function. In: Utley JR, ed. *Pathophysiology of Cardiopulmonary Bypass.* Baltimore, MD: Williams and Wilkins; 1983:164-169.
140. Pennock JL, Pierce WS, Waldhausen JA. The management of the lungs during cardiopulmonary bypass. *Surg Gynecol Obstet* 145:917-927, 1977.
141. Ratliff NB, Young WB, Hackel DB, et al. Pulmonary injury secondary to extracorporeal circulation. *J Thorac Cardiovasc Surg* 65:425-432, 1973.
142. Baier RE, Dutton RC. Initial events in interaction of blood with a foreign surface. *J Biomed Mater Res* 3:1919, 1969.
143. Campbell FW, Jobes DR, Ellison N. Coagulation management during and after cardiopulmonary bypass. In: Henesley FA, Martin DE, eds. *The Practice of Cardiac Anesthesia.* Boston, MA: Little Brown and Company; 1990:547-579.
144. Karpatkin S. Heterogenicity of human platelets. II. Functional evidence suggestive of young and old platelets. *J Clin Invest* 47:1083-1087, 1969.
145. Teoh K, Van Christakis GT, Weisel RD, et al. Dipyridamole preserved platelets and reduced blood loss after cardiopulmonary bypass. *J Thorac Cardiovasc Surg* 96:332-341, 1988.
146. Addonozio VP Jr, Macarak J, Nicolaou KC, et al. Effects of prostacyclin and albumin on platelet loss during in vitro stimulation of extracorporeal circulation. *Blood* 53:1033-42, 1989.
147. Holmson H, Karpatkin S. Metabolism of platelets. In: Williams WJ, Beutler E, Erslev AJ, et al., eds. *Hematology.* 3rd edition. New York, NY: McGraw-Hill; 1983:1157-1176.

148. Aster RH. Thrombocytopenia due to sequestration of platelets. In: Williams WJ, Beutler E, Erslev AJ, et al., eds. *Hematology*. 3rd edition. New York, NY: McGraw-Hill; 1983:1338-1340.
149. Bick RL. Hemostasis defects associated with cardiac surgery, prosthetic devices, and other extracorporeal circuits. *Semin Thromb Hemostas* 11:249-280, 1985.

Chapter 4

Optimal Flow During Cardiopulmonary Bypass

Bennett A. Mitchell, CCP,
and Pierre A. Casthely, MD

Although perfusion during bypass is a function of both flow and pressure, the optimal flows and perfusion pressures remain controversial. The subject of "optimal perfusion flow rates" for cardiopulmonary bypass (CPB) must be examined from the point of view of flow rate, arterial pressure, hemodilution, and hypothermia.

The oxygen requirements of the human body are based on weight, surface area, and age in both physiologic studies and clinical practice. The oxygen requirements for infants and children per kilogram of body weight is twice that of an adult. For newborn infants between 1 and 3 weeks old, the minimum oxygen consumption is approximately (7.6 mL/O_2/kg/min), it then rises to approximately (9 mL/kg/min) by the age of 2 months. It has been suggested that their enormous consumption of oxygen per unit of body weight may be due to the metabolic requirements of the brain, which is disproportionately larger than the rest of the body and is

From Casthely PA, Bregman D, (eds): *Cardiopulmonary Bypass: Physiology, Related Complications, and Pharmacology.* Mount Kisco, NY, Futura Publishing Company, Inc., © 1991.

developing at a faster rate. (Average adult oxygen consumption is approximately 250 mL/min (4 mL/kg/min)). Therefore, a higher flow rate is needed in children than in adults (Table I).

Table I
Ideal Perfusion Flow (mL/kg/min)

Normothermia (whole blood)	
Body Weight (kg)	*Flow (mL/kg/min)*
5	200
5–10	170
10–20	135
20–30	100
30–60	85
60 and over	60–70

Because it is firmly established that estimated oxygen requirements of the body at resting conditions, based on weight, surface area, and age are over 4 mL/kg/min, or 125 to 130 $mL/m^2/min$, Clark formulated a perfusion flow rate chart from theoretical equations derived from the Fick principle. By adding a few essential variables, such as hemoglobin content, coronary sinus, and bronchial return blood flow, etc., he made it applicable to CPB.

The theory suggests that the perfusion flow rate should be indicated by the ratio of oxygen needed by the organism to the oxygen supply expected per unit of blood flow; and the oxygen need determined by the basal requirement per unit of weight or surface area (Table II) The "ideal" perfusion flow rate was then calculated in the following way:

Table II
Total Body Perfusion Supplied by the Left Ventricle, an Extracorporeal Pump, or Both

Normal value: Flow	3.2 $L/M^2/min$
Oxygen uptake (VO_2)	100–130 $mL/m^2/min$
Hemoglobin value	15 gm%
Hematocrit value	45%
Normal systemic transport (SOT).	
20 vol. % $\times$ 32 $L/m^2/min$ or (640 $mL/O_2/min$)	

$$P = \frac{7.46\ W\ R}{H\ (A\text{-}V)} + C \quad \text{or} \quad P = \frac{25.8\ S\ R}{H\ (A\text{-}V)} + C$$

Perfusion Flow Rate:

Where: P = Perfusion flow rate (liters per minute)

7.46 and 25.8 are numerical constants related to the units chosen

W = Body weight (kg)

S = Surface area (m^2)

R = Basal oxygen requirement (in mL/kg/min); and Ca1/sq.m/h)

H = Hemoglobin (gm%)

A = Arterial blood saturation (in %)

V = Venous blood saturation (in %)

C = Coronary sinus and bronchial return blood in 1/min, is added to the equation, because it is blood aspirated from the field that did not perfuse peripheral tissues. Coronary sinus blood may reach very high values in sinus rhythm or fibrillating hearts. In these cases, the flow is increased by one half of the coronary sinus return volume

The above formula is an expression of the Fick principle where hemoglobin and percent of venous saturation is substituted for the usual denominator.

Thus: perfusion flow rate = oxygen need divided by the oxygen supplied in a given volume of blood

Because hemoglobin is of such importance in the computation of flow rates and because it varies as a result of the prime and additions of solutions, it was assumed that the arterial blood from the oxygenator would be 100% saturated.

Cerebral and Whole-Body Oxygen Consumption Versus Flow Rates

Despite the experience gained in over 35 years of CPB in humans, we are still not fully knowledgeable of the precise relationship between oxygen consumption, oxygen availability, and perfusion flow rates. This is due to our inability to measure accurately the above parameters continuously during CPB. A number of studies indicate that modern methods of anesthesia tend to reduce whole-body oxygen consumption especially when muscle relaxants are used. Moreover, information concerning patients undergoing CPB have been based on indirect calculations, using the product of perfusion flow rate and the arteriovenous oxygen difference. With the advent of in-line blood-gas monitoring electrodes, we will now be able to monitor oxygen consumption versus flow rates at various hypothermic levels very precisely.

During hypothermic and hemodiluted perfusions, the relationship between oxygen consumption and flow rate is very important, because the ultimate goal in CPB is the restoration of normal cardiac function in a cerebrally intact patient. Oxygen consumption by the brain is very important, because it is the organ most susceptible to hypoxia in the shortest time.

Distribution of Blood Flow to Organs

At basal conditions, blood flow to various organs differs due to their weight, or metabolic activity. During CPB, when perfusion flow rate is increased or decreased, the variations in flow are not equal in all organs because of pressure-flow relationship. Each organ (heart, kidney, skin, skeletal, splanchnic organs, and brain) reacts differently in its vasomotion to subtle changes in blood gases that accompany changes in flow rates (Table III).

For example, low flow to the kidney over a short period of time will cause a marked diminution in urine output, but the kidney's oxygen uptake would not be seriously impaired because of its enormous blood flow and minimal $(A-V)_{O_2}$ difference. When blood flow to the skin, skeletal muscle, and splanchnic organs is reduced, even over a long period of time, the organs are not seriously affected.

The brain and the heart are the best protected organs by what is termed "protected redistribution". During protective redistribution, vital organs such as the brain, heart, and kidneys receive more blood than nonvital organs. When the brain is affected by

Table III
Organ Blood Flow Rates During Profoundly Hypothermia (20°C), Nonpulsatile, Hemodiluted Cardiopulmonary Bypass.

	Organ Blood Flow Rate (mL.min^{-1}.100 gm^{-1})		
Organ	*1.5**	*1.0**	*0.5**
Whole body	10.29 ± 0.080	6.86 ± 0.053	3.44 ± 0.026
Brain	45 ± 6.3 (5.4%)	41 ± 7.9 (7.1%)	23 ± 2.8 (8.2%)
Heart	280 ± 84	170 ± 48	52 ± 9.3
Lung	3.8 ± 0.96	2.8 ± 0.75	1.0 ± 0.28
Liver	70 ± 36	36 ± 8.4	12 ± 2.5
Kidney Medulla	55 ± 14.2	18 ± 5.7	8.4 ± 1.52
Cortex	580 ± 112	410 ± 63	220 ± 22

Figure in parenthesis indicate the brain blood flow as percent of total body blood flow.
*Perfusion flow rate (L.min^{-1}.m^{2}).

hypoxemia, it vasodilates in order to maintain its oxygen supply, thus protecting itself despite alterations in cardiac output or changes in flow rates at the expense of other organs. The mechanisms that shunt blood from a less favored organ to one that is more vital are autonomous. Hypoxemia and probably local tissue acidity in the vessels leading to the organs involved stimulates preferential perfusion. For example, redistribution of blood flow in certain circumstances goes directly to the brain and heart. The brain averages only 2% of the total body weight, but it receives 14% of the cardiac output and consumes 20% of the total body oxygen. Because the oxygen requirements of the brain are disproportionate to its blood supply, it is very sensitive to oxygen deprivation. This sensitivity can be seen by the oxygen delivery to the oxygen consumption ratio of the brain compared to the kidney: 2:8 for the brain and 14:0 for the kidney.

The brain has the shortest tolerance for anoxia and generally sustains irreversible damage within 5 minutes of oxygen deprivation. During acute periods of hypoxemia, regional blood flow is increased to the cerebral vessels as much as 35% more than can be achieved by the increasing cardiac output alone.

The oxygen delivery to oxygen consumption ratio of the myocardium is even less. The heart consumes all of the oxygen perfusing its vasculature, and at rest, it consumes approximately 9% of the total oxygen available to the whole body just to sustain basal myocardial function. The coronary vessels, then, must be even more responsive than the brain to redistribution of blood flow.

It has been reported that what is perceived to be the "ideal perfusion flow rates" for normothermic CPB (2.2 to 2.4 L/m²/min), is in fact not enough to clear acid metabolites that apparently accumulate at this level and below. Even at (28°C to 30°C) flow rates below (2.0 L/m²/min) might not meet the tissue metabolic demands, and if perfusion flow is allowed to fall below (1.5 L/m²/min) for more than a short period of time, a progressive metabolic acidosis ensues, despite a fully saturated arterial blood. Venous oxygen tension falls because of the enormous tissue oxygen consumption. Hydrogen ions and organic acids increase resulting in metabolic acidosis.

Animal studies by Cheng and Starr[1,2] show that at normothermia, a minimum flow rate of (2.4 L/m²/min) is required to achieve 85% of the estimated maximum oxygen uptake. When the flow rate is reduced below this level, areas of microcirculation shut down and whole body oxygen uptake falls.

Hagerdal, et al.[3] in an animal study reported that, for each degree fall in temperature, oxygen consumption is reduced by 10% and metabolic rate decreases linearly in a temperature range between 22°C to 37°C, during which time cerebral blood flow (CBF) is not altered or reduced. However, when the temperature falls below 22°C, CBF is reduced to 15% of its normothermic level. Even at a temperature of 20°C and a flow rate below 1.2 L/m²/min, cerebral blood flow still remains approximately 15% of normal and cerebral oxygen uptake ($CMRO_2$) is unchanged as a result of autoregulation. Normal autoregulation is a result of what is called flow-metabolism coupling.

One study indicates that there is a significant decrease in regional CBF during hypothermic CPB, probably due to the effects of anesthetic agents being used, or the acid-base management strategy that is used.[4] Normal CBF is about 45–50 mL/100 g/min and $CMRO_2$ is about 3 mL/100 g/min. Changes in CBF that occur are directly related to temperature changes and cerebral metabolism. In regard to the effects of "optimal perfusion flow rates" during hypothermic CPB, Govier et al.[4] found a marginally significant ($p = 0.06$) relationship between regional CBF and perfusion flow rates in a study of 67 patients. They also examined the influence of flow rates in ten patients by randomly varying perfusion flow rates and keeping the mean arterial pressure, nasopharyngeal temperature, and $PaCO_2$ relatively constant. The results indicated that there was no significant change in regional CBF during hypothermic CPB 29.3°C to 25.6°C when flow rates were varied between 1.0 to 2.0 L/m²/min.

Miyamoto et al.[5] conducted an experimental study on the relation between perfusion flow rate and cerebral oxygen consumption during hypothermic CPB at 20°C. The perfusion flow rates were reduced in steps from 100, 60, 30, and 15 mL/kg/min every 30 minutes. Although CBF decreased as perfusion flow decreased, the ratio of CBF to perfusion flow rate increased significantly ($p = 0.05$) at 15 mL/kg/min, compared to flow rates of 100 or 60 mL/kg/min. In 50% of their experiments, the perfusion flow rate was reduced in one step from 100 to 15 mL/kg/min, and after 60 minutes at 15 mL/kg/min, the flow rate was returned to 100 mL/kg/min. Cerebral oxygen consumption decreased significantly during 60 minutes of perfusion at a flow rate of 15 mL/kg/min and did not return to its initial value after the flow rate was returned to 100 mg/kg/min. This data indicated that the "optimal perfusion flow rate" for the brain during CPB at 20°C, appears to be 30 mL/kg/min, with a possible oxygen debt in the brain resulting in anaerobic metabolism if the perfusion flow rate is kept at 15 mL/kg/min or less.

Okuda et al.[6] also studied the relationship between perfusion flow rate and whole body oxygen consumption at 20°C CPB. The study revealed that an oxygen debt and metabolic changes could possibly occur if CPB at 20°C was continued at a flow rate of 30 mL/kg/min; thus, the "optimal perfusion flow rate" at 20°C is considered to be 60 mL/kg/min. It was suggested that a relatively high flow rate is necessary to compensate for an increase in oxygen affinity for hemoglobin because of the shift to the left in the oxygen dissociation curve and to prevent shut down of the microcirculation, uneven distribution of the blood stream, and an increase of the arteriovenous shunt during CPB at 20°C.

Pump Flow During Bypass

In the late 1950s, flow rates of 2.4 L/m²/min were established for cardiopulmonary bypass. Many institutions still use flows of

2.0–2.4 $L/m^2/min$ during CPB. At Stanford, flows of approximately half these levels, namely 1.0–1.2 $L/m^2/min$ have been utilized. Neurologic results are not obviously different between institutions using these quite different flow rates. Well-controlled neurologic testing has not yet been performed using the low flow rates mentioned above. There are many centers in which different surgeons use different flows and perfusionists must keep track of each individual surgeon's preferences! Clearly definitive studies need to be done; although this may be difficult because neurologic outcome is probably the most important outcome criterion. Because this is true, the performance of these types of animal studies will probably not give us the answers we need. It is clear that "low-flow" bypass does result in less blood trauma, less noncoronary collateral flow, and might therefore be expected to result in better myocardial protection. Nonetheless, neurologic and neuropsychiatric damage following CPB is a major ongoing and continuing problem associated with these procedures. It was thought for many years that some of the neuropsychiatric and neurologic damage was related to flow and pressure, although many surgeons now believe that most damage is related to various types of emboli of various sorts. Maybe in the future, many centers may come to a compromise between the "high" and the "low" flow recipes, and use flow rates of 1.6 $L/m^2/min$.

Perfusion Pressure

The relation of arterial pressure to "optimal perfusion flow rates" is of major importance, but the prevailing opinions are diverse and contradictory.

At one time it was commonly believed that pressure was not so critical, as long as the calculated flow rate was maintained (2.2–2.4 $L/m^2/min$) during normothermic CPB. Several factors influence the perfusion pressure (Table IV).

In examining the role of arterial blood pressure during CPB, pressure can be defined as:

$$I = E/R \text{ (ohm)}$$

Where: (I) = blood flow is equal of the quotient between the

Table IV
Factors That Influence the Arterial Blood Pressure

1. Alteration in vascular response
2. Anesthetic agents
3. Operative trauma
4. Perfusion flow rate
5. Priming hemodilutional factor
6. Perfusate colloidal osmotic pressure
7. Temperature
8. Anatomic factor, such patent ductus arteriosus or a large bronchial collateral return in patients with tetraology of Fallot

pressure head necessary for flow; (E) & (R) is resistance of the vasculature.

In other words, perfusion pressure is directly related to the product of vascular resistance and blood flow. It is an approximate linear function of perfusion flow rate.

Perfusion pressures between 30 and 100 mm Hg are commonly used during CPB. A direct and linear relationship exists between blood flow and arterial blood pressure during total perfusion at rates ranging from 0.6 to 1.0 $L/min/m^2$. At higher flows, pressure increases, but to a lesser extent. Pressures greater than 100 mm Hg increase the amount of collateral bleeding into the heart, but more importantly, increase the possibility of component rupture in the extracorporeal circuit. Increased arterial pressure may also be a sign of increased systemic vascular resistance that, if uncorrected, reduces tissue perfusion.

Several studies have reported a definite correlation between low mean arterial pressure (MAP) and numerous neurologic deficits. Javid et al.[7] reported on neurologic damage when MAP was allowed to fall below 50 mm Hg duirng CPB. Juenga et al.[8] reported that even with moderate hypothermia (28°–30° C), pressure below 50 mm Hg for a protracted period will result in severe neurologic damage; especially if there are pre-existing cerebrovascular disorders. Kavan et al.[9] and Van Bergen et al.[10] reported that an arterial pressure below 50 mm Hg is the critical level at which neurologic dysfunction occurs during CPB. It was crucial to maintain arterial pressure above 50 mm Hg to avoid adverse postoperative neurologic sequelae.

The major concern about perfusion pressures of 30 to 40 mm Hg is inadequate organ perfusion, particularly of the brain. Early studies by Stockard et al.[11] (1970 to 1971) correlated the duration of low-pressure perfusion with postoperative neurologic deficits in 6 of 25 consecutive patients undergoing open heart surgery (hypothermia to 28–32°C), femoral arterial cannulation, arterial filtration of the extracorporeal circuit, and morphine or meperidine anesthesia. Neurologic deficits were correlated with the number of millimeters of mercury minutes of MAP below 50 mm Hg as well as with electroencephalographic (EEG) changes occurring at those times. Two patients who had irreversible coma and died had moderate-to-severe cerebrovascular disease. There were many problems with this study including its size, retrospective data analysis, correction of blood gases for temperature, long duration of bypass (137 versus 84 minutes in patients without neurologic deficit), and morphine anesthesia.

Stockard et al.[11] developed a scoring system showing the correlation between the depth and the duration of hypotension, and the degree and severity of the postoperative cerebral dysfunction.

In a subsequently larger prospective study of 75 patients, 15 patients had severe hypotension, 8 of whom had neurologic deficits correlating with EEG changes, and 7 were without neurologic deficits. In the patients with deficits, the investigators noted that pressures and cardiac output after reperfusion, advanced age, and history of cerebrovascular disease were the most important risk factors. Although this study was prospective, data were analyzed retrospectively, and no changes in management were made when hypotension occurred.[12]

Stockard's report concluded that during CPB: (1) perfusion pressures below 50 mm Hg can result in ischemic brain damage and postoperative central nervous dysfunction; (2) the risk of these complications is roughly proportional to the depth and duration of hypotension, but also varies with the extent of cerebral atherosclerosis and the age of the patient; (3) the deliberate use of pressor agents to prevent MAP from falling below 50 mm Hg can reduce central nervous system (CNS) morbidity and mortality after CPB. Higher minimum pressures are more desirable; thus, "optimal flow rates" become an important factor during CPB.

Recent human studies failed to confirm an association between hypotension and postoperative neurologic deficits.[13] Using a bubble oxygenator with arterial filtration, systemic hypothermia of 30°C during diazepam, morphine anesthesia, 30 to 50 mL/kg/min flow rates, and 30 to 50 mm Hg pressures, 41 of 204 patients developed neuropsychologic deficits (six motor deficits). However, MAPs were similar in both groups and the only factors to which neurologic deficits were attributable were age and prolonged duration of CPB. The EEG, however, was not monitored by Kolkka and Hilberman. To date, there has been no study comparing different flow rates at different pressures with multilead compressed spectral-array EEG analysis and testing of postoperative neuropsychologic function.

Although changes in myocardial perfusion also occur at lower flow rates, the heart is usually excluded from the circulation and perfused for only brief periods of time. In the presence of coronary occlusive disease, flows to 50 to 70 mL/kg/min at 50 mm Hg decrease endocardial flow. Renal plasma flow also decreases at total flows of less than 2 L/min/m^2 (about 60 mL/kg/min). Glomerular function is usually measurable at pressure over 30 mm Hg.

It is important to note that Ellis, et al.[14] and Govier disagree with Stockard to some extent. Ellis reported that a reduction in perfusion flow rates and arterial pressure does not result in cerebral dysfunction.[14] Govier reported that their study showed no evidence that a MAP lower than 50 mm Hg is accompanied by a decrease in regional CBF during CPB.[4] However, if cerebral autoregulation is deranged during CPB, then hypotension associated with decreased cerebral perfusion could produce central nervous ischemic injury.

The association between regional CBF and MAP is consistent with preserved autoregulation. During hypothermic CPB, the lower limit of autoregulation appears to be as low as 30 mm Hg, according to Govier. This is in contrast to normotensive, normothermic, human beings with normal cerebrovascular status in whom autoregulation maintains a constant CBF between 50 to 150 mm Hg. The most likely reason for the lower limit (30 mm Hg) of autoregulation is that less CBF is required during profound hypothermia.

Govier concludes that the lower limit of cerebral autoregulation is extended during hypothermic CPB at a flow rate of 1.6 L/min/m^2. Also pharmacologic support is not necessary to maintain a constant CBF between a MAP of 30 to 110 mm Hg. Furthermore, reducing perfusion flow rates to as low as 1.0 L/min/m^2 did not significantly reduce regional CBF, at least during the short intervals in which it was measured in their study.

In summary, it appears that moderate hypothermia (28° to 30°C) in conjunction with hemodilution (Hct 20% to 25%), regardless of the CPB flow rate necessary to achieve a blood minimum, a MAP between 65–75 mm Hg will confer protection in most patients regardless of age or pre-existing cerebrovascular conditions.[15]

Where should the arterial pressure and flow rate be during bypass? It is important to state again that there is no solid body of experimental evidence, in either animals or man, with respect to either cerebral or cardiac or any other vital organ outcome, that would strongly dictate any arterial pressure at any time during bypass. There is evidence that the lower limits of cerebral autoregulation are extended downward during CPB and that CBF is reasonably well maintained at arterial pressures greater than 30 mm Hg.

Hemodilution Versus Optimal Flow Rates

Hemodilution has been a most important adjunct to CPB for many reasons. In most instances, it obviates the need for donor blood with its attendant risks. It decreases colloid osmotic pressure dependent on the degree of hemodilution. It enhances the clotting mechanism by decreasing antithromboplastins; it improves perfusion to the microcirculation by reducing perfusate viscosity.

The viscosity of blood during CPB is very important. There are two factors that control viscosity: hematocrit and temperature. Gollan in 1954[16] reported that the viscosity of whole blood increases about 5% per degree decrease in temperature. The relationship between hematocrit and viscosity is proportional. A 50% decrease in hematocrit is approximately a 50% reduction in viscosity that offsets the rheologic effects of hypothermia. Reduced viscosity results in decreased resistance to blood flow through the capillaries, thus improving tissue perfusion to a degree that will compensate for the reduction in red cell concentration. Postoperative problems related to organ perfusion are somewhat lessened. It enhances renal perfusion, evidenced by an increase in glomerular filtration and an increase in diuresis. There is also evidence that suggests that there is a reduction in protein aggregates at the blood-gas interface in the bubble oxygenator and less blood loss in the postoperative phase. This reduction in viscosity may also allow a calculated flow rate to be achieved with a lower perfusion pressure. These considerations are applicable to CBF as well as the periphery. It is, therefore, necessary to reduce a normal hematocrit of (45%) to approximately (25%) to maintain a constant viscosity during CPB at 20°C. However, if the hemodiluted perfusate has a hematocrit greater than 25% of normal at 20°C, it leads to increased viscosity, decreased tissue blood flow at the same perfusion flow rate, arterial pressure, and systemic vascular resistance.

During hemodilution CPB, there are several determinants that affect the "calculated flow rate" because of the constant rheologic changes that occur. When the perfusate temperature falls, viscosity rises, systemic vascular resistance rises as diuresis occurs and subsequently the hematocrit rises; these determinants give rise to resistance of the "calculated flow rate". Consequently, flow rates must be constantly adjusted to meet these variances.

Hemodilution is used universally, but the degree and composition of the priming solutions vary widely among institutions. Hematocrits also vary, ranging from 15% to 30%. Theoretically, a hematocrit between 15% to 20% of normal can transport adequate oxygen but at severely reduced levels. It is sufficient to maintain CNS function if the hemoglobin is fully saturated and if the CBF can be increased through higher flow rates than calculated or hypercarbia is used to compensate for the reduced oxygen content. Studies have shown that hemodilution progressively increases CBF.

Siejo et al.[17] state that as long as cerebral perfusion pressure can be maintained, the brain can tolerate severe reduction in hemoglobin content.

There is a definite relationship between hemodilution and "optimal perfusion flow rates." Because hemodilution reduces the hemoglobin level and its oxygen carrying capacity, it is essential to raise the perfusion flow rate as well as the PO_2 especially during the warming phase of CPB in order to increase gas transfer through the capillary walls into the tissue fluids and cells.

Optimal Flow Rates in Profound Hypothermia and Circulatory Arrest Hypothermia

Hypothermia causes a variety of physiologic, hemodynamic, and rheologic changes. Hypothermia induces three basic changes in gas transport:

1. The solubility of gases in liquids is inversely related to temperature and therefore substantially more oxygen and carbon dioxide will be carried in physical solution in the blood under hypothermic conditions.
2. As the blood temperature is lowered, the oxyhemoglobin dissociation curve shifts to the left so that for a given partial pressure of oxygen in the tissues, less of the gas is unloaded from the hemoglobin.
3. Decreasing temperatures increase the carrying power of blood for carbon dioxide through an increased activity of the blood buffers.

The animal cell depends upon the utilization of energy for its viability. This energy is supplied by a complex breakdown of several organic molecules that require a constant supply of oxygen. The molecular chemical breakdown evolves in the formation of carbon dioxide and water, together with smaller metabolites of other end products that are immediately excreted from the cell. This process depends upon the circulation of oxygen to enhance the removal of waste products. However, under certain conditions, the lack of oxygen does not stop the production of energy that can continue for a protracted period by chemical reactions.

Anaerobic conditions are limited because of an accumulation of metabolites in the breakdown process. The buildup of these metabolites is mainly acid in origin, and without oxygen to reverse the chemical reactions, it leads to a state of metabolic acidosis.

In brief, hypothermia retards the metabolic breakdown process in cells, and protects them from anoxic death dependent on the degree of hypothermia. The metabolic rate of various organs varies, and their anoxic survival times are related to the duration and depth of temperature.

Oxygen Transport

The transport of gases during hypothermia is of great significance for several reasons.

1. The solubility of gases in liquids is inversely related to temperature, therefore more oxygen and carbon dioxide is carried in the physical solution in blood during hypothermia.
2. The dissolved oxygen content in plasma increases as the temperature is decreased. The amount dissolved at 38°C is approximately 0.3 vol%; at 30°C, 1.6 vol%; at 25°C, 2.0 vol%; at 10°C, 2.5 vol%, and at 0°C it is more than 4 vol%.
3. The oxyhemoglobin dissociation curve shifts to the left as the temperature is lowered.

In 1909, Barcroft[19] and Hill demonstrated how hypothermia shifted the oxygen (O_2) dissociation to the left and upward, thereby making less oxygen available at a given tension and therefore being the probable cause of tissue hypoxia during hypothermia.[18] This simply means that blood arriving at the tissue having an oxygen saturation of 100%, and a tension of 40 mm Hg at 38°C, will unload approximately 25% of its oxygen, whereas, at 10°C it will unload less than 10% because of a greater affinity of hemoglobin for the oxygen.

When hypothermia and hemodilution are used in conjunction with CPB, at temperatures of 22°C–25°C and high flow rates, no metabolic acidosis will occur. In other words, during CPB with hypothermia and hemodilution, sufficient blood and oxygen are available provided that the flow rate is adjusted according to the metabolic rate.

The reversal of hypothermia has the opposite effect. During rewarming, if the oxygen tension is not increased proportionally with the oxygen consumption of the tissues, PO_2 will fall. Therefore the amount of oxygen released by the hemoglobin will increase resulting in a metabolic acidosis. Thus arterial blood flow and gas flow must be increased to meet the metabolic demand. This is one concept that describes the importance of optimal flow rate during CPB.

Carbon Dioxide

Carbon dioxide (CO_2) is the major end product of cellular metabolism; it is continuously being produced by all cells. It also plays an important role in hypothermia. Decreasing temperatures increased the carrying power of carbon dioxide by the blood through an increased ability of blood buffers.[19] For example: if arterial blood at normal temperature (38°C) has a carbon dioxide tension of 40 mm Hg it will carry as dissolved gas 2.7 mL per 100 mL blood. However, at 10°C the amount of dissolved gas will be 5.4 mL per 100 mL blood.

The carbon dissociation curve is not like the oxyhemoglobin dissociation curve that is sigmoid in shape. The relationship between carbon dioxide tension in blood and the carrying capacity of carbon dioxide by the hemoglobin is relatively linear in the physiologic ranges (Hb = 15 g). Carbon dioxide has a reciprocal relationship with oxygen, in that a decreased PO_2 aids in the loading of carbon dioxide and an increased PCO_2 aids in the unloading of oxygen at the tissues. This enhancement of carbon dioxide transport by hemoglobin as it loses oxygen is known as the Haldane effect.

During hypothermia there is: (1) increased solubility of carbon dioxide which is twenty times more soluble in an aqueous media than is oxygen; (2) decreased dissociation and reduction of hydrogen ion activity; (3) increased carrying power of blood for carbon dioxide; (4) decrease in the base-binding capacity of proteins. Proteins are amphoteric and act as acids in an alkaline medium. Decreased ionization produces a decrease in the amount of dissociated hydrogen ion and an increase in the amount of free base or hydrogen ion acceptor. This free base is readily available to combine with carbonic acid and thus the carbon dioxide combing power of blood and, to a lesser extent, plasma is increased at low temperatures.

Buffers

The buffer system in various parts of the body, depending on its cellular content, behaves in a similar manner during hypothermia.

The red blood cell contains a high concentration of hemoglobin, which acts as a buffer since it ionizes as a weak acid under physiological conditions. As a buffer, the hemoglobin is capable of "absorbing" the hydrogen ions formed by the carbonic acid. The buffering power of hemoglobin is changed by certain physiological circumstances. As the removal of oxygen from hemoglobin decreases its acidity, the buffering power increases, thus enabling venous blood to carry more carbon dioxide. The lowering of blood temperature also diminishes the ionization of acid groups of the hemoglobin molecule, thus increasing its buffering capacity and its carrying power.

Metabolism

The relationship between metabolic rate and temperature is neither a linear nor an exponential function. However, the relationship between oxygen consumption and temperature is roughly exponential. In mammals, the decrease in oxygen consumption as the temperature is lowered can be transposed into a reduction of metabolic rate of approximately 7% per degree.

In practice, the metabolic rate for a given temperature is an empirical relationship determined experimentally once a steady state at the required temperature has been attained. Various investigators have given approximations of temperature versus metabolic rate.

Gollan[20] states that oxygen consumption is reduced about 50% between 28°C to 30°C; 80% between 18°C to 20°C, and 90% between 8°C to 10°C.[20] Brewin observed that the metabolic rate is reduced to about 60% to 70% of normal at 30°C; 25% at 20°C, 15% at 15°C, and 5% at 5°C.[21] Bjork states that he found a very different range, 16% to 39% at 18°C to 20°C, in three subjects, and 1% to 11% at 10°C to 13°C in 13 subjects.[22]

In infants and children with cyanotic heart disease, it is mandatory in many instances to reduce flow substantially for adequate surgical exposure. However, the controversy still exists as to the preferred flow rate during profound hypothermia, and the safe limits of circulatory arrest.[21,22] Does very low perfusion flow rate (0.5 $L/m^2/min$) or lower (0.25 $L/m^2/min$) provide more protection to the patient than total circulatory arrest? The answer lies somewhere among the divergence of opinions. Sixty minutes or less has been advocated by some as the safe limit (Table V). However, brain damage has still occurred in a number of reported cases. Kirklin and Miyamoto and colleagues both recommend low flow during profound hypothermia, instead of total circulatory arrest.[23,24] Kirklin has pointed out the need to avoid total circulatory arrest for any protracted period and suggests trying to maintain a low flow (.05 $L/m^2/min$) because of the possibility of introducing air into the arterial system.[25] This approach seems prudent, because it provides some blood flow to the brain and other vital organs. Moreover, after circulatory arrest, air may enter the system circulation and cause embolization when perfusion is restarted.

The measurement of brain tissue pH, PO_2 and PCO_2 have been examined during profound hypothermia and circulatory arrest by Watanabe et al.[25A] Their results have indicated that at a temperature of 20°C, and a total circulatory arrest for a period of 30 minutes, brain tissue PCO_2 increased. In another study by Katogi[26] during 45 minutes of low flow perfusion (25 mL/kg/min) at 20°C, the brain tissue PCO_2 increased without a decrease in brain tissue PO_2. The tissue values for pH, PO_2, and PCO_2 are thought to indicate their mean values in extracellular fluid in a limited tissue area.

Using brain tissue pH, PO_2, and PCO_2 measurements as an indicator of brain damage resulting from 60 minutes of circulatory arrest, (120 minutes of nonpulsatile and pulsatile low flow perfusion) arterial blood-gas analysis demonstrated that the blood base excess decreased the least during pulsatile flow. A significantly high rate of whole blood oxygen consumption, 10 minutes after circulatory arrest is attributed to the result of an acquired oxygen

Table V
Safe Duration of Circulatory Arrest

Temperature C°	*Oxygen Consumption*	*Circulatory Arrest*
37	100%	4–5
29	50%	8–10
22	25%	16–20
16	12%	32–40
10	6%	64–80

debt during the circulatory arrest period. Pulsatile blood flow also reduces the risk of brain damage even during low flow perfusion.

Pulsatile Flow

Controversy still exists about using pulsatile flow during CPB. However, pulsatile flow can be achieved by special roller pumps, intra-aortic balloon pump or pulsatile assist devices.[27] Advantages ascribed to pulsatile flow during CPB are shown in Table VI.[28]

Pulsatile flow enhances subendocardial perfusion in fibrillating hearts. In beating hearts, coronary flow and pressure and subendocardial flow decreased with pulsatile CPB. Pulsatile reperfusion after 60 minutes of ischemic arrest enhances ventricular performance over nonpulsatile reperfusion.[29]

Cerebral blood flow-glucose metabolism coupling in ten regions of the brain during pulsatile and nonpulsatile flow has been evaluated in one study.[30] Although both flow and metabolism decreased, the ratio remained normal, about 2 mL/μmol, with pulsatile flow (animals not on bypass). With extracorporeal nonpulsatile flow, the ratio became 3 mL/μmol, indicating perfusion in excess of metabolic demand. Possible explanations include effects of nonpulsatile flow on myogenic contractility of cerebral arterioles, interference with metabolic flow regulation, or interruption of flow to a portion of the capillary bed by microemboli.

However, other investigators have not been able to confirm the previously described advantages of pulsatile perfusion.[31,32] Also, the high-pressure jet of blood traversing the arterial inflow to pro-

Table VI
Advantages of Pulsatile Flow

Increased urine volume
Normal stress response
Less metabolic acidosis
Lower peripheral resistance
Smaller transfusion volumes
Increased oxygen consumption
Better myocardial perfusion and reperfusion

duce pulsation may increase aortic trauma.[33] Similar increases in corticotropin (ACTH), insulin, and glucose occur with either perfusion method while cortisol is unchanged.[34-36] Neither renal cortical flow, nor its distribution, differ with pulsatile or nonpulsatile flow.[37] The reported advantages are applicable only during CPB with long-term benefits still under investigation.

Conclusion

The controversy of "optimal flow rates for cardiopulmonary bypass", profound hypothermia and total circulatory arrest, or continuous low flow, will continue for a long time to come. The evidence covered in this chapter seems to indicate that there is not enough objective evidence showing that one method is superior to another. Quite a number of infants survive profound hypothermia with circulatory arrest, but some degree of CNS dysfunction occurs that cannot be measured scientifically or objectively.

The overwhelming evidence appears to indicate that there is no definite prescribed flow rate, but a range of physiologic parameters within which one can perfuse with a relative margin of safety, depending on the prevailing circumstances (hypothermia, hemodilution).

REFERENCES

1. Cheng H, Kusunoki T, Bosher LH, et al. A study of oxygen consumption during extracorporeal circulation. *Trans Soc Art Int Organs* 5:273-276, 1959.
2. Starr A. Oxygen consumption during cardiopulmonary bypass. *J Thorac Cardiovasc Surg* 38:46-56, 1959.
3. Hagerdal M, Harp J, Hilson L, et al. The effect of induced hypothermia upon oxygen consumption in the rat brain. *J Neurochem* 24:311, 1975.
4. Govier AV, Reves JG, McKay RD, et al. Factors and their influence on regional cerebral blood flow during non-pulsatile cardiopulmonary bypass. *Ann Thorac Surg* 38(6): 592-600, 1989.
5. Miyamoto K, Kawashima Y, Matsuda H, et al. Optimal perfusion flow rate for the brain during deep hypothermic cardiopulmonary bypass at 20°C. *J Thorac Cardiovasc Surg* 92:1065-1070, 1986.

6. Okuda A, Hirose H, Ohnishi K, et al. Experimental studies on the relationship between whole body oxygen consumption and perfusion flow rate. *Nippon Kyobu Geka Zasshi* 31(7): 1049-56.
7. Javid H, Tufo HM, Najafi H, et al. Neurologic abnormalities following open-heart surgery. *J Thorac Cardiovasc Surg* 58:502-509, 1969.
8. Juenga I, Flynn RE, Berger RL. The arterial and venous pressure and the electroencephalogram during open-heart surgery. *Acta Neurol Scand* 48:163-168, 1972.
9. Kavan EM, Brechner VL, Walter RD, et al. Electroencephalographic patterns during intracardiac surgery using cardiopulmonary bypass: a comparison of two anesthetic agents. *Arch Surg* 78:151, 1959.
10. Van Bergen FH, Buckley JJ, French LA, et al. Physiologic alterations associated with hexamethonium-induced hypotension. *Anesthesiology* 15:507, 1964.
11. Stockard JJ, Bickford RG, Schauble JF. Pressure dependent cerebral ischemia during cardiopulmonary bypass. *Neurology* 23:521-529, 1973.
12. Stockard JJ, Bickford RG, Meyers RR, et al. Hypotension-induced changes in cerebral function during cardiac surgery. *Stroke* 5:730-746, 1974.
13. Kolka R, Hilberman M. Neurological dysfunction following cardiac operation with low flow, low pressure cardiopulmonary bypass. *J Thorac Cardiovasc Surg* 79:432-437, 1980.
14. Ellis RJ, Wisniewski A, Potts R, et al: Reduction in flow rate and arterial pressure at moderate hypothermia does not result in cerebral dysfunction. *J Thorac Cardiovasc Surg* 79:173-180, 1980.
15. Kolka R, Hilberman M. Neurologic dysfunction following cardiac operation with low-flow, low pressure cardiopulmonary bypass. *J Thorac Cardiovasc Surg* 79:432-437, 1980.
16. Gollan F, Hoffman JE, Jones RM. Maintenance of life of dogs below 10°C without hemoglobin. *Am J Physiol* 179:640, 1954.
17. Seijo BK. Brain Energy Metabolism. New York, NY: Wiley; 1978: 446-449.
18. Barcroft J, Hill AV. The nature of oxyhemoglobin, with a note on its molecular weight. *J Physiol* 39:411, 1909-1910, 1984.
19. Bohr X, Hasselbalch K, Krough A. Uber einen in biologischer Belihung Wichtigen Einfluss den die Kohlensauerspanning des Blutes auf dessen Sauerstoffbindurg ubt, Skand. *Arch Physiol* 16:402, 1904.
20. Gollan F, Hoffman JE. Maintenance of life of dogs 10°C without hemoglobin. *J Physiol* 179:640, 1954.
21. Rittenhouse RA, Mohri H, Dillard DH, et al. Deep hypothermia in cardiovascular surgery. *Curr Rev* 17:63-98, 1974.
22. Haneda K, Sands M, Thomas R, et al. Prolongation of the safe interval of hypothermic circulatory arrest: 90 minutes. *J Cardiovasc Surg* 24:15-21, 1983.
23. Kirklin JW. Advances in Cardiovascular Surgery. New York, NY: Grune and Stratton; 1973:89-90.

24. Miyamoto K, Kawashime Y, Matsuda H, et al. Optimal perfusion flow rate for the brain during deep hypothermic cardiopulmonary bypass at 20°C. *J Thorac Cardiovasc Surg* 92:1065-1070, 1986.
25. Kirklin JW, McGoon DC, Theye RA. What is adequate perfusion? In: Allen JG, ed. *Extracorporeal Circulation.* Springfield, IL. Thomas, 1958: 125-138.
25A. Watanabe T, et al. Brain tissue PH, Oxygen tension and Carbon dioxide tension in profoundly hypothermic cardiopulmonary bypass. *J Thorac Cardiovasc Surgery* 97:396-401, 1989.
26. Katogi T. Analysis of brain tissue gas tension during hypothermia low-flow perfusion. *J Japan Assoc Thorac Surg* 31:1505-1512, 1983.
27. Shevde K, DeBois WJ. Pulsatile flow is preferable to non-pulsatile flow during cardiopulmonary bypass. *J Cardiothorac Anesth* 1:165-168, 1987.
28. Williams GD, Seifen AB, Lawson NW, et al. Pulsatile perfusion versus conventional high flow nonpulsatile perfusion for rapid core cooling and rewarming of infants for circulatory arrest in cardiac operation. *J Thorac Cardiovasc Surg* 78:667-677, 1979.
29. Habal SM, Weiss MB, Spotnitz HM, et al. Effects of pulsatile and non-pulsatile coronary perfusion on performance of the canine left ventricle. *J Thorac Cardiovasc Surg* 72:742-745, 1976.
30. Andersen K, Waaben J, Husum B, et al. Non-pulsatile cardiopulmonary bypass disrupts the flow metabolism couple in the brain. *J Thorac Cardiovasc Surg* 90:570-579, 1985.
31. Frater RWM, Wakayama S, Oka V, et al. Pulsatile cardiopulmonary bypass: failure to influence hemodynamics or hormones. *Circulation* 62 (Suppl): 19-25, 1980.
32. Kono K, Philbin DM, Coggins CH, et al. Adrenocortical hormone levels during cardiopulmonary bypass with and without pulsatile flow. *J Thorac Cardiovasc Surg* 85:129-133, 1983.
33. Finlayson DC. Non-pulsatile flow is preferable to pulsatile flow during cardiopulmonary bypass. *J Cardiothorac Anesth* 1:169-170, 1987.
34. Ogata T, Ida Y, Nonoyama A, et al. A comparative study of the effectiveness of pulsatile and non-pulsatile blood flow and extracorporeal circulation. *Nippon Geka Hokan* 29:59-66, 1960.
35. Taylor KM, Wright GS, Bain WGH, et al: Comparative studies of pulsatile and non-pulsatile flow during cardiopulmonary bypass. III. Response of anterior pituitary gland to thyrotropic releasing hormone. *J Thorac Cardiovasc Surg* 75:579-584, 1978.
36. Taylor KM, Wright GS, Reid JM, et al. Comparative studies of pulsatile and non-pulsatile flow during cardiopulmonary bypass. II. The effects on adrenal secretion of cortisol. *J Thorac Cardiovasc Surg* 75:574-478, 1978.
37. Sink JD, Chitwood WR, Hill RC, et al. Comparison of non-pulsatile and pulsatile extracorporeal circulation on renal cortical blood flow. *Ann Thorac Surg* 29:57-62, 1980.

Chapter 5

Anticoagulation for Cardiopulmonary Bypass

Sheldon Goldstein, MD
and Alexander W. Gotta, MD

In 1916, while studying procoagulants, McClean fortuitously found a phospholipid anticoagulant; subsequently Howell discovered heparin in 1922.[1] The discovery of the anticoagulant effect of heparin and the subsequent determination that protamine reverses this effect made possible the routine use of cardiopulmonary bypass (CPB). Adequate anticoagulation is necessary in order to prevent thrombus formation on the foreign surfaces of the extracorporeal circuit as well as secondary fibrinolysis. Controversy exists regarding many of the details of anticoagulation for CPB as well as its reversal. These issues include the required dose of heparin, accuracy of laboratory evaluation to assess anticoagulation, heparin titration during CPB, protamine dose for reversal, and assessment of adequate reversal of heparin effect. More complex issues include heparin resistance, heparin rebound, and complications of heparin therapy.

From Casthely PA, Bregman D, (eds): *Cardiopulmonary Bypass: Physiology, Related Complications, and Pharmacology.* Mount Kisco, NY, Futura Publishing Company, Inc., © 1991.

Chemistry and Pharmacology of Heparin

Heparin consists of a group of glycosaminoglycans with molecular weights from 3,000 to 30,000 d. Commercial heparin is comprised of two repeating dissacharide units, is strongly acidic, and is produced either from bovine lung or porcine intestinal mucosa. A USP unit of heparin is the amount that prevents 1 mL of citrated sheep plasma from clotting for 1 hour after the addition of 0.2 mL of 1:100 calcium chloride solution.[2] Heparin should be prescribed on a unit basis because potency varies between preparations. Though dosage has been described in milligrams, this is inaccurate and may lead to under or overdosage by a factor of ten. High-dose heparin is administered before CPB, usualiy in a dose of 300 U/kg. The anticoagulant activity of heparin seems to disappear from the blood according to first-order kinetics, yet the half-life is dependent on the dose. Intravenous bolus injection of 100, 400, or 800 U/kg will produce anticoagulant activity half-lives of approximately 1, 2.5, and 5 hours, respectively.[2] The half-life of heparin is significantly prolonged by hypothermia. Heparin clearance is described by the formula:

$$\frac{1}{(0.65 + 0.008D) +/- 0.1} \text{(mL)(min } -1\text{)(kg } -1\text{)}$$

where D represents the dose in IU/kg.[3] The volume of distribution is 0.058 ± 0.011 L/kg.[3]

Heparin is removed from the circulation primarily by the reticuloendothelial system, and from there it may be returned to the circulation.[4] It is inactivated in the liver by heparinase and its inactive metabolic products are excreted in the urine.[2] Heparin results in prolonged anticoagulation in patients with liver disease due to decreased metabolism. Prolonged heparin effects in patients with renal disease are explained by the fact that nonmetabolized heparin does appear in the urine after intravenous administration of large doses, such as those used for CPB. In patients with cirrhosis or renal failure, the half-life of heparin is significantly prolonged.[2]

Blood clotting in vitro is prevented by a whole blood heparin concentration of 1 U/mL.[2] For a 70-kg patient, intravenous injection of 10,000 units of heparin will produce a plasma heparin concentration of approximately 3 U/mL. However, not all patients will achieve a predictable heparin level nor will a given heparin level reflect an exact state of anticoagulation in any particular patient. Extravascular depots, hemodilution, and hypothermia all affect the anticoagulant effect of heparin. Patients who manifest heparin resistance or antithrombin III deficiency will vary greatly from predicted responses. These variations in response to heparin have made it necessary to employ the activated coagulation time (ACT) to determine the coagulation status of the patient prior to CPB. This test will be discussed at length.

Heparin Administration

Heparin administration usually precedes placement of the aortic cannula. This prevents formation of clot at the site that could subsequently embolize resulting in focal ischemia in the distribution of the involved artery. When a central line is present, heparin should be administered directly into the central circulation after aspiration assures blood return. Though rapid injection is usually tolerated, some recommend slow injection as histamine release may manifest as hypotension due to a decrease in systemic vascular resistance.[5] or a decreased inotropic state.[6] Blood should again be aspirated via the central line and flush solution administered. Administration in this manner accomplishes the following goals. First, it is known that heparin has entered the central circulation. Second, it is known that the full dose of heparin has been administered. This is important in the occasional patient who becomes hemodynamically unstable and must be placed on CPB immediately. This instability may be caused by arrhythmias provoked during atrial manipulation or cannulation, or less commonly by heparin itself. Though it is recommended to document adequate anticoagulation before CPB is initiated, arrhythmias or severe ischemia may preclude waiting for laboratory evaluation. The scenario to avoid is administration of heparin into a peripheral line that may have infiltrated (out of view of the anesthesiologist) or whose tubing length may prevent the full dose of heparin from reaching the patient. Initiating CPB in such cases may result in catastrophic thrombosis or secondary fibrinolysis, respectively. It is wise to adhere to a protocol for heparin administration, such as the one presented in Table I. Attention to the details described above will ensure adequate anticoagulation for those cases that require urgent initiation of bypass before documentation of adequate anticoagulation, except in the rare case of antithrombin III deficiency or perhaps heparin resistance.

We prefer to obtain a baseline ACT shortly after the anesthetic has begun. This affords time to repeat the value should it be unexpectedly elevated. We then obtain an ACT 3 minutes after heparin as this approximates its maximum effect. This usually provides adequate time to evaluate an unexpectedly low ACT value. Assuming an uneventful prebypass period, documentation of adequate anticoagulation should be obtained by measurement of the ACT before initiating CPB. If it becomes necessary to institute CPB immediately, one should check the ACT, even if incomplete. Moderate elevation of an ACT still in progress in a patient with no history suggesting heparin resistance is a good indicator that a safe level of anticoagulation is present. If the patient has been on heparin, it is reasonable to administer an additional 5,000 units of heparin empirically, because of the possibility of heparin resistance, and then to initiate CPB. The same could be done if the patient has become unstable and the ACT after heparin administration has not yet begun.

The most serious concern is the patient in whom a completed ACT has elevated only minimally after heparin administration. Obviously, heparin should be readministered, and the second dose should be from a different lot. It is likely that the patient has anti-

Table I
Suggested Protocol For Heparin Administration

1. A baseline ACT should be obtained before heparin administration.
2. Heparin should be administered via a central line that does not contain anesthetics, vasopressors, vasodilators or inotropes.
3. Aspirate the line until blood returns, then administer heparin slowly, to decrease the possibility of significant hypotension.
4. The ACT should be measured 3 minutes after the heparin has been administered.

thrombin III deficiency. A second full dose of heparin still may not provide adequate anticoagulation. The appropriate therapy is administration of fresh frozen plasma, which contains antithrombin III. The management of heparin resistance and antithrombin III deficiency will be discussed.

The Activated Coagulation Time

The activated coagulation time (ACT) is the test currently used to document a safe level of anticoagulation prior to proceeding with bypass. It was introduced by Hattersley in 1966 and is a rapid determination of the Lee-White whole blood clotting time.[7] Although manual rotation of the test tube and inspector visualization for presence of clot was initially described, the test is presently performed via an automated method and is known as the Hemochron (International Technidyne, Edison, NJ, USA). The ACT was an important advance because it is not reasonable to wait 20 or 30 minutes during cardiac surgery for the results of a whole blood clotting time. Automation allows the anesthesiologist to pay undivided attention to the patient. The anesthesiologist only needs to read the result when the audible timer indicates completion of the test. The Hemochron is performed as follows. Two cubic centimeters of whole blood are obtained after adequate removal of volume from the line to ensure a pure sample. Simultaneously, the blood is placed in the ACT tube and the timer is begun. The tube is vigorously shaken to mix the blood with celite, a diatomaceous powder that promotes coagulation by increasing surface area for contact activation. The tube is then placed in the well that is warmed by the heating block to 37°C. The tube contains a magnetic rod that maintains its position as noted by a magnetic detector. However, when fibrin strands form, they displace the magnetic rod from its position. The magnetic detector notes the change in the position of the rod and the timer releases an audible signal, indicating completion of the test. Normal range for the ACT has been reported as 107 seconds ± 13 seconds.[7] Common causes of an artificially prolonged ACT include inadequate warming of the heating block or the use of an ACT tube that has been in a cold operating room overnight. Alternatively, a sample drawn from an arterial line may contain a small amount of heparin flush solution. It is recommended that before drawing an ACT from an arterial line, a sample equivalent to twice the dead space be removed.[8] Additional reasons for artifactually prolonged ACT values include the following: diatomaceous earth has lot-to-lot variability or there is a lack of adherence to a strict protocol in performance of the test.[9] It is important to keep these concerns in mind when performing the ACT. Quality control kits are available to document normal values as well as elevated values for both low-dose therapy (CPL 1) such as that used in angiography suites and high-dose heparin therapy (CPL 2) as used for CPB (Hemochron QC, International Technidyne, Edison, NJ, USA).

The relationship between the whole blood clotting time and the ACT is expressed by the formula[10]

$$\text{WBCT (min)} = \frac{\text{ACT (secs)}}{2.5} - 45$$

If a patient has an ACT of 130 seconds 7 minutes are needed to obtain a whole blood clotting time. The quickness of the ACT is most appreciated though when patients are anticoagulated. A blood sample producing an ACT of 450 seconds would require 135 minutes to offer the same information! It is quickly apparent that in the cardiac surgical suite, where anticoagulation and its reversal need to be rapidly assessed, the ACT offers a major advance.

However, the ACT does not provide all the answers. It is a gross test of coagulation and as such is affected by essentially all aspects of the coagulation cascade, except factor XIII. Therefore, an elevated ACT after heparin reversal with protamine does not necessarily indicate that residual heparin is the cause of the elevated ACT. In addition to residual heparin, destruction of serine proteases, hypofibrinogenemia, fibrinolysis, and platelet abnormalities, both qualitative and quantitative, can all influence the ACT. Still, it is reasonable to say that the ACT is the best available test to assess heparin effect and its reversal in the operating room. One need only become knowledgeable regarding the limitations of the ACT in order to apply it in an appropriate manner in the clinical setting.

Heparin Concentration

Although heparin levels of 2 U/mL or greater frequently correlate with adequate anticoagulation for CPB, the ACT has become the preferred test of anticoagulation. Because occasional patients may be heparin resistant or antithrombin III deficient, knowing the heparin concentration does not guarantee appropriate anticoagulation in any given patient. The ACT, as a gross test of clotting, serves this purpose.

However, documentation of heparin concentration by performance of a Hepcon (HemoTec Inc., Englewood, CO, USA) is useful to support a diagnosis of heparin rebound. The Hepcon consists of four chambers that contain specific amounts of protamine, thromboplastin, and diluent. Air bubbles percolate through the blood in each chamber until a photocell detects clot formation in one of the chambers. Based upon the patient's height and weight, the device computes the heparin level.

Documentation of Anticoagulation

Now that we are convinced of the quickness and ease of use of the ACT, the real issues come to bear. What is an adequate ACT to commence CPB? Jobes et al.[11] reported that an automated ACT of greater than 300 seconds is adequate anticoagulation for CPB. Young et al.[12] did work on monkeys and children and reported that the automated ACT should be maintained at greater than 400 seconds, based upon measurement of elevated fibrin monomer in plasma and abundant fibrin, platelet debris, and cells noted with scanning electron micrographs of oxygenator filter mesh when the ACT fell below 400 seconds. They also noted a significant decrease in platelet counts and fibrinogen when the ACT fell below 400 seconds. Their work supports the concept that unless an adequate level of anticoagulation is obtained the patient is at risk of consumption of coagulation proteins and platelets. Not to leave the topic without a modicum of controversy, Metz and Keats[13] reported that for 20 years they used a single 300 U/kg dose of heparin, a pump prime of 20 mL/kg with 2,500 U/L of heparin, and never noted clot formation in the oxygenators for pump runs up to 2 hours. They then studied this regimen by measuring ACT serially as well as heparin levels and found that in more than 25% of their patients the ACT was less than 400 seconds at some time during the study, including four samples less than 300 seconds. They did not note clots in any perfusion circuit and no patient had a heparin level less than 2 U/mL at any time in the study. The patients with low ACT values did not bleed any more than their counterparts with ACT values greater than 400 degrees. They concluded that the minimum ACT value required for adequate anticoagulation for CPB is less than 400 seconds but that the absolute minimum has not been defined.

Though a low ACT value for a short time may not represent a great risk, a longer period may result in a consumptive coagulopathy. The time required for inadequate anticoagulation to result in consumption of serine proteases and platelets is not known, but it is generally agreed that to be on the safe side it is preferable to maintain the ACT at a minimum of 400 seconds at all time during cardiopulmonary bypass. Indeed, some have advocated that an adequate ACT is 480 seconds.[14]

Guidelines for Heparin Dosage

Before 1975, institutional protocols for the administration of heparin prior to cardiopulmonary bypass varied greatly. In that year Bull et al.[15] published two articles that shed a great deal of light on this issue. They studied several protocols in use at that time and found problems including under- and overheparinization. It became obvious that heparin doses and protamine reversal needed to be individualized. They showed that heparin effect varies threefold in sensitivity and fourfold in duration between patients, and presented a technique whereby a dose-response curve could be drawn for each individual patient.[14]

Bull's work has clearly established the importance of titrating the dose of heparin to the individual patient. Though extreme sensitivity to heparin is uncommon, it certainly would be detected by those using the dose-response curve, as manifested by an unusually high ACT after the original low dose. In the occasional patient who displays marked sensitivity to heparin, knowledge of this increased sensitivity would prevent excessive heparin administration. Excess heparin may worsen or prolong heparin-induced thrombocytopenia in the susceptible patient. It could also induce heparin rebound which may be related to heparin stores in the extravascular compartment. However, the most consistent benefit of avoiding excessive heparin administration is the decreased requirement for protamine reversal of anticoagulation, which may result in decreased risk of undesirable reactions to protamine.

Heparin Resistance

Decreased sensitivity to heparin, also called "heparin resistance" is a common problem encountered during cardiac surgery. Possible etiologies are listed in Table II.

Because hemodynamic instability requiring initiation of CPB may occur during or after placement of the atrial/venous cannulae, it is best to document an adequate ACT before this surgical maneuver. Though catastrophic thrombosis is not likely with inadequate anticoagulation, low grade coagulation with consumption of the serine proteases and platelets may produce a hemorrhagic diathesis in the post-CPB period.[12,16] This occurrence, known as secondary fibrinolysis because it is felt to be a response to ongoing coagulation, is probably less of a problem than in the past, because it is now routine to monitor anticoagulation with the ACT. However, this disorder still occasionally occurs, though perhaps there are other causes in addition to inadequate anticoagulation, such as deep venous thrombosis, etc. Though immediate laboratory confirmation is not obtainable, some cardiac anesthesiologists will send a battery of coagulation tests, i.e., PT, PTT, platelet count, fibrinogen

Table II
Causes of Heparin Resistance

1. Ongoing heparin therapy
2. Marked thrombocytosis
3. Anti-thrombin-III deficiency
4. Coronary artery disease
5. Ongoing coagulation
6. Heparin-induced thrombocytopenia
7. Disseminated intravascular coagulation
8. The patient did not receive an appropriate dose of pharmacologically active heparin. The wrong drug was administered or an outdated preparation used (not true heparin resistance)

level, and fibrin split products or d-dimer levels, and then treat the patient empirically for fibrinolysis with ϵ-aminocaproic acid.[17] As this disorder is not a complication of heparin per se, it will not be discussed further. Suffice it to say inadequate anticoagulation may result in a post-CPB coagulopathy.

Assuming a protocol such as proposed in Table I is in use, one should know with some time to spare that the patient exhibits heparin resistance. If careful attention is paid when preparing the heparin syringe the likelihood of the patient not having received heparin or having received an outdated preparation will have been decreased. Assuming then that the patient did in fact receive heparin, the most common cause of heparin resistance is the patient on heparin therapy. Heparin resistance may be due to decreased levels of antithrombin III or increased levels of platelet factor 4.[18] Indeed, we routinely give patients 350 units of heparin/kg, if they have been on heparin within the 24 hours prior to surgery. This will almost always result in adequate anticoagulation. Cloyd et al.[19] evaluated heparin resistance in patients on heparin preoperatively, both with and without intra-aortic balloon pumps. They concluded that patients on preoperative heparin therapy were at an increased risk of inadequate anticoagulation during cardiopulmonary bypass. They reported that neither baseline ACT, duration, nor total dose of heparin predicted which patients would have a decreased response to heparin. They recommended that patients on heparin preoperatively should receive a minimum of 400 U/kg of heparin as their initial dose and a rapidly performed ACT to document heparin effect.

Thrombocytosis

Marked thrombocytosis is not a frequent cause of heparin resistance in the cardiac surgical suite. Presumably, this is because patients who display this laboratory abnormality frequently have serious underlying medical disease and do not undergo surgery. It is due to high levels of platelet factor 4 (heparin neutralizing factor).[20] Platelet factor 4 is cationic and binds to heparin. This results in neutralization of heparin similar to the mechanism by which protamine neutralizes heparin. The treatment for heparin resistance secondary to thrombocytosis is the same as the patient on heparin. i.e., more heparin! Again, the total dose is titrated to the response as measured by the ACT.

Antithrombin III Deficiency

Heparin exerts its anticoagulant effect by enhancing the action of antithrombin III, the major naturally circulating inhibitor of coagulation. Heparin binds antithrombin III causing a conformational change that exposes additional binding sites on the antithrombin III molecule. This increases the ability of antithrombin III to bind with factors XIIa, XIa, IXa, and Xa thus accelerating their inhibition[21] and preventing the formation of fibrin. Although the presence of antithrombin III deficiency cannot be confirmed rapidly, any patient who displays a significantly decreased elevation of the ACT in response to two subsequent doses of heparin, should be suspected of this disorder. A blood sample should be obtained to document antithrombin III levels.

Anticoagulation has been obtained in patients with this disorder by giving excessive doses of heparin, but this raises associated problems such as increased bleeding, heparin rebound, and the need for large doses of protamine, with its associated complications. In one such reported case the patient received 1,380 U/kg of heparin.[22] The preferred treatment is fresh frozen plasma, which contains antithrombin III, as this will prevent the problems associated with excessive heparin administration. For a 70-kg patient who is antithrombin III deficient, two units of fresh frozen plasma will usually be sufficient to obtain an ACT greater than 400 seconds after 300 U/kg of heparin.

Coronary Artery Disease. Ongoing Coagulation and Disseminated Intravascular Coagulation

While coronary artery disease has been discussed as a cause of heparin resistance,[16] there is no known indicator by history or laboratory evaluation to predict this occurrence or its severity.

Similarly, while ongoing coagulation and disseminated intravascular coagulation (DIC) have been associated with heparin resistance, there is no method to predict which patient with a coagulation abnormality will manifest heparin resistance, nor what dose of heparin will be required. Once again the ACT will prove to be the end point to which we titrate heparin.

Heparin-Induced Thrombocytopenia

Heparin-induced thrombocytopenia may be associated with heparin resistance due to antibody-induced platelet aggregation with release of granule contents. As platelet factor 4 has heparin neutralizing activity, it may be responsible for the increased heparin requirements in many of these patients.[23,24] Platelet aggregation may also lead to a DIC-like disorder.[23,24]

Drug-induced immune thrombocytopenia is not an uncommon occurrence. Many offending agents have been identified, heparin included. It is due to the drugs' ability to cause IgG to bind to platelets.[25] Diagnostic assays involve coincubation of the drug, the patient's serum, and washed normal platelets. Antibody bound to the surface of platelets with negative controls is diagnostic of drug-induced thrombocytopenia.[26] Difficulties may arise in implicating a specific agent, because most patients on heparin have underlying medical diseases and therefore are on multiple drugs. Additionally, heparin-induced platelet aggregation studies are not particularly sensitive nor specific.[27] Though testing is improved by using a serotonin release assay[28] this test is neither in widespread use nor does it offer rapid results.

There are three forms of heparin-induced thrombocytopenia that have been described. Up to 40% of patients on heparin will develop a transient decrease in platelet count felt due to reversible clumping and sequestration of platelets.[18] This is not a clinically significant phenomenon[16] and is not associated with any other problems. The acute decrease in platelet count is seen immediately after a bolus injection of intravenous heparin.[29] That the thrombocytopenia is due to the heparin is supported by Gollub and Ulin's demonstration that reversal of heparin rapidly restores the platelet count.[30] This form of heparin-induced thrombocytopenia was described in dogs in 1939[31] and subsequently in man in 1948.[32]

The second (severe) form of heparin-induced thrombocytopenia is not seen frequently by the anesthesiologist, but a full discussion follows because it is a serious disorder when it does occur, especially in a patient about to undergo cardiopulmonary bypass. The incidence is just 0.6% and the disorder presents approximately 7-10 days after the initiation of therapy, presumably the time required for the immune system to generate antiplatelet antibodies.[16] Since most patients on intravenous heparin for control of unstable angina will be operated upon in a short period of time, it would be a rare patient who manifested this disorder during cardiac surgery. It would be more likely in a patient receiving continued heparin therapy after surgery for valve replacement or simply deep venous thrombosis prophylaxis, who returned to the operating room for postoperative problems such as ischemic bowel, etc. Though some drugs may be continued if the platelet count does not decrease below 60,000,[33] this possibility does not apply to heparin, as heparin-induced thrombocytopenia can result in arterial thrombosis due to intravascular platelet agglutination.[34] While a thrombotic event usually makes one consider inadequate anticoagulation, in a patient on heparin it should warn of possible heparin-induced thrombocytopenia.

The main concern in this syndrome is development of arterial thromboses. The first cases of arterial embolism during systemic heparinization were described in 1958 by Weismann and Tobin.[35] They reported complications including aortic thrombosis, myocardial infarction, cerebral emboli and femoral thromboses.[29] These events occurred between the 7th and 15th days of heparinization. Heparin was continued and resulted in further thrombotic events and six deaths. Platelet counts were not monitored in the series by Weisman and Tobin nor in that described in 1964 by Roberts et al.[36] However, Rhodes et al.[37] subsequently measured platelet counts of 8,000 and 10,000 per cubic millimeter in two patients who developed myocardial infarctions on days 8 and 10 of sytemic heparin therapy. The thrombocytopenia in the cases described by Rhodes et al.[37] developed on days 9 and 10 of therapy. Bone marrow revealed increased megakaryocytes. Platelet aggregation studies documented increased aggregation of normal platelets with patient serum in the presence of heparin. When heparin was stopped, platelet counts increased rapidly. Heparin was readministered several weeks later and produced a rapid and prolonged decrease in platelet counts. In 1977 Rhodes also reported a series of patients with delayed-onset heparin-induced thrombocytopenia who developed arterial thromboses.[38] The reported platelet counts ranged from 5,000 to 54,000 per cubic millimeter. The complications reported in this series were myocardial infarction, recurrent pulmonary embolism, and aorto-iliac occlusion. Many cases have now been reported although some have referred to this as the "white clot syndrome" due to the pale histologic appearance of these arterial emboli that contain platelet-fibrin-leukocyte material.

In 1987 Cines et al.[39] described endothelial cell injury as having a possible role in the development of arterial thromboses. They reported a series of 27 patients with heparin-dependent antiplatelet antibodies who deposited more than the usual amount of IgG, IgA, or IgM on human endothelial cells. They obtained serum from the same patients after heparin was discontinued and binding of immunoglobulin to endothelial cells was no longer present. This work suggests that the antiplatelet antibodies in this disorder may interact with heparin or heparin sulfate on the endothelial cell surface, in addition to causing platelet aggregation.

While heparin-induced skin necrosis, thought to be due to localized platelet aggregation and thrombosis, is a complication of subcutaneous administration, it is important to identify any patient with this history, as it may predict thrombosis after intravenous heparin. White et al.[40] reported two patients with heparin-induced skin necrosis who later received intravenous heparin and both became thrombocytopenic. One developed a myocardial infarction and a cerebral infarct. The second developed respiratory failure, peripheral cyanosis and necrosis of the skin of the feet.

While low molecular weight heparins are thought to have reduced platelet activating activity, results with them have been variable. While most patients with heparin-induced thrombocytopenia who were changed to low molecular weight heparin fractions recovered, some did not. Still this seems a reasonable alternative for the patient with this syndrome in whom reversal of anticoagulation can lead to life-threatening events. Leroy et al.[41] reported a series of 34 patients of whom 31 had positive heparin-induced platelet aggregation studies. When the diagnosis was suspected, the patients were changed to low molecular weight heparin preparations. Thirty-one patients recovered, but three died. Three patients required amputations and four became hemiplegic.

Nelson[42] has suggested there may be a third form of heparin-induced thrombocytopenia. It is a more mild disorder with platelet counts from 100,000-150,000 per cubic millimeter. The onset is 2 to 4 days after heparin is begun. The platelet count returns to normal within 1-5 days even if heparin is continued. This form of heparin-induced thrombocytopenia is not associated with arterial thromboses.

While there is disagreement in the literature regarding the frequency of heparin-induced thrombocytopenia, severe thrombocytopenia probably occurs in less than 5% of patients on heparin, while mild thrombocytopenia may be as frequent as 10%-20%. There is probably an equal frequency of severe thrombocytopenia (platelet count less than 100,000) with both bovine and porcine heparin.[43] Overall, the reported frequency of thrombocytopenia with bovine heparin varies from 2%-31%, while reports with porcine heparin vary from 0% to 24%. These differences in frequencies may be somewhat accounted for by different criteria used to define thrombocytopenia.

Management of Heparin-Induced Thrombocytopenia During Cardiopulmonary Bypass

Because full arrest of the coagulation mechanism is required for safe extracorporeal circulation, patients with heparin-induced thrombocytopenia are at serious perioperative risk. Several approaches have been used successfully on the day prior to surgery.

Long[44] reported the use of aspirin and persantine in a patient with the severe form of heparin-induced thrombocytopenia who was safely heparinized for cardiopulmonary bypass. He pretreated his patient with 325 mg of aspirin and 75 mg of dipyridamole the evening prior to and the morning of surgery. Cardiopulmonary bypass with heparin anticoagulation was uncomplicated. Makhoul et al.[45] reported two cases where cardiac surgery was necessary while heparin-induced platelet aggregation studies were still positive. Both patients displayed aspirin inhibition of heparin-induced platelet aggregation in vitro. Aspirin and dipyridamole were given preoperatively. Full heparinization was used for CPB and there were no hemorrhagic or thrombotic complications. Smith[46] had reported the first account of the severe form of heparin-induced thrombocytopenia in a patient undergoing cardiac surgery in 1985. Although this patient had postoperative bleeding despite dipyridamole and aspirin, a decreased dosage of these agents or the use of warfarin may have contributed to the postoperative bleeding.

Kappa et al.[47] have used iloprost (ZK36374), a synthetic analogue of prostacyclin, to increase intracellular cyclic adenosine monophosphate (AMP) thus inhibiting piatelet aggregation. They began a continuous intravenous drip of iloprost, 10-30 ng/kg/min, 1 hour before heparin was administered and continued the infusion until 15 minutes after protamine was given. Intraoperative heparin-induced platelet aggregation studies were negative. Kraenzler and Starr[48] have also reported the successful use of iloprost for this disorder in patients requiring heparinazation for cardiopulmonary bypass. As the half-life of this drug is 15-30 minutes, platelet function returns rapidly enough to permit hemostasis before leaving the operating suite. This seems the logical choice of therapy as persantine and aspirin can inhibit platelet aggregation for hours and days, respectively. Therefore, use of iloprost may significantly decrease the postoperative requirement for platelet transfusion, with an associated decrease in risk of infection transmission.

Kappa[49] has reported that in four of nine patients studied, aspirin failed to prevent in vitro heparin-induced platelet aggregation. Of more concern is one patient who underwent heparinization during carotid endarterectomy resulting in the loss of circulating platelets and spontaneous aggregation despite the fact that aspirin had inhibited in vitro platelet aggregation.

The literature to date supports the view that iloprost by itself or dipyridamole and aspirin together may both be acceptable regimens to approach patients with this disorder. Time will tell if one approach proves safer or more reliable than the other.

Recently, heparin-free CPB has been performed in a patient with heparin-induced thrombocytopenia, with anticoagulation induced by heparinoid (Org 10172).[50] Heparinoids are nonheparin glycosaminoglycans with molecular weights of 1,200-15,000 d, produced as a byproduct of heparin production. Low molecular weight heparins and heparinoids inhibit factor Xa to a greater extent than factor IIa, and are less likely to interact with platelets. The patient described had persistent in vitro platelet aggregation in the presence of heparin, but not in the presence of Org 10172. Fibrin deposition was noted in the cardiotomy suction apparatus upon initiation of cardiopulmonary bypass at which time additional heparinoid was administered. The authors reported that no more fibrin deposition or clots were noted until just before coming off bypass, but they do not detail the extent of the problem at that time. The patient's platelet count decreased to 117,000/mm^3 at the end of CPB from a baseline of 325,000/mm^3. He was transfused with ten units of platelets and four units of fresh frozen plasma, yet continued to bleed at an average rate of 300 mL/h for several hours postoperatively, and required 6 more units of fresh frozen plasma and a total of 16 units of packed red blood cells. The authors attributed this to prolonged antifactor Xa activity that is especially likely to be seen with the doses of heparinoid required for hemostatic paralysis. However, they did not report serial coagulation measurements to rule out the possibility of DIC or fibrinolysis secondary to fibrin deposition. Clearly, more work needs to be done before heparinoid can be recommended to effect anticoagulation for cardiopulmonary bypass. One clear indication might be in a patient who demonstrates in vitro heparin-induced platelet aggregation despite treatment with aspirin and dipyridamole, but in whom heparinoid does not induce platelet aggregation.

One final option available for the patient with heparin-induced thrombocytopenia is the use of Ancrod that is produced from the venom of the Malayan pit viper. It exerts its anticoagulant effect by decreasing the fibrinogen level. It has been used to provide anticoagulation for CPB, but its use may be limited by the fact that it requires a long infusion time preoperatively.[51]

Heparin Rebound

While high-dose heparin may increase the risk of bleeding, generally speaking the risk of underheparinization is much greater than that of overheparinization. Though Bull[15] proposed that excessive heparin use might increase the risk of intracranial bleeding among patients with unusually prolonged ACTs, there have not been reports to support this concern. In fact, intracranial bleeding after CPB is not a common occurrence. Though patients with lesions such as an unknown friable colon carcinoma may bleed secondary to heparin, the risk is there as long as the anticoagulation needed for CPB is present.

Concerns regarding an overdose of heparin are whether it will exacerbate or prolong thrombocytopenia, heparin rebound, protamine reactions or allergic reactions. Still, the most common clinical problem is that excessive doses of heparin require conjoined doses of protamine. Side effects and complications of protamine are numerous and some are potentially life-threatening. As we do not wish to administer excessive protamine, it is wise to titrate heparin appropriately. Measuring the ACT to prevent excessive heparin administration ensures documentation of adequate anticoagulation, while decreasing protamine dose and postoperative bleeding.[52]

Heparin rebound is a term used to describe a phenomenon that includes worsening of bleeding and prolongation of the ACT after the initial dose of protamine is administered. It is likely due to the fact that protamine effect is shorter than that of heparin or that an extravascular depot of heparin has formed. Still, numerous other etiologies have been postulated, as noted in Table III. Regardless of the exact pathophysiology, it is apparently due to heparin effect that is present after protamine reversal, and it has been shown quite clearly that heparin rebound can be prevented by administering additional protamine.[53] It is our opinion that heparin rebound can be prevented by administering an adequate dose of protamine. We recommend 1.3 mg of protamine for each 100 units of heparin given as the original dose by the anesthesiologist. Though it is wise not to give excess protamine routinely, occasionally additional doses are required even after an effective original dose that returned the ACT to normal. One cause may be that after protamine administration heparin may be reintroduced by blood transfused from the pump. Similarly, cell-saver blood may cause the same problem. Though cell-saver blood can be made "heparin free", occasional patients seem to have an increase in bleeding after cell-saver blood is administered. We believe we have decreased this problem by maintaining our wash cycle in the cell saver at 100-150 mL/min of saline solution and by using 1,000 mL of saline for each bowl in the cell saver, even though the supernatant is frequently clear before 1,000 mL of saline wash have been used. Still, we occasionally note a delayed elevation of the patient's ACT associated with the presence of heparin as documented by a heparin

Table III
Theories Proposed To Explain Heparin Rebound

1957	Heparin may be released by red blood cell breakdown.
1958	Heparin may escape from the circulation into the extravascular space and return via the lymphatics and thoracic duct to the circulation many hours later, after protamine has been administered and cleared.
1959	Heparin may be injected into tissues instead of intravenously, forming a depot source for prolonged absorption.
1961	A part of the heparin level may be temporarily neutralized by an endogenous antagonist, not otherwise specified. When this antagonist is cleared from the blood, heparin activity is then demonstrated.
1962	Protamine may be metabolized or combined with other plasma proteins before heparin is removed.
1966	Protamine chloride does not produce heparin rebound, although protamine sulfate does. This may be due in part to the more rapid metabolism of protamine sulfate.
1970	Heparin rebound is seen more commonly with hypothermia. It had previously been shown that heparin levels do not decay as rapidly during hypothermic perfusions.
1974	For a given heparin level, low levels of platelets result in a more pronounced effect of that heparin level on the coagulation mechanism. Since thrombocytopenia is a common occurrence following open heart surgery, it is quite possible that heparin activity may be enhanced.
1981	Monitoring post-cardiopulmonary bypass with an automated protamine titration will detect heparin rebound more frequently.

Adapted from Ellison N, Beatty CP, Blake DR, et al. Heparin rebound, studies in patients and volunteers. *J. Thorac Cardiovasc Surg* 67:723–729, 1974.

concentration (Hepcon, HemoTec Inc., Englewood, CO, USA) performed on remaining cell-saver blood. Certainly if increased bleeding is noted after cell-saver blood is administered, the ACT should be repeated and a heparin concentration should be simultaneously performed to help determine if residual heparin is the cause of the bleeding.

However, return of the ACT and Hepcon to normal do not guarantee maintenance of the normal coagulation state. Data obtained by combining the ACT and Hepcon in the intensive care unit document the existence of heparin rebound as a clinically important problem, and support the concept that improved protamine titration decreases postoperative blood loss.[54] These authors proposed that more exacting titration of protamine may have decreased postoperative bleeding by decreasing the associated antithromboplastin effect.[55] Although concern has been raised regarding the possible anticoagulant effects of protamine, it has been thought that this effect requires much larger doses of protamine than usually used. Ellison et al.[56] have shown that 600 mg of protamine in 70-kg unheparinized volunteers increased the whole blood clotting time from 6.7 to 8.2 minutes, with return to baseline values within 30 minutes, with similar effects noted in patients undergoing CPB. As the effects of protamine in clinical doses acting as an anticoagulant are likely to be minimal, another cause of heparin rebound in the postoperative period should be entertained. This may be postoperative transfusion, which may result in elevation of the ACT due to the effects of minimal residual levels of heparin on antithrombin III contained in blood products.[22] Regardless of the etiology of heparin rebound, it may be useful to repeat the ACT and Hepcon at clinically indicated intervals in the postoperative intensive care unit.

Allergic Reactions

Side effects of commercially prepared heparin are uncommon. Because heparin is produced from animals, patients with allergic histories may be prone to reactions. Local and systemic reactions to the preservative in multidose vials have been reported. Hypersensitivity reactions may manifest as fever, chills, urticaria, or anaphylactic shock.[2] Low molecular weight heparins range from 1,200 to 15,000 d and are thought less likely to produce allergic reactions.[57]

Though decreased blood pressure is frequently seen at the time of heparin administration, it is usually attributed to blood loss associated with placement of vascular cannulae or the adjustment of anesthetic or vasodilator infusions intended to decrease blood pressure prior to placement of the aortic cannula. However, heparin can decrease blood pressure independent of these variables[58] via a decreased systemic vascular resistance, likely due to histamine release,[51] or via the negative inotropic effects mediated by H2 receptors.[6] Heparin has also been reported to form a complex with calcium thus inducing hypocalcemia, and this has been touted to be another mechanism whereby heparin may cause hypotension.[59]

Finally, though the preservative benzyl alcohol has been raised as a possible cause of hypotension, a recently reported small series of patients support a vasodilatory effect of heparin independent of benzyl alcohol preservative.[60] Though allergic reactions to heparin do occur, most commonly they manifest as mild hypotension and are easily controlled with small doses of a vasoconstrictor, or volume infusion via the aortic cannula. At worst, if cardiovascular instability occurs, CPB should be instituted as soon as possible.

Protamine Reactions

The relative ease and safety of heparin administration are offset by the problems inherent in protamine reversal. Reactions range from those that are easy to treat to those that are life threatening. Though reviews have been presented elsewhere,[61,62] we will discuss protamine reactions briefly so one will not conclude that anticoagulation for CPB is benign. A knowledge of the different types of reactions combined with a high index of clinical suspicion should permit rapid diagnosis and treatment, resulting in good patient outcome. Whether hexadimethrine bromide (polybrene), a synthetic heparin antagonist, will be reintroduced in the United States remains to be seen. However, reactions to this drug may be at least as severe as those seen with protamine.[63]

Protamine is a protein isolated from salmon sperm and is the only clinically available antidote to heparin. Protamine is polycationic and forms a complex with heparin, thus reversing its effects. Concern has been raised regarding administration of protamine to insulin dependent diabetics who are receiving protamine containing insulin preparations,[64] and in fact diabetics do have a higher incidence of protamine reactions than the general population. Sharath et al.[65] reported that diabetic patients who have received protamine have high levels of antiprotamine immunoglobulin E, as compared to patients who have never received protamine. They also reported the first fatal case of anaphylaxis due to protamine. However, many diabetics have circulating antiprotamine IgE[62] or antiprotamine IgG,[64] and yet only one of 25 insulin dependent diabetics followed by Levy prospectively had a protamine reaction, and it was of the pulmonary vasoconstrictive type (type III).[66] Similar concerns have been raised for patients allergic to fish and salmon in particular, as well as patients who have had a vasectomy. Yet patients with fish allergies tolerate protamine quite well and among six patients with fish allergies followed prospectively, none developed adverse cardiopulmonary effects from protamine administration.[67] However, there is one reported case of a patient who had a severe protamine reaction and had a positive skin test to protamine, a codfish allergy documented by RAST testing, and increased levels of IgE, IgM, and IgG titers.[68] Theoretically, patients who have had a vasectomy have had disruption of the blood-testes barrier resulting in production of antisperm antibodies, which may produce a reaction upon administration of protamine. However, there has only been one reported reaction in a vasectomized patient, which manifested as hives and pruritis after protamine administration during cardiac catheterization performed 15 years after vasectomy.[69] Though the patient subsequently tolerated protamine well during cardiac surgery, he had been pretreated with antihistamines and corticosteroids. Despite these questionable predisposing problems, many patients with these conditions tolerate protamine well, and many patients without them have serious and sometimes life threatening reactions. It is therefore necessary to be especially vigilant during the administration of protamine in all patients.

Protamine reactions are divided into three types. The salient features of the different types of reactions are summarized in Table IV, while theorized pathophysiological mediators are summarized in Table V.

The first and most common reaction is manifested as systemic hypotension and is frequently worsened by rapid injection. It is due to release of mast cell mediators including histamine.[70] With rapid injection it is quite common. The hemodynamic changes most frequently seen are a decrease in mean arterial pressure, a decrease in systemic vascular resistance and an increase in cardiac index if filling pressures are maintained.[71] Anaphylactoid reactions may be divided into three groups: true anaphylaxis, immediate anaphylactoid reactions, and delayed anaphylactoid reactions. Antibodies mediate true anaphylaxis. Complement activation is felt to be the mediator of immediate anaphylactoid responses not mediated by antibodies. Complement activation occurs secondary to cardiopulmonary bypass as well as protamine administration.[72]

Table IV
Salient Features of the Various Protamine Reactions

Response type	*I Rapid administration*	*IIA Anaphylaxis*	*IIB Immediate anaphylactoid*	*IIC Delayed anaphylactoid*	*III Pulmonary vasoconstriction*
Distinguishing features	Transient ↓ SVR	↓ SVR, flushing, edema, and bronchospasm		Massive edema, insidious onset	Dilated right heart, ↑ PAP, ↓ SBP
Treatment	Fluid or none	O_2, fluid, epinephrine, steroids, antihistamines, positive pressure ventilation			Isoproterenol or epinephrine
Diagnosis	By history	Skin tests, RAST, immunoglobin electrophoresis	Serial serum levels of complement fragments	?	PA catheter and time course
Prevention	Use slow injection	Antihistamine and steroid preparation		?	?Slow administration
Incidence	Common	Uncommon	Uncommon	?	Rare

Reprinted with permission from Horrow JC. Protamine: a review of its toxicity. *Anesth Analg* 64: 348–361, 1985.

Table V
Pathophysiologic Pathways of Protamine Reactions

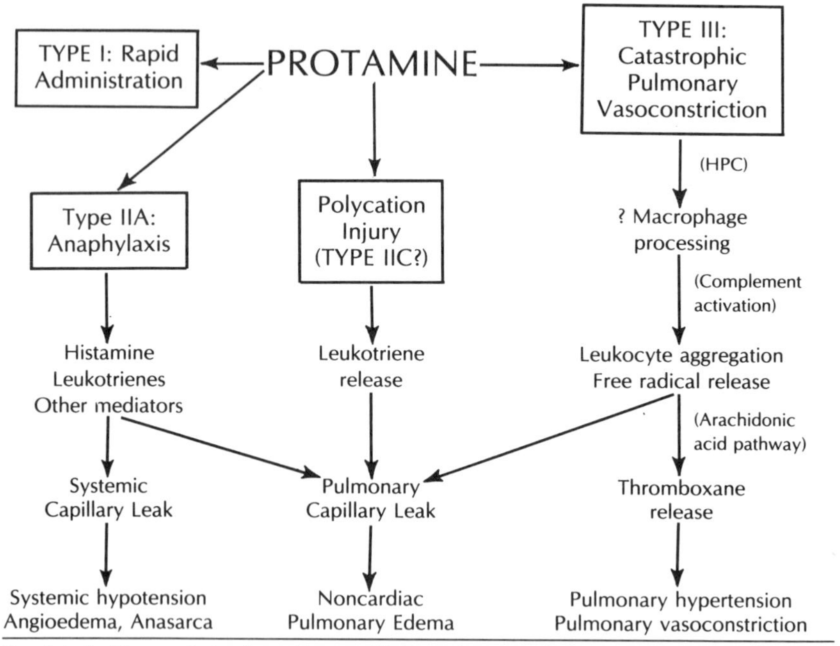

Reprinted with permission from Horrow JC. Heparin reversal of protamine toxicity: have we come full circle (editorial). *J Cardiothorac Anesth* 4:539–542, 1990.

Delayed anaphylactoid reactions may be due to polycation injury and leukotriene mediated capillary leak.[73]

Both anaphylactic and immediate anaphylactoid reactions usually present under anesthesia with a decrease in blood pressure, due to a decrease in systemic vascular resistance, while approximately 25% of these reactions have associated bronchospasm. Often, increased airway pressures are noted to be the first sign of the reaction. Prospective studies of anaphylactoid reactions have reported frequencies as low as one in fifteen[74] or one in seventeen patients.[75] These reactions are treated with antihistamines and steroids. Still occasional patients develop severe hypotension that does not respond to vasopressors or catecholamines. Reheparinization and reinstitution of cardiopulmonary bypass may be necessary.

There is then time to finish the administration of antihistamines and steroids and begin an intravenous infusion of epinephrine. The authors have treated patients with severe anaphylactoid reactions with benadryl, hydrocortisone, and ranitidine followed by an infusion of epinephrine. The patients subsequently received protamine with simultaneous calcium chloride infusion without incident. Indeed, Kambam et al.[76] have recently reported two patients who had anaphylactoid responses to protamine. They did not respond to therapy with benadryl, epinephrine, steroid preparations, calcium chloride, and volume infusions. Both patients then received 300 mg of cimetidine by infusion and improved dramaticaily. Though no one has compared the efficacy or hemodynamic effects of cimetidine versus ranitidine to treat anaphylactoid reactions, the authors have administered 50 mg of ranitidine over 3-5 minutes when anaphylactoid reactions have occurred. We have observed good responses to ranitidine and have not noted adverse hemodynamic effects.

Type III pulmonary vasoconstrictive reactions are rare, but potentially catastrophic. Increasing airway pressures may also be the first indicator of a type III reaction. They seem to occur more frequently in patients with baseline elevations of pulmonary artery pressures, regardless of the etiology. The right heart dilates and the pulmonary artery pressure rises while left-sided filling pressures decrease, resulting in decreased systemic blood pressure. The treatment should combine inotropes with pulmonary vasodilators. Calcium alone may be efficacious, though many other drugs have been used including dobutamine, epinephrine, and isuprel. For catastropic reactions it may be necessary to infuse a pulmonary vasodilaor via a central venous line while simultaneously infusing inotropes and or vasoconstrictors via a left atrial line. Though the etiology of this reaction has not been clearly defined, thromboxane A2, a potent vasoconstrictor, has been implicated[77] and in pigs a thromboxane receptor antagonist was shown to prevent the effects of thromboxane A2 release,[78] as did indomethacin, a cyclooxygenase inhibitor.[79] Still, protamine does not consistently raise thromboxane levels in humans.[80] Even if certain agents are proven to block pathways of injury in humans effectively, we will still need methods to predict which patients will require pretreatment with these agents, in order to justify the risk of any associated side effects.

A syndrome of noncardiogenic pulmonary edema (type IIC-delayed anaphylactoid) has been associated with protamine administration after cardiopulmonary bypass,[81,82] but several etiologies have been proposed to explain this reaction.[61] Protamine may be an innocent bystander as it is the only agent currently available to reverse heparin and, in fact, a case has been reported in a patient before protamine was administered.[83] Still, polycations can cause pulmonary and vascular damage and may be the underlying mechanism if protamine-induced type IIC reaction is proven to exist.[84] Lock and Hessell[85] have reported what may represent reversal of protamine reactions with heparin. The proposed mechanism is heparin reversal of protamine-induced inhibition of plasma carboxypeptidase N, an enzyme that inactivates bradykinin, and anaphylatoxins C'3a, C'4a and C'5a.[86] The size of heparin-protamine complexes may determine the manifestations of protamine reactions and variations in human lung macrophage populations may explain the idiosyncratic nature of these reactions.[73]

Type I reactions may be prevented or attenuated by changing the site of injection or slowing the rate of administration. Frater et al.[70] showed that the site of injection is related to both hemodynamic changes and histamine release. They showed that plasma histamine levels were significantly higher in patients who received protamine via the right atrium as compared to patients who received left-sided injections. Though they noted no significant hemodynamic changes during left-sided administration, right-sided injections produced a significant decrease in systolic blood pressure and systemic vascular resistance as well as a transient increase in cardiac index. Similar findings were reported by Casthely et al.[87] who reported significant hemodynamic changes in dogs that received protamine injections via a central venous line, as compared to dogs that received injections via the left atrium or a peripheral vein.

Though the potential for protamine reactions exists in all patients they may be prevented or attenuated by slow peripheral infusion of a dilute solution. A recommended protocol for protamine administration is presented in Table VI. With this technique, the authors have noted a very low incidence of reactions, with only one being accompanied by significant hypotension. Whether this is because this method results in a minimum of large heparin-protamine complexes remains to be seen. Some administer calcium chloride simultaneously with protamine as it seems to attenuate

Table VI
Recommended Method of Protamine Administration

1. The patient should be off CPB and hemodynamically stable.
2. 1–1.3 mg of protamine is administered for each 100 units of heparin given prior to CPB.
3. The protamine is added to 50 cc of D5W, that contains 5 mg/kg of calcium chloride.
4. The labelled reversal solution is administered over 10–15 minutes as a piggyback over a well running peripheral line, thus diluting the solution further.

the hypotension that frequently occurs. In the rare patient with a known history of an anaphylactic reaction to protamine the possibility of letting heparin wear off over time may be considered. Obviously, this may result in increased transfusion requirements. Although the use of thromboxane or cyclooxygenase inhibitors has not been clinically evaluated, pretreatment with H1 and H2 receptor blockers is relatively benign and has been documented to be an effective regimen to attenuate the hemodynamic eifects of histamine during morphine anesthesia.[88] Also, it has been shown that H1 receptor blockade is not sufficient to prevent the cardiovascular effects of histamine and that H2 receptor blockade prevents the negative inotropic effects of histamine.[6] Because a single dose of an H1 receptor blocker may only block 30% of available H1 receptors,[89] the authors prefer to treat patients with known allergic reactions with 3 or 4 doses of H1 antagonists beginning the day prior to surgery. We initiate H2 receptor blockade simultaneously because though combined H1 and H2 receptor antagonist therapy has itself been shown to release histamine, significant clinical symptoms are unlikely to occur when administered simultaneously, presumably because the receptor blockade prevents the effects of endogenous histamine.[90] Because of concern for sternal dehiscence and infection, the authors reserve the use of preoperative steroid preparations for patients with known anaphylactic reactions to protamine.

Summary

In a modern cardiac surgical suite, heparinization and protamine reversal are usually accomplished uneventfully. Still, occasional patients have unusual problems that present clinical management dilemmas. Monitoring the ACT and Hepcon at appropriate intervals should permit early identification of patients with unusual responses to heparin or protamine. This may result in improved hemostasis and decreased transfusion requirements. Careful attention to hemodynamic parameters will almost always allow the clinician to manage even life-threatening complications successfully. Hopefully further research identifying the mediators of these reactions and preventative agents or the development of new anticoagulant and reversal agents will allow anticoagulation for CPB and its reversal to become benign therapies.

Acknowledgments: The authors wish to thank David R. Jobes, M.D. and Joseph I. Simpson, M.D. for their review of the manuscript and invaluable suggestions.

REFERENCES

1. Howell WH. Heparin: an anticoagulant. Preliminary communication. *Am J Phys* 63: 434-435, 1922.
2. O'Reilly RA. Anticoagulant, antithrombotic and thrombolytic drugs. In: Gilman AG, Goodman LS, Rall TW, et al. eds. *The Pharmacological Basis of Therapeutics*. New York, NY: MacMillan Publishing Company; 1985:1338-1344.
3. Pharmacokinetic data. Appendix II. In: Gilman AG, Goodman LS, Rall TW, et al. eds. *The Pharmacological Basis of Therapeutics.* New York, NY: MacMillan Publishing Company; 1985:1689.
4. Fox ML. Anticoagulants. In: Attia RR, Grogono AW, Domer FR. *Practical Anesthetic Pharmacology.* Englewood, NJ: Appleton-Century Crofts; 1987:291.
5. Green JP, Day M, Roberts M. On the smooth-muscle stimulating activity of preparations of heparin. *J Pharmacol Exp Ther* 132:58-64, 1961.
6. Powell JR, Brody MJ. Identification and specific blockade of two receptors for histamine in the cardiovascular system. *J Pharmacol Exp Ther* 196:1-14, 1976.
7. Hattersley PG. Activated coagulation time of whole blood. *J Am Med Assoc* 196:150-154, 1966.
8. Clapham MCC, Willis N, Mapleson WW, et al. Minimal volume of discard for valid blood sampling from indwelling arterial cannulae. *Br J Anaes* 59:232-235, 1987.
9. Jobes DR, Ellison N, Campbell FW. Limit(ation) for ACT (letter). *Anesth Analg* 69:142-143, 1989.
10. Schriever HG, Epstein SE, Mintz MD. Statistical Correlation and heparin sensitivity of activated partial thromboplastin time, whole blood

coagulation time and an automated coagulation time. *Am J Clin Pathol* 60:323-329, 1973.

11. Jobes DR, Bikhaze G, Ellison N. Rapid assessment of heparin anticoagulation and reversal. In: *Abstracts of American Society of Anesthesiologists*. San Francisco, CA, 1976:437-438.
12. Young JA, Kisker CT, Doty DB. Adequate anticoagulation during cardiopulmonary bypass determined by activated clotting time and the appearance of fibrin monomer. *Ann Thorac Surg* 26:231-240, 1978.
13. Metz S, Keats AS. Low activated coagulation time during cardiopulmonary bypass does not increase postoperative bleeding. *Ann Thorac Surg* 49:440-444, 1990.
14. Bull BS, Huse WM. Heparin therapy during extracorporeal circulation II. The use of a dose-response curve to individualize heparin and protamine dosage. *J Thor Cardiovasc Surg* 69:685-689, 1975.
15. Bull BS, Korpman RA, HUse WM, et al. Heparin therapy during extracorporeal circulation 1. Problems inherent in existing heparin protocols. *J Thor Cardiovasc Surg* 69:674-684, 1975.
16. Ellison, N. Heparin-protamine monitoring and cardiovascular effects. In: Estafanous FG, ed. *Anesthesia and The Heart Patient*. Stoneham, MA: Butterworths; 1989:143-149.
17. Lambert CJ, Marengo-Rowe AJ, Leveson JE, et al. The treatment of postperfusion bleeding using epsilon-amonocaproic acid, cryoprecipitate, fresh-frozen plasma and protamine sulfate. *Ann Thorac Surg* 28:440-444, 1979.
18. Esposito RA, Culliford AT, Colvin SB, et al. Heparin resistance during cardiopulmonary bypass: the role of heparin pretreatment. *J Thorac Cardiovasc Surg* 85:346-353, 1983.
19. Cloyd GM, D'Ambra MN, Akin CW, et al. Diminished anticoagulant response to heparin in patients undergoing coronary artery bypass grafting. *J Thorac Cardiovasc Surg* 94:535-538, 1987.
20. Burns ER. Characteristics and use of antithrombotic drugs. In: *Clinical Management of Bleeding and Thrombosis*. Cambridge, MA: Blackwell Scientific Publications; 1987:175-178.
21. Damus PS, Hicks M, Rosenberg RD. A generalized view of heparin's anticoagulant action. *Nature* 246:355-357, 1973.
22. Soloway HB, Christiansen TW. Heparin anticoagulation during cardiopulmonary bypass in an anti-thrombin III deficient patient: implications relative to the etiology of heparin rebound. *Am J Clin Path* 73:723-725, 1980.
23. Ansell J, Deykin D. Heparin-induced thrombocytopenia and recurrent thromboembolism. *Am J Hematol* 8:325-332, 1980.
24. Kelton JG. Heparin-induced thrombocytopenia. *Hemostasis* 16:173-186, 1986.
25. Kelton JB, Meltzer D, et al. Drug-induced thrombocytopenia is associated with increased binding of IgG to platelets both in vivo and in vitro. *Blood* 58:524-529, 1981.

26. Burns ER. Approach to the medically ill patient with bleeding. In: *Clinical Management of Bleeding and Thrombosis*. Cambridge, MA: Blackwell Scientific Publications; 1987:75-76.
27. Kelton JG, Bain H, Powers P, et al. Ciinical usefulness of testing for a heparin-dependent platelet-aggregating factor in patients with suspected heparin-associated thrombocytopenia. *J Lab Clin Med* 103:606-612, 1984.
28. Sheridan D, Carter C, Kelton JG. A diagnostic test for heparin-induced thrombocytopenia. *Blood* 67:27-30, 1986.
29. Cola C, Ansell J. Heparin-induced thrombocytopenia and arterial thrombosis: alternative therapies. *Am Heart J* 119:368-373, 1990.
30. Gollub S, Ulin AW. Heparin-induced thrombocytopenia in man. *J Lab Clin Med* 59: 430-435, 1962.
31. Jaques LB. The effect of intravenous injections of heparin in the dog. *Am J Phys* 125:98, 1939.
32. Wessler S, Gitel SN. Low-dose heparin: is the risk worth the benefit. *Am Heart J* 98:94-101, 1979.
33. Burns ER. Approach to the medically ill patient with bleeding. In: *Clinical Management of Bleeding and Thrombosis*. Blackwell Scientific Publications; 1987:71-87.
34. Chong BH, Pitney WR, Castaldi PA. Heparin induced thrombocytopenia: association of thrombotic complications with heparin-dependent IgG antibody that induces thromboxane synthesis and platelet aggregation. *Lancet* 2:1246-1249, 1982.
35. Weismann RE, Tobin RW. Arterial embolism occurring during systemic heparin therapy. *Arch Surg* 76:219-227, 1958.
36. Roberts B, Rosato FE, Rosato EF. Heparin—a cause of arterial emboli? *Surgery* 55:803-808, 1964.
37. Rhodes GR, Dixon RH, Silver D. Heparin induced thrombocytopenia with thrombotic and hemorrhagic manifestations. *Surg Gynecol Obstet* 136:409-416, 1973.
38. Rhodes GR, Dixon RH, Silver D. Heparin induced thrombocytopenia: eight cases with thrombotic-hemorrhagic complications. *Ann Surg* 186:752-758, 1977.
39. Cines DB, Tomaski A, Tannenbaum S. Immune endothelial cell injury in heparin-associated thrombocytopenia. *N Engl J Med* 316:581-589, 1987.
40. White PW, Sadd JR, Nensel RE. Thrombotic complications of heparin therapy including six cases of heparin-induced necrosis. *Ann Surg* 190:595-608, 1979.
41. Leroy J, Leclerc MH, Delahousse B, et al. Treatment of heparin-associated thrombocytopenia and thrombosis with low molecular weight heparin (CY216). *Semin Thromb Hemostasis* 55:90-93, 1986.
42. Nelson JD, Lerner RG, Goldstein R, et al. Heparin-induced thrombocytopenia. *Arch Intern Med* 138:548-552, 1978.
43. Ansell JE, Price JM, Shah S, et al. Heparin-induced thrombocytopenia: what is its real frequency? *Chest* 88:878-882, 1985.

44. Long RW. Management of patients with heparin-induced thrombocytopenia requiring cardiopulmonary bypass. *J Thorac Cardiovasc Surg* 89:950-951, 1985.
45. Makhoul RG, McCann RL, Austin EH, et al. Management of patients with heparin-associated thrombocytopenia and thrombosis requiring cardiac surgery. *Ann Thorac Surg*43: 617-621, 1987.
46. Smith JP, Walls JT, Muscato MS, et al. Extracorporeal circulation in a patient with heparin-induced thrombocytopenia. *Anesthesiology* 62:363-365, 1985.
47. Kappa JR, Ellison N, Fisher CA, et al. The use of Iloprost (ZK 36 374) to permit cardiopulmonary bypass in patients with heparin-induced thrombocytopenia. *Anesthesiology* 63:A32, 1985.
48. Kraenzler EJ, Starr NJ. Heparin-associated thrombocytopenia: management of patients for open heart surgery. *Anesthesiology* 69:964-967, 1988.
49. Kappa JR, Fisher CA, Berkowitz HD, et al. Heparin-induced platelet activation in sixteen surgical patients: diagnosis and management. *J Vasc Surg* 5:101-107, 1987.
50. Doherty DC, Thomas LO, Norbert de Bruijn, et al. "Heparin-free" cardiopulmonary bypass: first reported use of heparinoid (Org 10172) to provide anticoagulation for cardiopulmonary bypass. *Anesthesiology* 73:562-565, 1990.
51. Zulys VJ, Glynn MFX, Tesdale S, et al. Ancrod (Arvin) as an alternative to heparin for anticoagulation for cardiopulmonary bypass. Abstracts of Ninth Annual Meeting of Society of Cardiovascular Anesthesiologists. 1987:81.
52. Verska JJ. Control of heparinization by activated clotting time during bypass with improved postoperative hemostasis. *Ann Thorac Surg* 24:170-173, 1977.
53. Ellison N, Beatty CP, Blake DR, et al. Heparin rebound: studies in patients and volunteers. *J Thorac Cardiovasc Surg* 67:723-729, 1974.
54. Pifarre R, Sullivan HJ, Montoya A, et al. Management of blood loss and heparin rebound following cardiopulmonary bypass. *Semin Thromb Hemostasis* 15:173-177, 1989.
55. Goldman BS, Joisen J, Austin WG. Cardiovascular effects of protamine sulfate. *Ann Thorac Surg* 7:459-471, 1969.
56. Ellison N, Ominsky AJ, Wollman H. Is protamine a clinically important anticoagulant? *Anesthesiology* 35:621-629, 1971.
57. Harenberg J, Heene DL. Pharmacology and special clinical appiications of low-molecular-weight heparins. *Am J Hematol* 29:233-240, 1988.
58. Seltzer JL, Gerson JI. Decrease in arterial pressure following heparin injection prior to cardiopulmonary bypass. *Acta Anaesth Scand* 23:575-578, 1979.
59. Urban P, Scheidegger D, Buchmann B, et al. The hemodynamic effects of heparin and their relation to ionized calcium levels. *J Thorac Cardiovasc Surg* 91:303-306, 1986.

60. Kelleher JF, Smith RC, Hull RL, et al. Role of benzyl alcohol preservative in heparin-lnduced hypotension prior to cardiopulmonary bypass. *Anesthesiology* 73:A130, 1990.
61. Horrow JC. Protamine: a necessary evil. In: Ellison N, Jobes DR, eds. *Effective Hemostasis in Cardiac Surgery. A Society of Cardiovascular Anesthesiologists Monograph.* Philadephia, PA: WB Saunders Co.; 1988:15-39.
62. Horrow JC. Protamine: a review of its toxicity. *Anesth Analg* 64:348-361, 1985.
63. Castaneda AR, Ganz H, Weber KC, et al. Heparin neutralization: experimental and clinical studies. *Surgery* 62:686-697, 1967.
64. Kurtz AB, Gray RS, Markamd S, et al. Circulating IgG antibody to protamine in patients treated with protamine-insulins. *Diabetalogia* 25:322-324, 1983.
65. Sharath MD, Metzger WJ, Richerson HB, et al. Protamine-induced fatal anaphylaxis: prevalence of antiprotamine immunoglobulin E antibody. *J Thorac Cardiovas Surg* 90:86-90, 1985.
66. Levy JH, Zaidan JR, Faraj B. Prospective evlauation of risk of protamine reactions in patients with NPH insulin-dependent diabetes. *Anesth Analg* 65:739-742, 1986.
67. Levy JH, Schwieger I, Faraj B, et al. Prospective evaluation of patients with fish allergies for anaphylaxis to protamine. Abstract Presented at Ninth Annual Meeeting of the Society of Cardiovascular Anesthesiologists 1987:82.
68. Knape JTA, Schullez JG, De Haan P, et al. An anaphylactic reaction to protamine in a patient allergic to fish. *Anesthesiology* 55:324-325, 1981.
69. Watson RA, Ansbacher R, Barry M, et al. Allergic reaction to protamine: a late complication of elective vasectomy? *Urology* 22:493-496, 1983.
70. Frater RWM, Oka Y, Hong Y, et al. Protamine-induced circulatory changes. *J Thorac Cardiovasc Surg*, 87:687-692, 1984.
71. Shapira N, Schaff HV, Piehler JM, et al. Cardiovascular effects of protamine sulfate in man. *J Thorac Cardiovasc Surg* 84:505-514, 1982.
72. Kirklin JK, Chenoweth DE, Naftel DC, et al. Effects of protamine administration after cardiopulmonary bypass on complement, blood elements, and the hemodynamic state. *Ann Thorac Surg* 41:193-199, 1986.
73. Horrow JC. Heparin reversal of protamine toxicity: have we come full circle (editorial). *J Cardiothorac Anesth* 4:539-542, 1990.
74. Conahan TJ, Andrews RW, MacVaugh H. Cardiovascular effects of protamine sulfate in man. *Anesth Analg* 60:33-36, 1981.
75. Masone R, Oka Y, Hong YW, et al. Cardiovascular effects of right atrial injection of protamine sulfate as compared to left atrial injection. *Anesthesiology* 57:A6, 1982.
76. Kambam JR, Merrill WH, Smith BE. Histamine 2 receptor blocker in the treatment of protamine related anaphylactoid reactions: two case reports. *Can J Anesth* 36:463-465, 1989.

77. Morel DR, Zapol WM, Thomas SJ, et al. C5a and thromboxane generation associated with pulomnary vaso- and bronchoconstriction during protamine reversal of heparin. *Anesthesiology* 66:597-604, 1987.
78. Conzen PF, Habazettl H, Gutmann R, et al. Thromboxane mediation of pulmonary hemodynamic responses after neutralization of heparin by protamine in pigs. *Anesth Analg* 68:25-31, 1989.
79. Hobbhahn J, Conzen PF, Zenker B, et al. Beneficial effect of cyclooxygenase inhibition on adverse hemodynamic responses after protamine. *Anesth Analg* 67:253-260, 1988.
80. Konstadt SN, Thys DM, Kong D, et al. Absence of prostaglandin changes associated with protamine administration in patients with pulmonary hypertension. *J Cardiothorac Anesth* 1:388-391, 1987.
81. Olinger GN, Becker RM, Bonchek LI., Noncardiogenic pulmonary edema and peripheral vascular collapse following cardiopulmonary bypass: rare protamine reaction? *Ann Thorac Surg* 29:20-25, 1980.
82. Culliford AT, Thomas S, Spencer FC. Fulminating noncardiogenic pulmonary edema. *J Thorac Cardiovasc Surg* 80:868-875, 1980.
83. Iglesias A, Nunez L. Pulmonary edema (letter). *Ann Thorac Surg* 33:304, 1982.
84. Chang SW, Voelkel NF. Charge-related lung microvascular injury. *Am Rev Resp Dis* 139:534-545, 1989.
85. Lock R, Hessell EA. Probable reversal of protamine reactions by heparin administration. *J Cardiothorac Anesth* 4:604-608, 1990.
86. Tan F, Jackman H, Skidgel RA, et al. Protamine inhibits plasma carboxypeptidase N, the inactivator of Anaphylatoxins and kinins. *Anesthesiology* 70:267-275, 1989.
87. Casthely PA, Goodman K, Fyman PN, et al. Hemodynamic changes after the administration of protamine. *Anesth Analg* 65:78-80, 1986.
88. Philbin DM, Moss J, Akins CW, et al. The use of H1 and H2 histamine antagonists with morphine anesthesia: a double-blind study. *Anesthesiology* 55:292-296,1981.
89. Personal communication, Jonathan Moss, MD, PhD. The University of Chicago, Department of Anesthesia and Critical Care.
90. Lorenz W, Doenicke A, Schoning B, et al. Histamine release, H1 and H2 receptor antagonists for premedication in anaesthesia and surgery: a critical view based on randomized clinical trials with haemaccel and various antiallergic drugs. *Agents Actions* 10:114-124, 1980.

Chapter 6

Myocardial Preservation

Charles A.S. Marrin, MB, BS
and William C. Nugent, MD

The authors make no apology for beginning with a brief account of the evolution of myocardial preservation. The novice might be forgiven for thinking that the deluge of publications on this subject over the last 20 years implies a broad understanding of the problem, but such is not the case. A daunting number of papers have been published describing many phenomena associated with myocardial injury and advancing various hypotheses. However, clinical reports frequently appear to refute experimental data, to contradict the results of other clinical investigators, and confound the theories of the physiologists. The science of myocardial preservation has deteriorated into phenomenology while the search continues for a unifying hypothesis. The bewildering literature, the variety of techniques still in use, and the continued (albeit much reduced) prevalence of perioperative myocardial infarction testify to the fact that no entirely satisfactory solution has yet been found. The subject will not make any sense without some historical background. A more extensive review may be found elsewhere.[1]

From Casthely PA, Bregman D, (eds): *Cardiopulmonary Bypass: Physiology, Related Complications, and Pharmacology.* Mount Kisco, NY, Futura Publishing Company, Inc., © 1991.

Historical Background

Early intracardiac operations such as closed mitral commissurotomy were performed "blindly" and without circulatory support. Surgical success depended almost entirely on the speed and dexterity of the surgeon and the major concern at that time was the risk of ischemic cerebral injury. However, following the introduction in the 1950s of the heart-lung machine and of hypothermia more complicated procedures such as repair of atrial septal defects became feasible. Two schools of cardiac surgery arose, one espousing hypothermia and the other the pump-oxygenator. Systemic hypothermia to 30°C offered the surgeon a bloodless, motionless heart for about 10 minutes while the venae cavae and aorta were occluded. Longer periods of circulatory arrest resulted in irreversible brain damage. Although a lower temperature was known to prolong the safe duration of circulatory arrest, the resulting increase in the incidence of spontaneous ventricular fibrillation, a dreaded complication, was unacceptable. Another drawback was the increased time necessary for cooling and rewarming.

As a result of refinements in the pump-oxygenator the two techniques were combined to increase the safe operating time. Nevertheless, surgeons were still obliged to work on a beating, distended heart in a pool of blood, resulting in a distressing incidence of errors in diagnosis and technique. Frustrated by these handicaps, surgeons continued the search for techniques to improve surgical exposure and operating conditions.

In this same era some surgeons began to induce ventricular fibrillation deliberately to avoid the dreaded complication of air embolism. They also realized that it afforded a quiet operative field and the technique became popular with surgeons mainly for this reason. Other surgeons developed doubts about the technique. In 1969 Najafi published a study of 31 patients who had died after valve replacement. Nearly all the patients had developed ventricular fibrillation in spite of attempts at coronary perfusion and all were found at autopsy to have hemorrhagic necrosis of the left ventricle in the absence of coronary disease. He speculated that the cause of the problem was ischemic necrosis of the myocardium. Others reported similar findings but they were largely ignored. Ultimately, induced ventricular fibrillation fell into disfavor following the publication of a classic series of papers in the early 1970s by Buckberg's group describing the adverse effects of ventricular fibrillation on myocardial perfusion, especially in hypertrophied hearts.[2–5] However, induced ventricular fibrillation is still routinely used at some centers with satisfactory results.

In 1956, Cooley and DeBakey took the daring step of occluding the ascending aorta for 31 minutes at normothermia.[6] They noted that cardiac arrest occurred after about 10 minutes of myocardial ischemia, that the heart fibrillated after removal of the clamp and was then successfully defibrillated. Surgeons were delighted by the quiet, fairly bloodless field and the technique of normothermic ischemic arrest became widely used. In 1969, Cooley's group reported 11.9% mortality in 636 patients undergoing valve replacement using normothermic ischemic arrest for periods between 26–90 minutes (average 38 minutes). However, other surgeons found that in their hands the technique carried a substantially higher operative mortality that could not be explained by underlying heart disease.

In 1972, Cooley[7] made what is probably the greatest of his many contributions to heart surgery when he described the so-called "stone heart" phenomenon in his own patients. He confirmed the impression of others that normothermic ischemic arrest produced substantial myocardial damage and brought the problem out into the open. The suggestion that it might be avoided by taking better care of the myocardium during surgery was adopted and the concept of myocardial preservation was born.

Other investigators had already embarked on a more scientific approach. In 1962, Gott[8] and coworkers demonstrated that the myocardial oxygen consumption of the arrested, vented left ventricle was reduced during cardiopulmonary bypass to 10% of control levels and that cooling the myocardium to 27°C further halved the oxygen consumption.

Reviving classic studies by Ringer, Melrose[9] had reported the experimental use of potassium citrate to induce cardiac arrest, a technique that was first used clinically by Effler's group in 1956. Many surgeons tried potassium cardioplegia, but abandoned it after reports of irreversible myocardial injury with this method too. Next, intermittent or continuous coronary perfusion came into fashion, with the addition by some surgeons of selective cardiac hypothermia, but the technique was cumbersome and time consuming. By 1973 no entirely satisfactory alternative had been found and the use of potassium cardioplegia was gradually resumed as a result of experimental studies demonstrating that lower concentrations of potassium in the cardioplegia solution were both safe and effective. In Europe, cardioplegia mixtures containing magnesium and procaine were adopted and remain popular there today.

In spite of the more scientific approach to myocardial preservation during the period of cardiac arrest, perioperative myocardial infarction remained a distressingly frequent complication of heart surgery. It was then realized that other factors may also be responsible and attention was then directed towards refining anesthetic techniques, especially the increased use of monitors and, more recently, to the management of reperfusion after the cross clamp is removed.

What distinguishes cardiac surgery from almost every other clinical discipline is the fact that a successful outcome depends not only on technical skill and judgement, but also (and probably more importantly) on the combined abilities of surgeon and anesthesiologist as clinical physiologists. The relevant physiology will therefore be briefly reviewed before discussing pathophysiological states.

Coronary Blood Flow

The heart's oxygen requirements vary enormously, necessitating an extremely efficient, demand-sensitive system for control of the coronary circulation. Myocardial oxygen extraction is very high, averaging 75% normally and increasing to almost 100% during stress. Thus, major increases in oxygen delivery can only be achieved by coronary vasodilation. At our present level of understanding the control mechanisms seem complicated. The interactions are confusing and research has been hindered by the difficulty of controlling the physiological variables, which will now be briefly reviewed. An excellent, more detailed account appears elsewhere.[10]

Perfusion Pressure

Coronary blood flow is determined by the pressure gradient between the aortic root and the right atrium (coronary sinus), and the extrinsic and intrinsic coronary vascular resistance. Coronary blood flow is phasic, especially in the left ventricle, being greater in diastole when ventricular pressures and wall stresses are less. During systole left ventricular coronary flow is only 7%–45% of diastolic flow. Thus the diastolic pressure in the aortic root and the duration of diastole are major determinants of coronary perfusion. Tachycardia, which mainly shortens diastole, may cause a profound decrease in coronary perfusion.

Extrinsic Coronary Vascular Resistance

The effect of systolic compression of the coronary arteries is not uniform. The thick muscular wall of the left ventricle, in particular, implies greater stresses in the inner layers than near the epicardium. Distortion of the coronary vessels may also occur in the inner layers. The subendocardium is thus notoriously vulnerable to ischemic injury, especially in the presence of increased left ventricular diastolic pressure or hypertrophy. Indeed, experimental studies of arrested hearts have demonstrated a 35% decrease in coronary resistance, presumably by eliminating systolic compression of the coronary arteries but ischemia and cardioplegia may account for some or all of the changes. In contrast in the thin-walled right ventricle coronary blood flow is more evenly distributed and the lower systolic pressure does not interfere with coronary perfusion to the same extent.

Intrinsic Coronary Vascular Resistance

Autoregulation is achieved by changes in coronary vasomotor tone which, in turn, is controlled by various feedback loops triggered predominantly by local metabolic stimuli but also by neurohumoral mechanisms. During basal metabolism there is substantial vasomotor tone in the coronary microvasculature, as may be inferred from the fivefold increase in coronary blood flow produced by maximal coronary vasodilation. At coronary perfusion pressures between 70–145 mm Hg constant flow is maintained by autoregulation, but outside this range coronary blood flow is no longer controlled by autoregulation, being almost entirely determined by perfusion pressure. Thus the myocardium is vulnerable to ischemic injury at lower pressures or microvascular injury at higher pressures.

Local Metabolic Control

Experimental evidence points to several chemical mediators. Adenosine, a byproduct of high-energy phosphate metabolism, is an extremely potent coronary vasodilator agent that is produced in large quantities by the myocardium during metabolic stress. Myocardial oxygen tension also plays an important part. A close, inverse correlation exists between the coronary sinus pO_2 and coronary blood flow; autoregulation is not observed when the coronary sinus pO_2 exceeds 32 mm Hg. The exact mechanisms have not yet been elucidated, however, and pH and even prostaglandins may play a role in the control of coronary blood flow.

Although local metabolism is the most important determinant of coronary blood flow, neural and humoral mechanisms also play an important, complementary role. Neural stimuli produce rapid changes in vasomotor tone augmented by humorally mediated effects that are of slower onset but more sustained duration.

Neurohumoral Mechanisms

In the normal heart, neural stimulation causes coronary vasodilation mediated largely by increased myocardial metabolism but, to a lesser extent, by direct activation of coronary β-adrenergic receptors. However, in the presence of coronary stenosis, sympathetic coronary activation causes coronary vasoconstriction, redistributing coronary blood flow from relatively overperfused regions to those that are underperfused. Moreover, after β-adrenergic blockade neural stimulation produces coronary vasoconstriction as a result of unopposed α-adrenergic activity. The clinical implications for the β-blocked patient with ischemic heart disease and a critical coronary stenosis are obvious; neural reflexes may further diminish an already tenuous blood supply causing myocardial ischemia. Coronary sympathetic nerve terminals contain various other neurotransmitters but their role in the regulation of coronary blood flow remains a matter for conjecture.

The effects of circulating sympathomimetic agents on the heart and on the coronary circulation have been studied in great detail. Elegant research has repeatedly refined Ahlquist's original classification of adrenergic receptors (the heart contains both α_1 and α_2 as well as β_1 and β_2 receptors) and has led to the development of increasingly specific "cardioselective" drugs for the treatment of heart disease but the exact physiological role of these mechanisms is not well understood.

Myocardial Oxygen Consumption

The heart is an extraordinarily efficient pump. By corollary, not only are the oxygen requirements of the heart high, but its energy reserves are minimal. Aerobic metabolism produces 36 molecules of adenosine triphosphate (ATP) from 1 molecule of glucose. Anaerobic metabolism of 1 molecule of glucose, however, produces only 2 molecules of ATP (3 per molecule of glucose 6-phosphate from glycogen). It has been estimated that anaerobic metabolism can provide only 65%–70% of the energy that the heart needs to sustain itself. Oxygen consumption is closely coupled to energy utilization in the myocardium and myocardial oxygen consumption has become accepted as an index of cardiac metabolism.

The principal determinants of myocardial oxygen consumption are heart rate, the contractile state of the myocardium and the developed tension in the myocardium. The simple concept of the double or triple product is familiar to everyone who deals with patients suffering from ischemic heart disease. It is useful, however, to consider the developed tension, a rather more nebulous concept, in more detail. The components of myocardial wall stress are simply expressed in the form of an equation derived by Badeer[11] from the Law of Laplace:

$$T = \frac{P \times Ri}{2h}$$

where T = mean myocardial wall stress, P = transmural left ventricular pressure, Ri = internal radius of the left ventricle and h = thickness of the left ventricular wall.

Taking this simple concept a step further we have:

$$T = \frac{P \times Ri}{2h}$$

T	=	mean myocardial wall stress	(myocardial oxygen consumption)
P	=	transmural LV pressure	(contractile state and afterload)
Ri	=	internal LV radius	(LVEDV or preload)
h	=	LV wall thickness	(LV hypertrophy)

The effect on myocardial oxygen consumption of left ventricular hypertrophy and of variations in preload, afterload and contractile state may be readily appreciated.

In cardiac surgery (but not in clinical medicine) one other variable may be manipulated. Myocardial oxygen consumption and, for that matter, total body oxygen consumption may be reduced by cooling, thereby slowing all metabolism in accordance with the equation of Arrhenius.

Pathophysiology of Ischemia

The confusion that bedevils our understanding of the pathophysiology of ischemia is due partly to the slipshod use of terminology and partly to the frequently unwarranted assumption that observations about regional ischemia may be applied to global ischemia and that observations from experimental animal models have immediate and direct applications in human heart surgery.

It is especially important to draw the distinction between anoxia and ischemia:

Ischemia (inadequate blood flow) implies not only an inadequate supply of nutrients but also the accumulation of potentially toxic metabolites such as lactate, carbon dioxide and protons. Total cessation of blood flow rarely occurs clinically or even experimentally unless the heart is excised. The problem confronting the clinician is usually one of *inadequate* blood flow that may occur even in the absence of coronary artery disease whenever demand exceeds supply, as in the hypertrophied left ventricle of aortic stenosis.

After the aortic cross clamp has been applied oxygen is still available, albeit in small amounts, from noncoronary collateral blood flow. Indeed, rewarming of the myocardium and washout of the cardioplegia solution by bronchial and mediastinal collaterals have been demonstrated in the clinical setting. The reinfusion of cardioplegia solution at intervals during the period of cardiac arrest serves mainly to maintain hypothermia and to wash out metabolites.

Hypoxia or anoxia, however, indicate inadequate or nonexistent oxygen delivery to the myocardium with an uninterrupted supply of blood and nutrients and continuing removal of metabolites. According to this strict definition anoxia is rarely observed clinically.

Biochemical Changes

Normally the energy requirements of the heart are met entirely by mitochondrial oxidative phosphorylation, for which glucose is the principal substrate. It has been shown that the maintenance of high-energy phosphate stores during ischemia is essential in order to sustain obligatory metabolism and preserve the structural integrity of the cellular organelles.

After the onset of ischemia, the amount of available oxygen dwindles rapidly (reserves are minimal because of high oxygen extraction) and anaerobic conditions develop. Whereas aerobic metabolism produces 36 molecules of adenosine triphosphate (ATP) from 1 molecule of glucose, anaerobic metabolism of 1 molecule of glucose produces only 2 molecules of ATP (3 per molecule of glucose 6-phosphate from glycogen). It has been estimated that anaerobic metabolism can provide only 65%–70% of the energy that the heart needs to sustain itself. Moreover, anaerobic metabolism is rapidly inhibited by intracellular acidosis. As a result the onset of ischemia initiates a rapid and progressive depletion of ATP, moderated only by the potential for collateral blood supply to sustain limited aerobic metabolism. A direct correlation has been established between ischemic contracture and decreased myocardial ATP. Two major factors determine the rate of loss of ATP: the duration of contractile events after the onset of ischemia (the energy consumed to perform external work) and the temperature of the myocardium (that determines the rate of energy consumption for obligatory metabolism).

Energy depletion leads to a disruption of the active transport mechanisms that control both cell volume and the ionic gradients of sodium, potassium, calcium, and magnesium. Failure of the sodium-potassium pump causes accumulation of sodium ions within the cell and potassium ions outside, leading to persistent depolarization of the cell membrane. The heart becomes asystolic. Although reperfusion after 1 hour of normothermic ischemic arrest reestablishes the sodium and potassium gradients across the cell membrane, longer periods of normothermic ischemia produce irreversible changes. Likewise, calcium ions are redistributed within the cell because energy is required to maintain the normal gradients by sequestering calcium ions in the sarcoplasmic reticulum. Magnesium ions, essential cofactors for cellular respiratory enzymes, leave the cell and all metabolism ceases. The net result is an accumulation of water and of sodium, chloride and calcium ions within the cell, and a loss of intracellular potassium, magnesium and phosphorus ions. The accumulation of protons within the cell and the calcium overload also set the stage for further injury which may occur during reperfusion. Total depletion of ATP can lead to the loss of its precursor, adenosine, by diffusion across the cell membrane. The restoration of ATP to normal levels is then impossible.

Structural Changes

As mitochondrial oxidative phosphorylation is the first casualty of ischemia, it is scarcely surprising that structural changes in the mitochondrion are early and sensitive indicators of ischemia and have been the subject of intense scrutiny.[12] Detectable changes do not occur immediately, however, and the picture is further confused by the fact that susceptibility to ischemic injury varies considerably among species. Early ischemic injury of the mitochondrion (manifested by disappearance of glycogen granules, lysis of the cristae, and swelling) has been demonstrated after 30–40 minutes of ischemia in the human myocardium during cardiac surgery.

Severe ischemic injury is characterized by extensive mitochondrial damage, nuclear pyknosis, cellular swelling, myofibrillar disruption, and the appearance of contracture bands. After 40 minutes of normothermic ischemia, irreversible changes take place and 50% of myocardial cells die. Reperfusion at this stage leads to explosive cellular swelling, deposition of calcium phosphate and intense ischemic contracture resembling rigor mortis.

Functional Changes

Experimental studies in dogs have demonstrated a significant, but largely reversible depression of cardiac output after 30 minutes of normothermic ischemia. After 60 minutes, cardiac output was depressed to 40% of control levels and failed to improve after reperfusion. The functional changes were correlated with myocardial rigor closely resembling the "stone heart" described by Cooley and only 30% of the animals survived. There were no survivors after 2 hours of normothermic ischemia. Other investigators have reported 45% survival in dogs after 1 hour of ischemia at 35°C. Survivors evaluated 5 months later were found to have reduced contractility, compliance and ejection fractions. Hypertrophied hearts exhibit more profound changes still.

Free Radicals and Reperfusion Injury

Oxygen-derived free radicals are now thought to be a factor in myocardial injury both during ischemia and reperfusion.[13] The interest in this area is relatively recent and the subject is still controversial. For reasons that are not immediately obvious but probably reflect the difficulties many clinicians had (have) with physical chemistry, the chemical principles involved have been made needlessly complicated; the chemistry is actually quite simple.

A free radical is simply a molecule that is very reactive by virtue of having an odd number of electrons, leaving it with an open or "unsatisfied" bond. In scientific notation the odd electron is denoted by a dot. A chemical reaction between a free radical ($R^{\bullet}$)

and a stable compound or molecule (AB) with an even number of electrons produces a stable compound (RA) and another free radical ($B^{\bullet}$):

$$R^{\bullet} + AB \dashrightarrow RA + B^{\bullet}$$

Similarly, a reaction between two free radicals eliminates both, producing a stable compound with no unpaired electron:

$$R^{\bullet} + B^{\bullet} \dashrightarrow RB$$

The implication is that because free radicals are highly reactive they may precipitate a chain reaction, producing increasingly reactive and possibly toxic free radicals. Moreover, free radicals may be either oxidizing or reducing agents. Oxygen normally undergoes tetravalent reduction, accepting four electrons simultaneously. However, as much as 2% of cellular oxygen undergoes univalent reduction, accepting one electron at a time and creating a superoxide anion ($O_2^{-\bullet}$):

$$O_2 \overset{e^-}{\dashrightarrow} O_2^{-\bullet}$$

The addition of another electron produces hydrogen peroxide, which may in turn break down to produce the hydroxyl free radical ($OH^{\bullet}$):

$$O_2^{-\bullet} \overset{e^- + 2H^+}{\dashrightarrow} H_2O_2 \overset{e^- + 2H^+}{\dashrightarrow} H_2O + OH^{\bullet}$$

The hydroxyl free radical is the most reactive of all and will oxidize almost instantaneously any organic molecule. The small quantities of free oxygen radicals produced normally are detoxified by the enzyme superoxide dismutase (SOD):

$$O_2^{-\bullet} + O_2^{-\bullet} + 2H^+ \overset{\text{Superoxide dismutase}}{\dashrightarrow} H_2O_2 + O_2$$

This protective enzyme occurs in all aerobic tissue but is found in substantial quantities only inside the cell. Free oxygen radicals are also detoxified by the naturally occurring enzymes catalase (CAT) and peroxidase. During ischemia the production of hypoxanthine is greatly increased as a result of the catabolism of ATP:

ATP ----//-----> AMP -----> adenosine -----> inosine -----> hypoxanthine

It has been established that hypoxanthine accumulates in the ischemic myocardium. In the absence of oxygen the enzyme xanthine dehydrogenase (type D) is converted to xanthine oxidase (type O) which converts hypoxanthine to xanthine. It appears that this conversion from type D to type O involves calcium. Although there is no evidence that oxygen-derived free radicals play a role in the injury of the "calcium paradox", the sudden influx of calcium during reperfusion may trigger the D to O conversion in tissue that is neither ischemic nor hypoxic.

When the ischemic tissue is again exposed to oxygen during reperfusion, xanthine oxidase catalyzes the reaction:

$$\text{xanthine} + H_20 + 2O_2 \xrightarrow{\text{xanthine oxidase}} \text{uric acid} + 2O_2^{-\bullet} + 2H^+$$

It is noteworthy that xanthine dehydrogenase found in the cells of skeletal muscle does not convert to the oxidase during ischemia, which may account for the resistance of skeletal muscle to ischemic injury. By contrast, in cardiac muscle the defense mechanisms against superoxide-mediated ischemic injury are well developed. They take the form of scavenging enzymes that may be antioxidants, such as glutathione peroxidase and catalase, or chain-breaking antioxidants, such as SOD, ascorbate (vitamin C) and α-tocopherol (from vitamin E). It has been observed that the myocardium of patients with cyanotic heart disease is particularly susceptible to damage by superoxide radicals during surgery and it may be that the defense mechanisms are not as effective in patients with chronic ischemia who are then exposed to higher oxygen tensions during cardiopulmonary bypass. There is strong circumstantial evidence that superoxides and probably hydroxyl free radicals are important in ischemic injury. Indeed, a question arises as to whether or not what has previously been called ischemic injury and has been thought to occur during ischemia is in fact a reperfusion injury that is initiated by ischemia but precipitated by reperfusion. It is this mechanism that has led to the concept of scavenging free radicals both during ischemia and reperfusion. The role of allopurinol, which inhibits xanthine oxidase, in preventing superoxide-mediated injury is obvious. Transition metals, such as iron found in heme may also react with hydrogen peroxide to produce hydroxyl free radicals:

$$H_2O_2 + O_2^{-\bullet} \xrightarrow{Fe^{++}} O_2 + OH^- + OH^\bullet$$

Chelating agents such as desferoxamine inhibit this reaction and have also been advocated in the prevention of superoxide-mediated injury. Other investigators have demonstrated that the administration of SOD, CAT, allopurinol and mannitol to ischemic myocardium before reperfusion is associated with a more rapid and complete recovery of ventricular function. Various techniques using antioxidant therapy to ameliorate superoxide-mediated injury are being investigated but the current vogue for blood cardioplegia may well completely prevent it, obviating the need for antioxidants altogether.

The Calcium Paradox

It is well established that calcium is essential to the interaction between actin and myosin and in the regulation of myocardial contraction. Although calcium homeostasis within the cell is not yet fully understood, a proper distribution of calcium within the cell is necessary to maintain the integrity of the cell membrane and other functions. Normally calcium is sequestered in the sarcoplasmic reticulum by an energy-dependent process, but failure of this pump as a result of depletion of ATP may cause an increase in cytosolic calcium which in turn, may increase the permeability of the cell membrane, allowing a rapid influx of calcium into the cell. Certainly, the characteristic histological change of the calcium paradox is separation of the basement membrane from the sarcolemma. It is thought that calcium leaks across the membrane when the extracellular calcium concentration is low, but a rapid influx of calcium back into the cell occurs when the extracellular calcium returns to normal. This situation typically arises during reperfusion following the administration of cardioplegia solutions that contain no calcium. The calcium paradox does not occur inevitably, however, implying that many of these changes are reversible. Nevertheless, in some cases the influx of calcium leads to preferential sequestration in the mitochondria (inhibiting the production of high-energy phosphates) and also to cellular swelling, rupture and the appearance of contracture bands, the hallmark of severe ischemic injury, in the myocardial fibers. Contracture bands are thought to be caused by abnormal overlapping of the actin and myosin filaments in the sarcomere as a result either of failure of relaxation or of a sort of tetanic contraction. A great deal of experimental work has been done over the last 10 years using calcium channel blockers in the hope of ameliorating the calcium paradox, but the results have been disappointing. The problem appears to occur only infrequently during surgery, presumably because wash-out of the cardioplegia solution by collateral flow provides small amounts of calcium to the myocardium. The phenomenon of calcium paradox is diminished by hypothermia that, interestingly enough, also appears to abolish the negative inotropic effects of the calcium channel blocking agents and implies that they may be unnecessary.

Summary

Ischemic injury increases exponentially with time. After 15 minutes of normothermic ischemia the changes in the myocardium are subtle and largely reversible. After half an hour, the metabolic and structural changes are obvious but functional recovery appears to occur before the structural and metabolic changes resolve. After 1 hour of normothermic ischemia, irreversible biochemical and cellular damage take place that are associated with substantial mortality and permanent ventricular dysfunction in the survivors.

Practical Considerations

It is a truth universally acknowledged that the likelihood of a successful outcome after heart surgery is directly proportional to the extent of correctable pathology and the completeness of the correction. Even after a prolonged but totally corrective procedure the heart is more likely to be forgiving of ischemic injury than after a short operation in which not all of the pathology is correctable or corrected. Indeed, the functional reserve of the heart frequently allows ischemic injury to be attended by surgical success. However, as the cardiac surgical patient population ages and the surgical indications are extended, fewer patients present with pathology that is totally amenable to surgical correction and the complexity and duration of procedures continue to increase. Scrupulous attention to myocardial preservation is therefore becoming the key to operative survival, especially in the frustrating but all too frequent situation in which there is minimal improvement after surgery.

Myocardial preservation is more than just a matter of choosing which cardioplegia solution to use. In fact the conduct of anesthesia and surgical strategy may play a far more important role, as may be surmised from the perfectly satisfactory results reported using any number of different cardioplegia mixtures. At its simplest, myocardial preservation means avoiding, detecting, and treating *unplanned* ischemia and the careful management of the period of planned ischemia and reperfusion.

Surgical Strategy

Surgical strategy involves devising a plan to minimize, or ideally to avoid completely, ischemic injury without unnecessarily compromising the conduct of the operation itself. Obviously the nature and magnitude of the planned procedure and the patient's condition are major factors in the decision. For example, few surgeons would approach a patient needing a single coronary bypass to the left anterior descending coronary artery as they would a patient with severe aortic stenosis, three vessel coronary artery disease, and impaired left ventricular function. The first case might involve only 15 minutes of cross clamp time and 25 minutes of perfusion at normothermia and few surgeons would use a vent. The second case, however, would certainly involve hypothermia, most surgeons would use a left ventricular vent and many would use retrograde cardioplegia or, at least, give more than one dose. Some would advocate the use of saphenous vein for all the grafts, rather than the internal mammary artery, in order to deliver cardioplegia down the grafts after each distal anastomosis is complete.

The presence of significant pulmonary hypertension might also militate in favor of using bicaval cannulation and tapes to avoid rewarming and subsequent dysfunction of the right ventricle during what would inevitably be a longer cross clamp time.

Similarly, in the stable patient who does not have a critical stenosis of the left main coronary artery it is feasible to construct the proximal anastomoses using a partial occlusion clamp on the ascending aorta before cardiopulmonary bypass is instituted. Nevertheless, it must be acknowledged that this is a compromise. The increase in afterload produced by partial occlusion of the aorta is bound to increase myocardial oxygen consumption and the fact that this approach is usually successful is a testament to the reserves of the myocardium rather than an endorsement of the technique.

Reoperations, especially valve reoperations, usually reward careful planning. In desperately ill patients it is wise to have a fall back position in order to deal with unforeseen contingencies arising during the procedure. Surgeon and anesthesiologist are wise to review the problems and strategy beforehand and to discuss and modify the plan in light of events during surgery.

Before Induction of Anesthesia

The main objective at this stage is to maintain myocardial oxygen supply and to minimize myocardial energy consumption so that the stores of ATP are not depleted before the aortic cross clamp is applied. Thorough preoperative evaluation may uncover anemia, acid-base, fluid and electrolyte disturbances that should be corrected. It may even be deemed prudent to insert an intra-aortic balloon preoperatively, but anesthetic and monitoring techniques have improved to the point where this is rarely necessary as a prophylactic measure. Myocardial oxygen consumption is increased by anxiety, excitement, tachycardia and systemic arterial hypertension. Careful attention to premedication will avoid the arrival in the operating room of an anxious, hypertensive patient with chest pain and ischemic changes in the electrocardiogram. The risks of discontinuing intravenous heparin therapy in order to facilitate safer insertion of monitoring lines must be carefully weighed. Certainly, any evidence of ischemia in a patient who had been receiving an intravenous infusion of heparin militates in favor of reinstituting it in the hope of averting acute coronary closure. Such patients frequently develop antithrombin III deficiency and develop a hypercoagulable state. Monitoring the ST segments of the electrocardiogram enables the anesthesiologist to promptly detect and treat ischemia. The routine use of pulmonary artery catheters and of transesophageal echocardiography (TEE) remains controversial. Nevertheless, in the high-risk patient both can be extremely useful monitoring techniques. The major disadvantage is the expense in both cases. There is some risk associated with the use of pulmonary artery catheters but, in experienced hands and provided certain simple precautions are observed, the risk should be minimal. However, the pulmonary artery catheter is not a therapeutic modality and it is useless as a monitoring device unless the operator knows enough physiology to interpret the data correctly and to make the appropriate intervention. Recent studies indicate that this can by no means be taken for granted. Continuous, online pulmonary arterial oximetry is an additional refinement that obviates the need for frequent determinations of cardiac output and is probably most useful in postoperative management in the intensive care unit. Transesophageal echocardiography is an extraordinarily useful technique but it is very operator-dependent. It is especially useful in the detection of changes in regional wall motion and ventricular contractility, volumes and compliance, to say nothing of its application in the detection and evacuation of intracardiac air and in the assessment of valve repair or replacement.

Before Bypass

It is at this stage that meticulous attention to the details on the part of the anesthesiologist can make an enormous difference, especially in the unstable patient. The surgeon's attention is frequently focused on the dissection of the internal mammary artery and preparation for bypass. Bearing in mind the relationship described earlier:

$$T = \frac{P \times Ri}{2h}$$

T	=	mean myocardial wall stress	(myocardial oxygen consumption)
P	=	transmural LV pressure	(contractile state and afterload)

Ri =	internal LV radius	(LVEDV or preload)
h =	LV wall thickness	(LV hypertrophy)

and also the factors governing myocardial oxygen supply and coronary blood flow, the ratio of supply to demand may be kept in balance by the appropriate therapeutic intervention including, if all else fails, instituting cardiopulmonary bypass, attention to the control of heart rate, the suppression of arrhythmias (and treatment of underlying acute ischemia) and to control of arterial blood pressure. In this regard it should be noted that in the anesthetized patient with coronary artery disease the double product (heart rate $\times$ systolic arterial blood pressure) is a poor index of myocardial oxygen consumption because the heart rate is a much more important determinant of myocardial oxygen consumption than the blood pressure in the anesthetized patient.

During Bypass

It has already been noted that the conduct of perfusion should, to some extent, be individualized. The patient's left and right ventricular function (i.e., tolerance for ischemic injury), the circumstances of the operation, the nature and duration of the planned procedure and the resulting change in physiology that is anticipated are factors that should be taken into account. Routines may then be modified by changing the cannulation scheme, the use of ventricular vent, the extent of cooling and so on.

Once cardiopulmonary bypass has been safely established, the patient is cooled. The extent of cooling will depend on the nature and magnitude of the procedure. Thus a short procedure may obviate the need for cooling altogether. Likewise, in a reoperation cooling may be deliberately delayed until the pericardial adhesions have been divided to avoid premature ventricular fibrillation.

Maintaining adequate coronary perfusion (i.e., 50 mm Hg mean arterial pressure) at this stage is extremely important. However, in cases of severe aortic insufficiency it is rarely possible to establish a satisfactory perfusion pressure until the aortic cross clamp has been applied and the operative strategy must be modified accordingly. Ventricular distension may interfere with subendocardial blood flow and should be avoided.

Ventricular fibrillation increases myocardial oxygen demand and periods of ventricular fibrillation should ideally be avoided altogether or at least minimized. The use of a ventricular vent offsets the increase in oxygen consumption to a certain extent, especially during hypothermia. The combination of ventricular fibrillation and aortic insufficiency is to be avoided at all costs because inadequate coronary perfusion is compounded by a dangerous increase in myocardial oxygen consumption as the heart fibrillates and then distends.

In practical terms myocardial oxygen consumption may be reduced in three ways during cardiac surgery, i.e., by inserting a left ventricular vent (eliminating external work), by stopping the heart beat (eliminating the work of contraction), and hypothermia (minimizing basal metabolic requirements). Similarly, coronary perfusion may be enhanced by maximizing the transmural gradient across the left ventricular wall, which is achieved by maintaining arterial perfusion pressure (by vasoactive agents, if necessary) and also by inserting a left ventricular vent.

The Left Ventricular Vent

The left ventricular vent, which is usually inserted via the right superior pulmonary vein and advanced across the mitral valve into the left ventricle, has various applications. The elucidation of the pathophysiology involved has been almost exclusively the work of Buckberg's group and the subject of an excellent series of publications.[2] The left ventricular vent serves:

(1) to minimize external work and thus myocardial oxygen consumption
(2) to maximize the transmural gradient and coronary perfusion
(3) to prevent distension of the left ventricle
(4) to prevent rewarming of the left ventricular subendocardium by noncoronary collateral blood flow
(5) to provide a dry operative field by minimizing back bleeding from the coronary arteries

The effect of decompression of the left ventricle on myocardial oxygen consumption in the beating heart is depicted in Figure 1. The elimination of external work reduces oxygen consumption to that required to maintain coordinated contractions and to sustain basal metabolism. The effect on myocardial oxygen consumption in the fibrillating heart is shown in Figure 2. It will be noted that the oxygen consumption of the fibrillating heart is higher than that of the beating vented heart. However, when the myocardium is cooled the vigor and rapidity of fibrillation decrease. At 32°C the oxygen consumption of the fibrillating, vented heart is less than that of the beating vented heart (Fig. 3). The necessity for decompression of the left ventricle during ventricular fibrillation is well established. In patients in whom a ventricular vent is not used the most dangerous period is immediately after the cross clamp is removed. The development of ventricular fibrillation at this stage is obviously highly undesirable. Similarly, ventricular asystole in the presence of aortic insufficiency will rapidly lead to ventricular distension and is best treated by using a pacemaker to enable the ventricle to "protect itself". The development of ventricular fibrillation in a patient with significant aortic insufficiency can rapidly

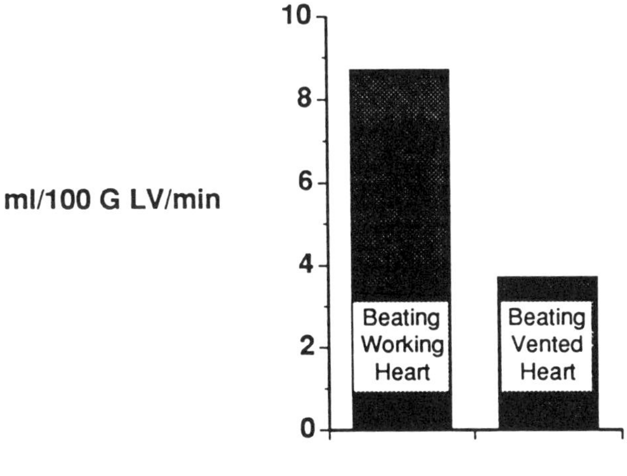

Figure 1. Left ventricular myocardial oxygen consumption. (Data from Hottenrot.[2])

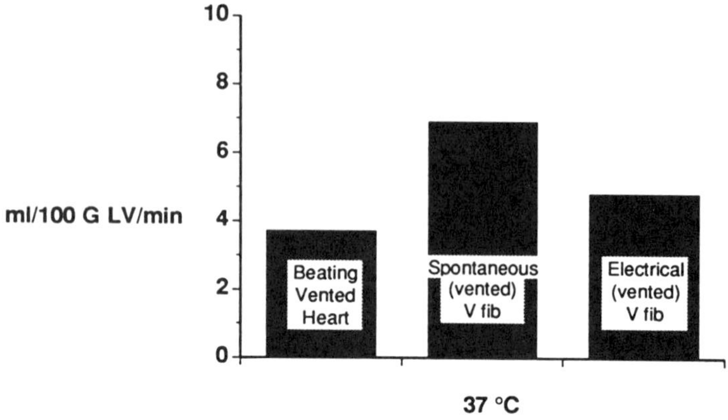

Figure 2. Left ventricular myocardial oxygen consumption. (Data from Hottenrot.[3])

produce a catastrophe. The dangers of acute ventricular distension cannot be overestimated and concerns about this very situation disturb heart surgeons more than almost any other. In such circumstances the vent is a comfort to surgeon and patient alike.

It is clearly not necessary to use a ventricular vent routinely in combination with cardioplegia. Many surgeons obtain excellent results by venting the aortic root, often through a "Y" on the cardi-

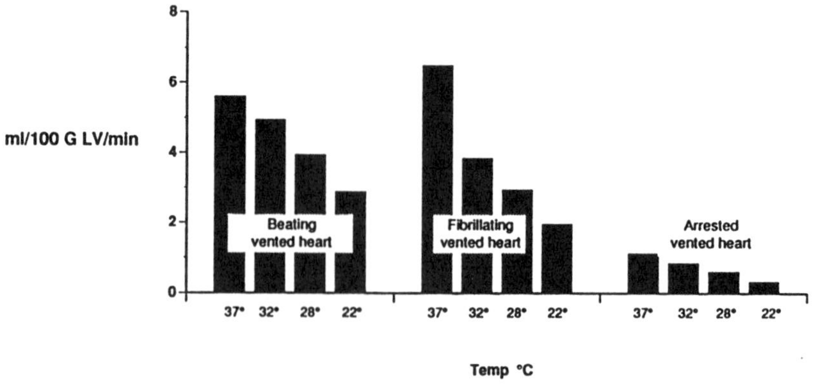

Figure 3. Left ventricular myocardial oxygen consumption. (Data from Buckberg.[14])

oplegia cannula, or by venting the main pulmonary artery. The aortic root vent serves mainly to provide a dry operative field and has little if any effect on the ventricle. Venting the pulmonary artery is a compromise between an aortic and a ventricular vent. Other surgeons dispense with the vent altogether. The arguments against the use of a ventricular vent include:

- the possibility of the introduction of air and subsequent air embolism
- the possibility of bleeding from the cannulation site
- the risk of perforation of the left atrium or left ventricle
- the additional time involved for insertion and removal

All of these objections are valid but none represents an overwhelming argument. If due care is taken, the use of a ventricular vent is quite safe. It is certainly unnecessary to use a ventricular vent in every case, provided that physiological principles are observed, but it offers an extra margin of safety. The dogmatic macho approach—"Real men don't need a vent"—has no place in modern cardiac surgery.

Hypothermia

A review of the physiology of hypothermia is beyond the scope of this chapter. According to the equation of Arrhenius the rate of a chemical reaction is directly proportional to the temperature at which it takes place. Hypothermia thus reduces the metabolic rate. Much of our understanding of this subject derives from the study of hibernating mammals and, from the earliest days of cardiac surgery attempts have been made to induce a state of hibernation.

Lowering the temperature protects the myocardium by reducing myocardial oxygen consumption by:

(1) reducing the rate of the beating heart
(2) reducing the vigor (wall tension) and rate of fibrillation in the fibrillating heart
(3) reducing the metabolic rate

Cooling causes a steady decrease in heart rate, albeit with a concomitant increase in the myocardial oxygen consumption per beat, probably as a result of the prolongation of systole. The net effect, however, is a reduction in myocardial oxygen consumption in the beating and in the fibrillating heart (Fig. 3). Although spontaneous ventricular fibrillation usually occurs when the myocardial temperature reaches 28°C, the heart may continue to beat at lower temperatures but electrical and mechanical activity ceases when the temperature falls below 16°C. Figure 3 clearly shows that oxygen consumption is least in the cold arrested heart.

Hypothermia may also decrease the oxygen supply by:

(1) altering the distribution of coronary blood flow
(2) increasing the viscosity of the blood
(3) shifting the hemoglobin-oxygen dissociation curve to the left

Coronary perfusion is evenly distributed across the myocardium of the beating empty heart at all temperatures. The fact that coronary blood flow is redirected towards the subendocardium of the fibrillating ventricle at myocardial temperatures above 32°C appears to present a paradox, implying improved subendocardial perfusion. In fact it indicates that oxygen requirements are higher in this region under these circumstances. As the heart is cooled the distribution of coronary flow in the fibrillating heart becomes more uniform, provided that perfusion pressures are adequate.

The increase in the viscosity of blood is rarely a problem clinically now that hemodilution is used universally for heart surgery. It is noteworthy that profound hemodilution occurs naturally in hibernating mammals. Increased viscosity may pose problems with the use of cold blood cardioplegia and also in patients with cold agglutinins.

Although the leftward shift in the dissociation curve leads to higher arterial oxygen saturation at a given oxygen tension, the amount of oxygen available to the tissue is correspondingly reduced.

Hypothermia also affects pH. It has been suggested that the ideal state for cellular metabolism is one of chemical neutrality, which implies that the extracellular fluid must be relatively alkaline to facilitate the elimination of acid metabolites from within the cell.[15] The dissociation of water is temperature dependent like all other chemical reactions. At 37°C neutral pH is 6.8, but at 0°C neutral pH is 7.5. Indeed, in poikilotherms pH is inversely proportional to temperature and increases to about 7.8 during hypothermia. Maintaining the pH in this range has been shown to produce more rapid and complete recovery of myocardial function and it is now customary to buffer cardioplegia solutions so as to maintain an alkaline pH.

The clinical application of hypothermia involves several complementary concepts:

Perfusion is the safest and most effective method of inducing hypothermia. However, it is slow because the rate of cooling is proportional to the mass of the tissue being cooled and the time consumed is doubled by the duration of rewarming. Moreover, perfusion may be uneven in the presence of arterial stenosis with the result that the most vulnerable tissue is the one that is slowest to cool. For procedures that do not involve the use of circulatory arrest it is impractical to cool the entire patient. Instead **differential hypothermia** is used, whereby the patient is cooled somewhat or not at all and the heart is cooled as much as possible. From what has been said so far it should be obvious that the objective is to cool the heart as much and as quickly as possible and to maintain the myocardial temperature as low as possible while the aortic cross clamp is on. The heart, then, is cooled to a certain extent by perfusion before the aortic cross clamp is applied. Cooling of the heart then continues by perfusion with cold cardioplegia solution (antegrade via the aortic root or down the vein grafts and/or retrograde via the coronary sinus), by **topical hypothermia,** by irrigation with cold saline, packing the heart in frozen saline slush or surrounding the heart with a special cooling jacket. Usually some combination of these techniques is used. Additional cooling of the subendocardium may be achieved during aortic and mitral valve replacement by irrigation of the inside of the ventricle with cold saline. Likewise, cooling of the interior of the right atrium and ventricle may be enhanced by local irrigation or by the indirect approach to retrograde infusion of cardioplegia (directly into the right atrium after snaring the superior and inferior vena cava and clamping the pulmonary artery). The measurement of myocardial changes in temperature may detect uneven cooling and rewarming of the myocardium from various sources[16] and may determine the need for further measures or even operative strategy (graft the warmest region first and give cardioplegia down the graft). However, recent studies have shown that the inverse correlation between myocardial temperature and myocardial metabolism is not universal. Placing an insulating pad between the heart and the pericardium serves both to prevent rewarming by conduction from the warm blood in the descending thoracic aorta and to reduce the incidence of cold-induced injury to the phrenic nerve.

At present there is no consensus about the ideal temperature for myocardial preservation. The linear relationship between oxygen consumption and temperature and the exponential relationship between the duration of ischemia and the extent of injury support the current orthodoxy of cooling the heart as much as possible and maintaining the temperature of the myocardium as low as possible. Damage caused by freezing of the myocardium is not a realistic concern in the clinical situation.

Stopping the Heart

The main reason for stopping the heart (by inducing fibrillation or asystole) is to provide adequate surgical exposure. Surgical exposure also demands a relatively bloodless operating field and therefore coronary perfusion is usually interrupted by applying the aortic cross clamp, but certain situations and techniques make this unnecessary. It is, of course, possible to perfuse the coronary arteries selectively while the aorta is occluded and this may be done intermittently or continuously by direct cannulation of the coronary ostia. However, this necessitates opening the aorta unless it has already been opened (for aortic valve surgery for example). Coronary perfusion may also be maintained while the aorta is occluded by means of coronary grafts, viz. internal mammary arteries, vein grafts or even Dacron grafts, as in the Cabrol procedure for replacement of the aortic root. Selective coronary perfusion was used with considerable success in the early days of heart surgery and was only abandoned when cold chemical cardioplegia was found to be safe as well as convenient. A skeptic might observe that we have now come full circle and that there is little difference between the use of blood cardioplegia, especially warm continuous blood cardioplegia, and coronary perfusion!

It is, likewise, possible to operate on or in the beating heart, as of old. Although it is not then feasible to construct microvascular anastomoses for coronary bypass surgery, the operating conditions are satisfactory, if not ideal, for valve surgery, correction of atrial and ventricular septal defects and for ventricular aneurysm resection. Indeed, for tricuspid annuloplasty and repair of ventricular septal defects, in which there is a significant risk of injury to the conducting system, many surgeons prefer to operate on the beating heart so that they can observe changes in conduction on the electrocardiogram. The same approach has been adopted in the burgeoning field of arrhythmia surgery. The major disadvantage of operating on the beating heart, apart from compromising surgical exposure, is the risk of air embolism.

Procedures requiring no more than 15 minutes of aortic cross clamp time may be performed without the use of cardioplegia (or indeed any adjuncts to myocardial preservation) with comparative safety. Such simple procedures are rare nowadays and the technique of normothermic ischemic arrest is infrequently used or justified.

There are four ways of stopping the heart, viz. electrically-induced ventricular fibrillation, ischemic arrest, cold cardioplegia and chemical cardioplegia. The last two techniques are usually combined.

Ventricular fibrillation

Applying a low-voltage alternating current (c. 5 V) to the surface of the heart induces ventricular fibrillation. The technique is an old one that has several advantages. It produces a relatively quiet heart without interrupting coronary perfusion, allowing the surgeon to proceed without having to worry about cross clamp time. It also avoids the risk of air embolism that attends surgery on the beating heart, although the ventricular vent may introduce air into the left heart.

At 37°C the oxygen consumption of the fibrillating, vented heart is actually higher than that of the beating, vented heart (Fig. 2). Although total myocardial oxygen consumption is lower during continuous, electrically maintained ventricular fibrillation than during spontaneous fibrillation (Fig. 2), excellent studies by Buckberg's group have shown that continuous electrical fibrillation impedes coronary blood flow to the subendocardium, causing ischemia. On the basis of these studies it is now generally agreed that the use of a ventricular vent is mandatory during prolonged ventricular fibrillation. Figure 3 shows that the addition of moderate hypothermia (32°C) has a salutary effect on oxygen consumption if a vent is used. Buckberg's studies also demonstrated the importance of maintaining adequate coronary perfusion pressure and the higher risk of ischemic injury in the hypertrophied heart.

By meticulous attention to these physiological principles, Akins[17] has obtained excellent results in coronary bypass surgery. He combines continuous fibrillation with the routine use of a left ventricular vent, regional coronary occlusion, moderate hypothermia to 28°C and pericardial cooling. His technique also stresses the importance of adequate coronary perfusion which he ensures by maintaining systemic perfusion pressure between 80 and 100 mm Hg.

Clearly, induced ventricular fibrillation is a viable technique but is used only rarely by most surgeons at present.

Cardioplegia

As noted originally by DeBakey and Cooley in 1956, interrupting coronary perfusion by cross clamping the aorta leads to ventricular fibrillation followed by asystole. It was nearly 20 years before it was realized that the heart stopped only when the supplies of ATP were no longer adequate for cardiac contraction. This is now referred to as ischemic (or occasionally, and incorrectly, anoxic) arrest.

Nowadays the objective is to stop the heart as quickly as possible in order to enjoy the benefits of a quiet, bloodless operative field without running the risk of significant ischemic injury. In spite of some evidence to the contrary, it is generally believed that cold chemical cardioplegia provides better protection than cold ischemic arrest (without a cardioplegic agent). There are almost as many cardioplegia solutions as there are heart surgeons and it is beyond the scope of this chapter to review all of them in detail. The discussion will therefore be confined to some of the salient points.

The ideal cardioplegia solution should be simple, cheap and easy to prepare. It should eliminate external cardiac work by the immediate induction of diastolic arrest, minimize the oxygen requirements for basal cardiac metabolism and cause no myocardial damage itself. It is almost universal practice to cool the solution, usually to about 4°C because hypothermia potentiates the protective effect of chemical cardioplegia.

Composition of cardioplegia solutions

Potassium chloride is the cardioplegic agent that is most frequently used in North America. The concentrations used range from about 10–30 mEq/L but there is evidence of a direct correlation between higher (20 mEq/L) potassium concentrations and postoperative cardiac arrhythmias, and concentrations of 5 mEq/L are both effective and less likely to cause arrhythmias. Other investigators attribute the high incidence of postoperative arrhythmias following the use of cardioplegia to inadequate cooling or rewarming of the right atrium resulting in ischemic injury to the conducting system. It appears that higher potassium concentrations (30 mEq/L) are necessary with blood cardioplegia.

The addition of **magnesium** to the potassium mixture appears to enhance postischemic recovery, possibly by blocking the phosphorylase activity of myosin and thus preserving high energy substrates. Magnesium, itself, induces cardiac arrest, albeit slowly, by inhibiting excitation-contraction coupling. It also appears to delay the influx of calcium ions into the cell by blocking receptor sites on the cell membrane. In Europe, magnesium (as magnesium-l-aspartate or magnesium sulphate in varying concentrations) is commonly used with **procaine** that both stabilizes the cell membrane and is, itself, a cardioplegia agent; it acts by decreasing the permeability of the membrane to sodium during depolarization. Moreover, it is common practice in Europe to use one solution for inducing arrest and a different solution for maintenance of arrest (e.g., St. Thomas' Hospital Solutions 1 and 2) but the technique, based as it is on entirely theoretical considerations, seems unnecessarily complicated. It is worth noting, in passing, the current vogue in North America for the use of a different solution immediately before or after reperfusion (secondary blood cardioplegia and the "hot shot") are open to similar criticism. The very name "hot shot" marks it as a fad of the silliest sort, there is little scientific evidence that the technique is beneficial and it is to be hoped that it will soon join other half-baked ideas in oblivion.

Ions, blood, and buffers

There are two schools of thought about the general composition of cardioplegia solutions. In North America, the consensus favors a solution that approximates the characteristics of the **extracellular** fluid in ionic concentration, osmolarity etc., whereas the European centers favor an **intracellular** composition. Comparable results are achieved on both sides of the Atlantic Ocean and the arguments pro and con must be considered moot. It is, however, generally agreed that the solution should be slightly **hypertonic** (315–350 mOsm/L) in order to avoid the myocardial edema that develops after the use of isotonic (310 mOsm/L) or hypotonic (270 mOsm/L) solutions. Hyperosmolar (400 mOsm/L) solutions may produce myocardial dehydration. Hypertonic solutions have for many years incorporated mannitol, originally because it was cheaper than albumin. Recent investigations have uncovered the fact that mannitol appears to scavenge free oxygen radicals, an additional benefit not afforded by other osmotic agents.

Because of changes in the dissociation constant of water (discussed above) at lower temperatures and because tissue acidosis may itself cause ischemic myocardial injury, it is usual to **buffer** the cardioplegia solution to a rather alkaline pH (7.6–7.8).

Although cold chemical cardioplegia reduces myocardial oxygen demand, it has no effect on supply. It makes intuitive sense to **incorporate oxygen** in the cardioplegia solution to address this issue. Three methods have been described. The simplest is to oxygenate a cold crystalloid cardioplegia solution, capitalizing on the increased solubility of oxygen at lower temperatures. At 10°C about 4 mL of oxygen will dissolve in 100 mL of crystalloid solution. The most physiological vehicle is, of course, blood (shades of cold coronary perfusion!) which, presumably, also offers ideal buffering capacity and ionic concentrations. In fact, little oxygen is released from hemoglobin during hypothermia because of the pronounced leftward shift of the hemoglobin-oxygen dissociation curve and only the oxygen dissolved in the plasma is actually available to the cell—approximately 3.6 mL of oxygen/100 mL plasma at a hemoglobin concentration of 5 G/100 mL.[18] The use of fluorocarbons, in which oxygen is very soluble, remains experimental.

After the publication by Buckberg's group of a report describing superior results a number of centers adopted the use of blood cardioplegia with or without the addition of oxygen to the mixture. Although other investigators have reported similar results, blood cardioplegia is used at only about half of the centers in North America and it should be added that oxygenation of cardioplegia solution is routine at fewer centers still. The simplest and most frequently used system for mixing blood cardioplegia involves sequestering blood from the oxygenator reservoir and adding the other ingredients favored by the surgeon.

Thus most surgeons merely "nod in the general direction" of blood cardioplegia, by using a solution that can more accurately be described as *red cardioplegia* by virtue of hematocrits approximating 5%. It may therefore be deduced that most surgeons do not believe that the benefits justify the extra trouble and expense.

From the results of an informal survey it appears that nearly half the surgeons in the U.S.A. are quite satisfied with the results obtained using cold crystalloid cardioplegia solutions. Moreover, as a result of the drive to reduce health care costs by limiting reimbursement, it seems likely that the simplest and cheapest approach will be adopted universally. A standard cardioplegia solution is available commercially (Plegisol, Abbott Laboratories) that certainly combines the advantages of convenience, simplicity, consistency of formulation and guaranteed sterility. It is also quite cheap (list price: $23.82/1,000 mL bag) but the "house mixture" can be produced more cheaply still by the hospital pharmacy ($8.59/1,000 mL bag at the authors' institution).

Additives to Cardioplegia Solutions

Calcium is essential to myocardial contractility and also to maintain the integrity of the cell membrane and other cellular functions. For this reason and because of concerns about reperfusion injury caused by calcium paradox (see above) most cardioplegia solutions include small amounts (1 mM/L) of calcium. It is not considered necessary to add calcium to blood cardioplegia mixtures. Indeed, some surgeons advocate the use of citrate to chelate the calcium in the blood. Although (slow) **calcium channel blockers** have been shown in experimental studies and in some clinical reports to be effective in preventing myocardial injury caused by ischemia and reperfusion, they have proved a disappointment in clinical use because of their negative intropic effect and especially because of the conduction disturbances that develop after reperfusion. The studies are open to criticism on several grounds. It has been discovered that the rapid influx of calcium responsible for the calcium paradox occurs via channels that are not affected by slow channel blockers and at temperatures below 27°C changes in the cell membrane decrease slow channel currents, obviating the need for calcium channel blockers. Magnesium also acts as a slow channel blocker, as does procaine. The clinical efficacy of administering calcium channel blockers before, during or after ischemia has not yet been proven.

Likewise, the exact role of **free radical scavengers** such as SOD, CAT, mannitol and allopurinol has yet to be defined. They offer tantalizing possibilities in preventing ischemic injury and are the focus of a considerable amount of research at present.

Reperfusion

Changes in cardiac surgery have strained current techniques of myocardial preservation to the limit. Confronted by this problem, surgeons have become resigned to accepting some degree of ischemic injury but the focus of attention in myocardial preservation has changed from devising methods of preventing ischemic injury to the development of techniques that are designed to reverse or at least ameliorate ischemic injury once it has occurred.

It has become clear that certain pharmacological interventions immediately before or during reperfusion together with meticulous attention to such details as coronary perfusion pressure, the transmural gradient, and avoiding or treating ventricular fibrillation may play a vital role. The objective at this stage is to rest the heart as much as possible while it is being perfused; the supply of oxygen and nutrients should be greatly in excess of demand, reversing the imbalance produced by ischemia. The ideal situation is the adequately perfused, beating, vented heart. Although there is still debate, most surgeons would accept an asystolic heart if vented and perfused. Pacing is mandatory for the unvented, asystolic heart during reperfusion as is prompt treatment for ventricular fibrillation. The development of ventricular fibrillation in the unvented heart with aortic insufficiency is a potential catastrophe.

The significance of the calcium paradox and free radicals has already been discussed. The administration of 200 mg of lidocaine immediately before removing the aortic cross clamp is a common practice and reduces the incidence of ventricular fibrillation. Bretylium has been used for the same reason but the resulting, profound and fairly prolonged decrease in perfusion pressure is far from ideal during reperfusion.

Direct metabolic interventions to minimize and/or reverse ischemic injury have been the subject of intense interest in recent times. The two main approaches have included substrate or enzyme inhibition that, to a certain extent occurs naturally because of tissue acidosis, and replenishment by the stimulation of anabolic enzymes or the administration of enzyme or substrate (**substrate enhancement**).

Attempts to modify carbohydrate metabolism have been made for many years. The use of glucose and insulin or glycogen for this purpose has not been shown to be beneficial and may even cause myocardial damage in higher concentrations. Preliminary reports suggest that the administration of glutamate and aspartate, substrates in the Krebs cycle, may also be beneficial but the results have yet to be confirmed.

Purine metabolism has been modified by reperfusing ischemic myocardium with adenosine, AMP, ADP and ATP and some improvement has been reported both in biochemical and functional recovery of ischemic myocardium. Other approaches have included blocking adenosine transport with pyridamole (reversing the tendency for adenosine to leak out of the cell), inhibition of the enzymes adenosine deaminase 5-nucleotidase and the use of inosine and ribose.

Lastly, there are advocates for the administration of warm blood cardioplegia (the "hot shot"), also known as secondary blood cardioplegia, immediately before reperfusion. It is held to eliminate the useless expenditure of mechanical energy during reperfusion while providing substrate for metabolic restoration. Although there is some evidence to support this contention as well as anecdotes about reduced incidence of reperfusion and postoperative arrhythmias, recent work indicates that it offers no advantages over more conventional approaches to reperfusion.

None of these techniques has yet emerged from the laboratory to enter the operating room, but they seem to hold promise for the future.

Delivery of Cardioplegia Solution

The technical details may be found in surgical texts. A few words about how cardioplegia is delivered are appropriate. The **antegrade** approach has been traditional. The solution is administered via a cannula placed in the aortic root between the aortic cross-clamp and the competent aortic valve. The solution is thus forced into the coronary ostia, the only egress, by the roller pump or pressure bag used for the infusion. The technique is simple, cheap and generally applicable. Nevertheless, there are some deficiencies. Although a mildly insufficient aortic valve can be rendered competent by digital pressure, significant insufficiency leads to ventricular distension, without perfusing the coronary arteries at all. The technique is also limited by the presence of significant coronary stenosis (especially of the left main coronary artery) or occlusion (as may occur after a failed PTCA) and by the presence of patent internal mammary artery bypass grafts during reoperations. Direct infusion into the coronary ostia, only really feasible if the aorta must be opened as part of the surgical correction, overcomes problems with aortic insufficiency but not the other drawbacks. Moreover there is some risk of injury to the coronary ostia themselves as a result of direct cannulation. Extremes of perfusion pressure are to be avoided (no more than 150 mm Hg in the aortic root), as is distension of the right atrium by return from the coronary sinus when the venae cavae have been snared. This is easily done by releasing one of the vena caval tapes while cardioplegia solution is being infused or by making an incision in the right atrium.

The use of **retrograde cardioplegia,** which is infused via the coronary sinus (by cannulation directly or via a special cannula placed in the right atrium after occluding the pulmonary artery), is a very useful adjunct in certain circumstances of which these are some examples. Any procedure involving a long period of ischemia, and in which interruptions to administer cardioplegia are undesirable, lends itself to the use of retrograde cardioplegia, which may be given continuously. The typical situation is that of a complex repair of the mitral valve, especially in the presence of coronary artery disease. Exposure of the mitral valve invariably causes aortic insufficiency, ruling out administration of additional doses via the aortic root without disturbing the surgical exposure. The composition of the solution used is identical but the technique is slightly different. The heart is slow to arrest by this technique which is more suitable for the maintenance of arrest. The heart should therefore be arrested first in some other way. Most surgeons give an initial antegrade infusion for this purpose before converting to retrograde infusion. The exact technical details of cannula insertion are of paramount importance in order to avoid injury to the coronary sinus, to the conducting system or venous infarction. The aortic root must be decompressed to allow escape of the solution returning via the coronary arteries and the infusion pressure must be monitored closely. It must not be allowed to rise above 40 mm Hg to avoid venous injury but higher pressures (60–80 mm Hg) are permissible if the solution is administered indirectly via the right atrium. Provided that these precautions are observed the technique is quite safe and affords excellent myocardial protection, especially in some tricky situations where other methods are inadequate.

Nevertheless the additional expense (the cost of the special cannulae varies from $50–75) and clutter associated with the use of retrograde cardioplegia mean that it is best reserved for selected cases.

Summary

Adequate myocardial protection may be obtained using many different techniques, which are most often used in combination and are properly individualized to address the particular situation.

The best results will only be obtained by the thorough understanding and application of basic physiological principles and there is no "right way to do it". It will not, however compensate for an operation that was either ill conceived or poorly executed in the first place.

REFERENCES

1. Marrin CAS, Spotnitz HM, Bregman D. Myocardial Preservation. *Curr Probl Surg* 18(8):477–538, 1981.
2. Hottenrott C, Buckberg G. Studies of the effects of ventricular fibrillation on the adequacy of regional myocardial blood flow. II. Effects of ventricular distention. *J Thorac Cardiovasc Surg* 68:626, 1974.
3. Hottenrott C, Maloney JV, Buckberg G. Studies of the effects of ventricular fibrillation on the adequacy of regional myocardial flow. I. Electrical vs. spontaneous fibrillation. *J Thorac Cardiovasc Surg* 68:615, 1974.
4. Hottenrott C, Maloney JV, Buckberg G. Studies of the effects of ventricular fibrillation on the adequacy of regional myocardial blood flow. III. Mechanisms of ischemia. *J Thorac Cardiovasc Surg* 68:634, 1974.
5. Hottenrott CE, Towers B, Kurkji HJ, et al. The hazard of ventricular fibrillation in hypertrophied ventricles during cardiopulmonary bypass. *J Thorac Cardiovasc Surg* 66:742, 1973.
6. Cooley DA, DeBakey ME. Resection of entire ascending aorta in fusiform aneurysm using cardiac bypass. *J Am Med Assoc* 162:1158, 1956.
7. Cooley DA, Reul GJ, Wukasch DC. Ischemic contracture of the heart: "stone heart." *Am J Cardiol* 29:575, 1972.
8. Gott VL, Bartlett M, Long DM, et al. Myocardial energy substances in the dog heart during potassium and hypothermic arrest. *J Appl Physiol* 17:815, 1962.
9. Melrose DG, Dreyer B, Bentall HH, et al. Elective cardiac arrest: preliminary communication. *Lancet* 2:21, 1955.
10. Feigl EO. Coronary physiology. *Physiol Rev* 63:1-205, 1983.
11. Badeer HS. Contractile tension in the myocardium. *Am Heart J* 66:432, 1963.
12. Jennings RB, Ganote CE. Mitochondrial structure and function in acute myocardial ischemic injury. *Circ Res* 38(Suppl I):80, 1976.
13. Shlafer M, Kane PF, Wiggins VY, et al. Possible role for cytotoxic oxygen metabolites in the pathogenesis of cardiac ischemic injury. *Circulation* 66(Suppl 1):I-85–92, 1982.
14. Buckberg GD, Brazier JR, Nelson RI, et al. Studies of the effects of hypothermia on regional myocardial blood flow and metabolism during cardiopulmonary bypass. I. The adequately perfused beating, fibrillating and arrested heart. *J Thorac Cardiovasc Surg* 73:87, 1977.

15. Rahn, H, Reeves RB, Howell BJ. Hydrogen ion regulation, temperature, and evolution. *Am Rev Respir Dis* 112:165, 1975.
16. Rosenfeldt FL, Watson DA. Interference with local myocardial cooling by heat gain during aortic crossclamping. *Ann Thorac Surg* 27:13, 1979.
17. Akins CW. Myocardial preservation with hypothermic fibrillatory arrest for coronary grafting. *J Mol Cell Cardiol* 22:S44, 1990.
18. Digerness SB, Vanini V, Wideman FE. In vitro comparison of oxygen availability from asanguinous and sanguinous cardioplegic media. *Circulation* 64(Suppl II):80, 1981.

Chapter 7

Partial Cardiopulmonary Support

John Dluzneski, MD, Pierre A. Casthely, MD, and John Niedzinski, CCP

Percutaneous coronary angioplasty has become widely used in the nonsurgical treatment of coronary artery disease. This procedure was initially limited to patients with single vessel coronary artery disease with well-preserved myocardial function.[1,2] During the past decade, however, coronary angioplasty ha been applied to patients with multivessel disease and patients with unstable angina with or without good left ventricular function.[2,3] Many patients with poor left ventricular function with lesions in arteries supplying a large amount of viable myocardium were not considered candidates for coronary angioplasty because it was felt that they could not tolerate the transient ischemia during balloon inflation.[2] Coronary angioplasty is also associated with a 5% risk of acute arterial closure,[4] with many of these patients requiring emergency coronary artery bypass graft surgery, which is associated with mortality rates between 2% and 12%.[5,6]

From Casthely PA, Bregman D, (eds): *Cardiopulmonary Bypass: Physiology, Related Complications, and Pharmacology.* Mount Kisco, NY, Futura Publishing Company, Inc., © 1991.

Intra-aortic balloon pumping has been used in select patients[7] in emergency situations during percutaneous transluminal coronary angioplasty (PTCA) and prior to emergency surgery.[8] However, its usefulness in each patient varies and it may be ineffective during total hemodynamic collapse.

Femoral-femoral cardiopulmonary bypass to prophylactically assist and also resuscitate high-risk patients undergoing coronary artery angioplasty is a newly accepted technique.[2,3,9-12] This support is an up-to-date nonsurgical interventional therapy available to patients with severe atherosclerotic heart disease.

History

The effectiveness of femoral-femoral cardiopulmonary bypass to provide cardiopulmonary support (CPS) was first demonstrated in the late 1960s following induced ventricular fibrillation.[13,14] Cardiopulmonary bypass was also used in an emergency room setting in patients in cardiogenic shock; and in patients with severe cardiac dysfunction including congestive failure and cardiac arrest; with a marked increase in survival rate for these otherwise terminal patients.[15-17] In 1983, several authors reported the use of percutaneous cardiopulmonary bypass for cardiac arrest patients. They cannulated the artery and vein with only a 12F cannula and consequently were only able to achieve flow rates of up to 2.5 L/min. Even with this low flow rate all five of their study patients were adequately resuscitated using this technique.[18]

The use of cardiopulmonary bypass in postcoronary angioplasty patients in shock or cardiac arrest was first reported in 1988.[19] These patients were refractory to the conventional means of resuscitation that included intra-aortic balloon pumping.[19]

In the same year, Vogel et al.[11] reported the successful use of semipercutaneous CPS for high-risk coronary angioplasty and aortic valvuloplasty. In this series of patients, the femoral artery and vein were surgically exposed under local anesthesia (semipercutaneous), and the support cannulae were placed under direct vision. Out of seven patients studied one expired 12 hours postvalvuloplasty due to sudden onset of ventricular fibrillation.

In 1989 total percutaneous CPS was used for coronary angioplasty in high-risk elective patients, "inoperable" patients, and patients in cardiogenic shock for elective coronary angioplasty.[20-22] Thirty-five patients were studied with 85 out of 86 lesions successfully dilated and a 3% mortality rate.[22] It was also used on an emergency basis in a group of eight patients with acute myocardial infarction in cardiogenic shock; one patient expired and seven were successfully dilated and remained asymptomatic 22 months after the procedure.[2]

Indications for the use of percutaneous CPS are, as with any newer procedure, in the evolution stage (Table I). They include: (1) abrupt vessel closure with associated hemodynamic collapse; (2) cardiac arrest in the catheterization laboratory; (3) high-risk coronary angioplasty; (4) high-risk valvuloplasty; and (5) cardiogenic shock due to acute myocardial infarction.

An ejection fraction of $\leq$ 25% in patients for elective coronary angioplasty should be the cutoff for use of CPS based on initial National Registry experience.[3,10] Clinically, percutaneous CPS has been used in emergency and elective settings, (such as elective and emergency angioplasty)[20] and in cardiogenic shock[21] with impressive results. It was successfully used in patient resuscitation even when conventional modes of resuscitation (including insertion of an intra-aortic balloon pump) were not effective. Cardiopulmonary support was also used in an emergency setting in patients with refractory cardiac arrest, as well as pulmonary emboli, hypothermia, trauma, and sepsis.[9] Percutaneous bypass support enabled Phillips et al.[9] to resuscitate almost all patients that were studied with the exception of the trauma patient who expired due to uncontrollable hemorrhage. With the amount of heparinization required for use of the CPS system, uncontrollable hemorrhage that occurs when CPS is used in trauma patients comes as no surprise. However, in almost all other cases the patients were successfully resusci-

Table I
Indications for Cardiopulmonary Support

— Abrupt vessel closure with cardiovascular collapse
— Cardiac arrest during P.T.C.A.
— High-risk P.T.C.A. (ejection fraction <25%)
— High-risk valvuloplasty
— Cardiogenic shock following acute myocardial infarction

tated when other modes of therapy were ineffective, making CPS a useful tool in heretofore hopeless cases.

Patients after failed angioplasty with refractory cardiac arrhythmia and cardiogenic shock can be sent directly to the operating room in a stable state, allowing better organ perfusion and a less stormy postoperative course when CPS is used.[2]

In cardiogenic shock, patients can also be stabilized using bypass support when conventional therapies (i.e., vasoactive drugs, intra-aortic balloon pump) fail, and then can undergo dilation of the most severe coronary lesions. If the duration of shock is less than 4 hours, the use of CPS to stabilize the patient for angioplasty may be the most effective treatment,[20,21] and by rapidly unloading the ventricles, the size of infarction may be reduced.[23]

Several complications following percutaneous CPS have been reported (Table II). They include femoral artery pseudoaneurysm, femoral artery thrombosis, infection and hematoma at the site of cannulation, and femoral nerve injury.[2,9]

Myler et al.[10] report that several centers are evaluating techniques with total open, total percutaneous, and semipercutaneous cannula introduction to determine any statistical differences in post-procedure complications. Higher cardiopulmonary flow rates (5-6 L/min) are usually not needed, allowing the use of the smaller 12-16F catheters that may further reduce complications.[2,10]

The CPS system is a more compact system than the extracorporeal bypass equipment that is used in the operating room during open heart surgery. The CPS system consists of a centrifugal, nonocclusive pump, a polypropylene hollow fiber membrane oxygenator, a heat exchanger and a temperature controller (Fig. 1). Setting up this support system until time of initiation of bypass support can be accomplished in under 10 minutes.[24] A flowmeter is usually added to the circuit between the centrifugal pump and the heat

Table II
Complications Following Partial Cardiopulmonary Support

— Femoral artery pseudoaneurysm
— Femoral artery thrombosis
— Femoral nerve injury
— Infection at the site of cannulation
— Hematoma at the site of cannulation

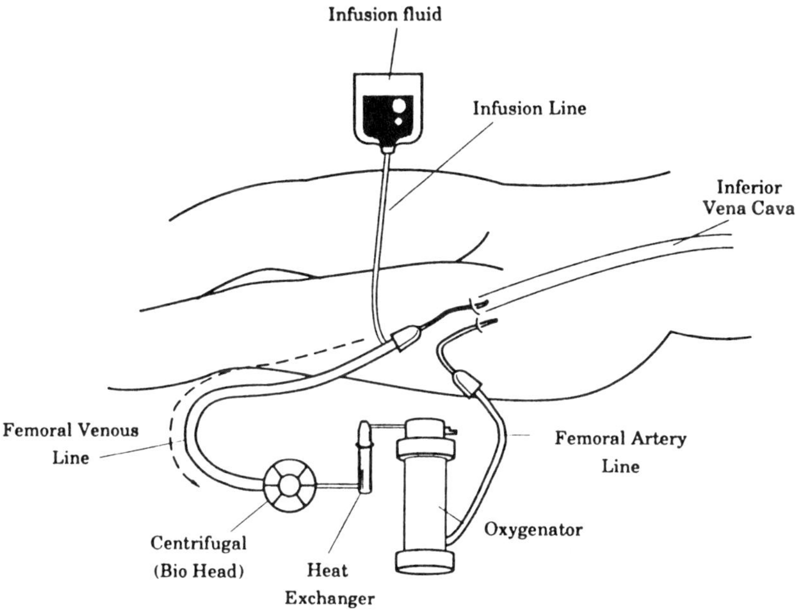

Figure 1. Essential components of the cardiopulmonary support system.

exchanger. A manometer is also added to the circuit after the oxygenator via a Y connector to monitor the pressure in the tubings that usually are 3/8 mm x 3 mm x 32 seconds (diameter x wall thickness x seconds).

Using this compact system, a vortex pump aspirates blood directly from the right atrium and vena cava. This offers advantages over traditional gravity drainage systems in that greater blood flow can be obtained using smaller cannulae, and the nonocclusive nature of the centrifugal pump does not allow excessive pressure to develop if an outlet of the pump is occluded.[2,25]

Other advantages to the use of this compact cardiopulmonary system are due to the hollow fiber membrane oxygenator. Gas exchange utilizing this oxygenator is relatively atraumatic when compared to other membrane oxygenators.[26,27] This oxygenator design has a very low pressure drop across the membrane (40 mm Hg with 6 L/blood flow) that allows higher flows at lower pressures, making the system safer from cavitation or explosion.[2]

A further advantage of this CPS system is in its safety regarding introduction of air into the patient. If any massive amount of air is introduced the centrifugal pump will stop and prevent its administration to the patient. When any smaller amount of air is present, it will be trapped in the membrane oxygenator and removed from the system, via diffusion.[4,5]

Monitoring

Monitoring used during the procedure include radial arterial line, pulse oximeter, ECG, temperature, and pulmonary artery catheter.

To utilize this system for CPS in the catheterization laboratory, the patient is prepped and draped. Either via surgical cutdown under local anesthesia, or percutaneously, femoral arterial, and venous sheaths are placed. The patients are then heparinized using 300 U/kg of heparin intravenously and blood is sent for activated clotting time (ACT). Guidewires are placed over cannulae into the right atrium via the femoral vein, and into the distal aorta via the femoral artery. The cannulae initially used were size 18-20 F, which deliver CPS flows of 4-6 L/min. In our institution we use smaller 16-18F cannulae, which deliver CPS flow of 3-4 L/min and provide adequate perfusion.[2,11]

The cannulae are then attached to the CPS system as shown in Figure 1. After adequate evidence of heparinization, (ACT > 350) CPS is initiated slowly with a gradual increase in flow rates. During CPS the pulmonary capillary wedge pressure can decrease to 0-5 mm Hg. Cardiopulmonary support may reduce systolic arterial pressure and slightly increase the diastolic blood pressure, depending on the patient's volume status at initiation of bypass support.[2] Most patients who develop hypotension respond to volume infusion. Certain patients with low systemic vascular resistance will also respond to a neosynephrine infusion.[2] The use of a cell saver may minimize the risk of blood transfusion.

Echocardiography performed on patients undergoing CPS shows a reduction in left atrial as well as left ventricular dimensions. Because of these reductions, CPS can then reduce myocardial oxygen demand so that these patients can undergo balloon inflation and angioplasty with little or no angina or electrocardiographic changes.

In managing CPS, baseline hemodynamic values should be obtained. These parameters include the systolic and diastolic arterial pressure, right atrial pressure, pulmonary capillary wedge pressure, cardiac output, and systemic and pulmonary vascular resistance. The elective patient should have adequate filling pressures and systemic vascular resistance optimized prior to initiation of bypass support. Cardiopulmonary support is then started slowly at a rate of 2 L/min and increased as necessary if PCW > 5 mm Hg. Chest pain, ECG changes, or hypotension during balloon inflation are usually treated by increasing the CPS flow rate.

It has been reported that most patients undergoing elective angioplasty may only need a flow rate between 2 and 3.5 L/min. However, patients with very poor left ventricular function or who are undergoing dilation of their only remaining open coronary artery may need higher flow rate. Calculations of flow rates are made according to body surface area (2.2- 2.4 L/min per square meter of body surface area) or to weight (50- 60 mL/kg body weight). Adequate CPS may be checked by measuring venous oxygen saturation (maintain above 65%).[2]

When the angioplasty has been successfully performed, CPS can be gradually weaned off. The filling pressure should be brought back to prebypass levels by volume infusion prior to clamping the support cannulae. The cannulae are removed only after the patient appears clinically stable. If the cannulae were placed by surgical cutdown, the vessels can be repaired under direct vision. If the percutaneous approach was used, an external clamp can be applied and adjusted so that the pedal pulse is present by palpation or Doppler. The heparin is usually not reversed and the ACT is checked frequently until it falls below 100 seconds at which point the external clamp is reduced gradually. If the ACT is very high (over 600 seconds) small doses of protamine are given slowly via the peripheral line to reverse the heparin. The pulmonary artery catheter and angioplasty sheaths can be removed in 24-48 hours depending on the patients' clinical situation. Most patients can be discharged in 3 to 5 days, and are placed on oral anticoagulants for 2-3 months to prevent deep vein thrombosis.

Anesthesia management of these patients is accomplished using small amounts of intravenous amnesics (i.e., benzodiazepines) while monitoring any hemodynamic changes that these agents can cause. The benzodiazepines possess the favorable qualities of sedation and an anxiolysis as well as anticonvulsant. The benzodiazepines most commonly used are diazepam, lorazepam and midazolam. Diazepam had been the standard benzodiazepine in clinical usage for many years. It works reasonably quickly and is approximately five times less potent than lorazepam and about one fourth as potent as midazolam. Specific disadvantages include venous irritation and a long terminal half-life that increases with liver and kidney failure. Lorazepam like diazepam cause venous irritation but has a longer duration of action. It is still clinically prudent to decrease lorazepam doses in the patient with liver disease. Midazolam has many advantages over the other benzodiazepines that include a lack of venous irritation, short elimination half-life, lack of accumulation in most patients. Short-acting narcotic analgesics like fentanyl, alfentanyl, and sulfentanyl may also be titrated, to produce sedation and have additional safety values of being reversible if the patient becomes too somnolent. The use of naloxone to reverse the respiratory effects of narcotics should be discouraged as much as possible since it may produce acute pulmonary edema.[28,29] Morphine sulfate is the old and reliable drug in this class. It can be given as a small bolus or via continuous infusion. Disadvantages include hypotension due to histamine release and direct vasodilatation and a long elimination half-life. Meperidine is another alternative drug with the disadvantages of tachycardia and potential for myocardial depression. Ideally, the patient should be kept calm but alert for questions and instructions. When CPS is initiated additional sedation may be required due to the expansion of intravascular volume through use of the bypass system. Patients with severe left ventricular dysfunction and valvular problems, however, do not require a large amount of sedation and adequate time should be allowed for its effect due to the prolonged circulation time.

Contraindications to the use of CPS are enumerated in Table III. Patients at risk for hemorrhage secondary to high doses of heparin (recent subdural, epidural or intracerebral hemorrhage, massive trauma, etc.) would have to have the risks versus benefits weighed before having elective CPS. Percutaneous CPS used as an emergency procedure in patients with cardiovascular collapse is more effective than the use of an intra-aortic balloon pump in acute

Table III
Contraindications for Cardiopulmonary Support

— Intracerebral hemorrhage
— Massive trauma
— Recent subdural hematoma
— Epidural hematoma

resuscitation as demonstrated by the overall patient outcome.[30] As bypass support is used in an emergency setting as the last possible effective mode of resuscitation, its contraindications will be outweighed by the patient survival rate. If all other attempts at resuscitation have failed any intervention with a chance of success should be instituted.

In conclusion, percutaneous cardiopulmonary bypass support for high-risk patients undergoing coronary angioplasty, a well as patients in refractory cardiogenic shock, appears to show great promise in the stable management of these patients. Other high-risk patients may be managed with an intra-aortic balloon pump alone, for example patients with good collateral flow to the myocardium served by the target artery. Risks of patient complications with CPS must be taken into consideration against the patients' possible benefits due to a 41% morbidity reported.[3,10] Several investigators have used CPS as a bridge between surgical and nonsurgical intervention in the care of select patients. Some patients previously not thought to be candidates for surgery or angioplasty may now undergo supported angioplasty. Studies are needed to further define the patient population best served by the use of CPS during angioplasty, as well as the ultimate role of this support in the catheterization laboratory.

As intracardiac interventions become more complex, percutaneous cardiopulmonary bypass support will have an expanding role in stabilizing these patients and allowing enough time to safely complete future interventions.

REFERENCES

1. Gruentzig AR. Transluminal dilation of coronary artery stenosis. *Lancet* 1:263, 1978.

2. Shawl FA. Percutaneous cardiopulmonary support in high-risk angioplasty. *Cardiol Clin* 7(4):865-875, 1989.
3. Vogel RA, Shawl FA, Tommaso C, et al. Initial report of the national registry of elective cardiopulmonary bypass supported coronary angioplasty. *J Am Coll Cardiol* 15:23-29, 1990.
4. Cowley MJ, Dorros G, Kelsey SF, et al. Acute coronary events associated with percutaneous transluminal coronary angioplasty. *Am J Cardiol* 53:12C-16C, 1984.
5. Parsonnet U, Gielchinsky I, Hochberg MS, et al. Emergency surgery after failed angioplasty (abstract). *J Am Coll Cardiol* 9:123A, 1987.
6. Roubin GS, Talley JD, Anderson HV, et al. Morbidity and mortality associated with emergency bypass graft surgery following elective coronary angioplasty (abstract). *J Am Coll Cardiol* 9:124A, 1987.
7. Alcan KE, Stertzer SH, Wallsh E, et al. The role of intra-aortic balloon counterpulsation in patients undergoing percutaneous transluminary angioplasty. *Am Heart J* 105:527-529, 1983.
8. Margolis JR. The role of the percutaneous aortic balloon in emergency situations following percutaneous transluminal coronary angioplaty. In: Kaltenbach M, Gruentzig A, Rentrop K, et al., eds. *Transluminary Coronary Angioplasty and Intracoronary Thrombolysis.* Berlin: Springer-Verlag; 1982:145-150.
9. Phillips SJ, Zeff RH, Kongtahworn C, et al. Percutaneous cardiopulmonary bypass: application and indication for use. *Ann Thorac Surg* 47:121-123, 1989.
10. Myler RK, Stertzer SH. Cardiopulmonary support: the risk and benefit of assisted coronary angioplasty. *J Am Coll Cardiol* 15:30-31, 1990.
11. Vogel RA, Tommaso CL, Gundry SR. Initial experience with coronary angioplasty and aortic valvuloplasty using elective semipercutaneous cardiopulmonary support. *Am J Cardiol* 62:811-813, 1988.
12. Gundry SR, Brinkley J, Wolk M, et al. Percutaneous cardiopulmonary bypass to support angioplasty and valvuloplasty. *Trans Am Soc Artif Intn Organs* 35:725-727, 1989.
13. Proctor E. Closed chest circulatory support by pump-oxygenator in experimental ventricular fibrillation at normal temperature. *Thorax* 21:385-390, 1966.
14. Proctor E, Kowalik TA. Circulatory support by pump-oxygenator in experimental ventricular fibrillation and acute left heart failure induced by coronary artery ligation. *Cardiovac Res* 1:186-193, 1967.
15. Lande AJ, Edwards L, Block JH, et al. Clinical experience with emergency use of prolonged cardiopulmonary bypass with a membrane pump-oxygenator. *Ann Thorac Surg* 10:409-423, 1970.
16. Baird RJ, Rocha AG, Miyagishima RT, et al. Assisted circulation following myocardial infarction: a review of 25 patients treated before 1971. *Can Med Assoc J* 107:287-291, 1972.
17. Mattox ICL, Beall AC. Application of portable cardiopulmonary bypass to emergency instrumentation. *Med Instrum* 11:347-49, 1977.
18. Phillips SJ, Ballentine B,Slonine D, et al. Percutaneous initiation of cardiopulmonary bypass. *Ann Thorac Surg* 36:223-225, 1983.

19. Kanter KR, Pennington DG, Vandormael M. Emergency Resuscitation with Extracorporeal Membrane Oxygenation for Failed Angioplasty (Abstract. *J Am Coll Cardiol* 11:149, 1988.
20. Shawl FA, Domanski MJ, Punja S, et al. Cardiopulmonary bypass supported coronary angioplasty in inoperable patients (abstract). *J Am Coll Cardiol* 13:53A, 1989.
21. Shawl FA, Domanski MJ, Punja S, et al. Emergency percutaneous cardiopulmonary (bypass) support in cardiogenic shock (abstract). *J Am Coll Cardiol* 13: 160A, 1989.
22. Shawl FA, Domanski MJ, Punja S, et al. Percutaneous cardiopulmonary bypass to support high risk elective coronary angioplasty (abstract). *J Am Coll Cardiol* 13:160A, 1989.
23. Lachinger JC, Grossi EA, Cunningham JN Jr, et al. Adjunctive left ventricular unloading during myocardial reperfusion plays a major role in minimizing myocardial infarct size. *J Thorac Cardiovasc Surg* 90:80-85, 1985.
24. Shawl FA: Use of percutaneous cardiopulmonary support: perfusion physiology. (In press)
25. Roberts C, Litziek F. *Cardiopulmonary Support System: Technical Specification Reference Manual.* Billerica, MA: Bard Cardiosurgery Division; CR Bard, 1986.
26. Clark RE, Beauchamp RA, Magrath RA, et al. Comparison of bubble and membrane oxygenators in short and long perfusions. *J Thorac Cardiovasc Surg* 78:655-666, 1979.
27. Volkmer I, Nienhaus KH, Meyers F, et al. Blood trauma during extracorporeal circulation: a comparison between two bubble and two membrane oxygenators in a standardized dog model. *J Thorac Cardiovasc Surg* 29:323-327, 1981.
28. Flacke JW, Flacke WE, Williams GD. Acute pulmonary edema following naloxone reversal for high-dose morphine anesthesia. *Anesthesiology* 47:376-378, 1977.
29. Partridge BL, Ward CF. Pulmonary edema following low-dose naloxone administration. *Anesthesiology* 65:709-710, 1986.
30. Smalling RW, Cassidy DB, Merhige M, et al. Improved hemodynamic and left ventricular unloading during acute ischemia using the hemopump left ventricular assist device compared to intra-aortic balloon counterpulsation (abstract). *J Am Coll Cardiol* 13(Suppl A):160, 1989.

Chapter 8

Hematologic Disorders Following Cardiopulmonary Bypass

Soomyung Lee, MD

Cardiac surgery requiring cardiopulmonary bypass (CPB) has been evolving in both number and safety over the last three decades. Although tremendous improvements in surgical, anesthetic, and perfusion techniques, as well as training of those personnel, have led to the increased safety of cardiac surgery, post-CPB bleeding continues to be a major cause of perioperative morbidity. Hemostasis is dependent on the integrity and normal function of three components: intact blood vessels or surgical control of bleeding vessels; platelets adequate in both number and activity to form a platelet plug; and normal coagulation cascades to form a stable clot (Fig. 1). A delicate balance exists between the coagulation system and the anticoagulating fibrinolysis system to maintain blood in the liquid form. Activation of any component of hemostasis will produce clotting, while deficiencies will result in bleeding.

Depending on the criteria for excessive bleeding, the incidence of post-CPB bleeding varies from 4%-32%,[1] with 3%-7% incidence

From Casthely PA, Bregman D, (eds): *Cardiopulmonary Bypass: Physiology, Related Complications, and Pharmacology.* Mount Kisco, NY, Futura Publishing Company, Inc., © 1991.

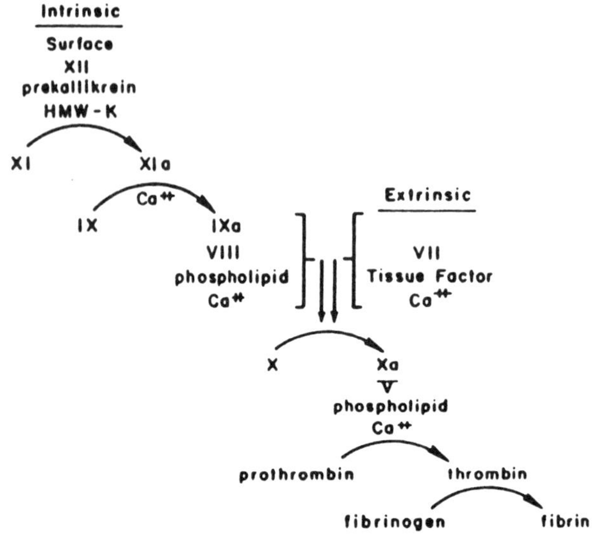

Figure 1. Normal coagulation cascade.

of reexploration for such bleeding.[2,3] In 1982, over 250,000 cardiac cases were performed in the United States.[4] As cardiac surgery accounts for over a quarter of all donor blood used, there is a tremendous burden on the blood bank supply and resources.[5] The etiology of nonsurgical hemostatic dysfunction is numerous and multifactorial. The effects of hemodilution, interaction of blood with extracorporeal circuit, effects of heparin and/or protamine, qualitative and quantitative platelet dysfunction, primary fibrinolysis, disseminated intravascular coagulation, coagulation factor deficiences, transfusion reaction, hypocalcemia, and hypothermia all may contribute to post-CPB bleeding. This chapter will review preoperative evaluation and specific hemostatic defects associated with cardiac surgery and extracorporeal circulation (ECC). Methods to decrease CPB alteration of the coagulation system, as well as specific therapies and risks of post-CPB bleeding, will also be discussed.

Preoperative Evaluation

History

As with all surgical patients, any patient undergoing cardiac surgery requires a detailed history, physical, review of drug therapy, and appropriate laboratory tests. Any preoperative coagulation deficits must be thoroughly investigated and its implication during cardiac surgery understood. Hematologic, renal, and hepatic diseases that may affect hemostatic homeostasis should be investigated. Many cases of cardiac surgical bleeding may be averted by eliciting a careful history including family history of bleeding diathesis; spontaneous or easy bruising; gingival bleeding with toothbrushing; excessive bleeding with previous surgery, menses or after tooth extraction; or any history of epistaxis, hemoptysis, hematemesis, hematochezia, or melena.[6]

Drug Therapy

A detailed drug history is of great importance in the cardiac surgery patient as many cardiac patients are on drugs with primary or incidental anticoagulant effects. The medications that affect platelets in a quantitative or qualitative fashion are very important (Table I). Cardiac surgery performed on patients taking aspirin increases blood loss and transfusion requirements.[7] As most drugs that inhibit platelets have a duration of 7-10 days, elective cardiac surgery should be delayed for 10-14 days. Warfarin depletes the vitamin K dependent coagulation factors II, VII, IX, and X. Because the anticoagulant effects of warfarin may last as long as 5 days after its discontinuation, warfarin should be changed to heparin if anticoagulation is required up to the time of surgery. For emergent situations, the effects of warfarin may be reversed by vitamin K or fresh frozen plasma. In patients receiving intravenous heparin for unstable angina, heparin is continued until the patient arrives into the operating room. Patients may present for emergency myocardial revascularization after thrombolytic treatment of acute coronary thrombosis and myocardial infarction. Streptokinase and tissue plasminogen activator (TPA) causes plasmin induced fibrinolysis to arrest and dissolve intravascular fibrin formation. Thrombolytic therapy depletes factors V, VIII:C, IX, X, and fibrinogen for 12-24 hours.

Physical Examination

Obvious physical signs of hemostatic defects include petechiae; ecchymoses; hematomas; hemarthroses; bruises; splenomegaly;

Table I
Drugs Inhibiting Platelet Function

(1) Antiinflammatory drugs	
	Aspirin
	Ibuprofen,qlIndomethacin
	Mefenamic acid
	Naproxen
	Phenylbutazone
	Sulfinpyrazone
(2) Cardiovascular drugs	
	Adenosine
	Diltiazem
	Dipyridamole
	Hydralazine
	Nitroglycerin
	Papaverine
	Propranolol
	Sodium nitroprusside
	Verapamil
(3) Antibiotics	
	Carbenicillin
	Nafcillin
	Penicillin G
	Ticarcillin
(4) Miscellaneous Drugs	
	Aminophylline
	Theophylline
	Halothane
	Local anesthetics
	Diazepam
	Chlorpromazine

and hepatomegaly. Careful examination of the skin, mucous membranes, nailbeds, and sublingual areas may reveal evidence of thrombocytopenia or platelet dysfunction. Any signs of hereditary and acquired connective disorders that are associated with platelet dysfunction must be sought.

Preoperative Laboratory Studies

In many institutions, a satisfactory and economical laboratory work-up for patients without positive history, physical, or drug ingestion, are limited to a platelets count, prothrombin time (PT), and an activated partial thromboplastin time (aPTT).[8] However, because the majority of bleeding episodes postcardiac surgery are due to platelet dysfunction, other institutions include a more thorough presurgical hemostatic screen (Table II). Patients who are taking platelet inhibiting medication should have a template bleeding time (TBT). Any positive history and/or physical findings of hemostatic defects may require any combinations of the following tests: thrombin time (TT); fibrinogen level; qualitative platelet screen; coagulation factors, and cryoglobulins for hypothermic CPB.

Cardiopulmonary Bypass

The mechanical and surgical aspects of the cardiopulmonary bypass (CPB) circuit are discussed elsewhere in this book. However, this section will discuss the physiology and the specific effects of the CPB circuit as it affects the coagulation system.

Different heparin anticoagulation and its neutralization with protamine is used following different institutional protocols. Unless there is preexisting anemia, most adult extracorporeal circuits are primed with 500-2000 mL of crystalloids and colloids. This hemodilution will cause an immediate reduction, approximately 30%, in red blood cells, platelets, and coagulation factors. The CPB circuit and blood oxygenator:blood element interface stimulates what has been described as a "whole blood inflammatory response" involving the coagulation, the complement, and the kallikrein/kinin systems.[9] Intraoperative blood loss is scavenged and trauma-

Table II
Presurgical Hemostasis Screen

Platelet count or blood smear
Prothrombin time
Activated partial thromboplastin time
Template bleeding time
Thrombin time
Cryogloblins

tized by cardiotomy suction of varying degree. Different degrees of hypothermia are utilized. The above variations in individual and institutional protocols contribute to different results regarding the etiology and incidence of postoperative bleeding. The same factors make comparative analysis of post-CPB bleeding extremely difficult. This section will describe the basic physiologic alterations of hemostatic function during CPB and review the experiences of different institutions.

Thrombocytopenia

Platelets initiate the process of clot formation by (1) adhesion to disrupted vascular endothelium; (2) aggregation to form a platelet plug; (3) secretion of pro-coagulating cofactors to facilitate coagulation cascades; and (4) inducing vasoconstriction. Proper platelet activity requires the presence of an adequate number of functional platelets.

A consistent finding of CPB is a reduction in the platelet count. Depending on the preoperative platelet count, decrease of 25%-60% from the baseline occurs. Dilution at the inititation of CPB will decrease the platelet count by approximately one third because prime solutions consisting of crystalloids, colloids, and blood do not contain platelets.[10] Mammen et al.[11] have shown that dilution accounts for 80%-90% of the decrease in the platelet count during CPB. The oxygenator, venous reservoir, the extracorporeal circuit, arterial line filters, and surgical wounds are all sources of platelet retention and fragmentation.[1]

There appears to be significant sequestration of platelets in solid organs, especially in the liver, within few minutes of inititation of CPB,[12] with increased platelet turnover and mobilization of platelet reserves in the spleen and marrow. In animals, hypothermia causes platelet sequestration in the liver that reverses with rewarming.[1] Transient thrombocytopenia due to sequestration occurs below 25°C[13] with in vitro platelet aggregation abolished below 33°C.[14] The shear stress of the cardiotomy suction and exposure of blood:air and blood:tissue interfaces causes both destruction and activation of the platelets. The volume and percentage of blood aspirated by cardiotomy suction correlate directly with platelet loss.[15,16]

There is controversy regarding effects of bubble oxygenators versus membrane oxygenators on platelet count. Initially, there is less thrombocytopenia with bubble oxygenators because there is less foreign surface. However, there is continued decrease in the platelet count with bubble oxygenators, while the platelet count is stable with membrane oxygenators. Membrane oxygenators are associated with: (1) less trauma to blood cells; (2) less thrombocytopenia; (3) less release of platelet release product β-thromboglobulin;[17] (4) less sequestration of platelets;[12,18] (5) reduced particulate microembolization; and (6) preservation of platelet function.[19] However, with bypass times less than 2 hours, the difference in bleeding between bubble oxygenators and membrane oxygenators may be insignificant.[17,20] Intravenous protamine reduces platelet count by one third within minutes. This effect lasts for less than 1 hour, probably from transient sequestration in the liver.[21]

Platelet Dysfunction

The interaction of blood and foreign surfaces is complex. Within seconds of contact, plasma proteins adhere to the surfaces, followed by cellular elements within minutes.[22] Fibrinogen has strong affinity to foreign surfaces and the bound fibrinogen in turn stimulates platelet adhesion via the platelet fibrinogen receptors with resultant loss of platelet membrane glycoprotein IIb/IIIa fibrinogen receptors.[23] Albumin coated surfaces reduce the binding sites of fibrinogen, reduce platelet granule release, and preserve functional and morphologic integrity of platelets.[24]

The stimulation of platelets occurs shortly after the initiation of CPB, possibly by release of adenosine diphosphate (ADP) from hemolyzed red cells or release of human neutrophil elastase by activation of the contact pathway[25] and a variety of humoral factors.[26] After few minutes of CPB, there is no further platelet adhesion, because fibrinogen is covered by platelet fragments, undergoes conformational change,[23] by activation of the foreign surface.[27] Activation of platelets causes a discoid to a spherical morphologic "platelet shape change".[28] With further stimulation, "primary" platelet aggregates form, which release PF4, B-TG, fibrinogen, and other substances from α granules.[29] Primary aggregation appears to be responsible for the decrease in circulating platelets during the first few minutes of CPB as there is no release of products in either bubble or membrane oxygenators.[27]

After initial activation, there is recovery of platelet morphology and function during CPB. However, prolonged bubble oxygenator CPB leads to further platelet dysfunction.[29] With strong or continued stimulation, these reversible "primary" aggregates transform into an irreversible "secondary" aggregates that secrete thromboxanes from dense granules. Once platelets are activated with loss of surface proteins and/or granules, platelets are not able to function normally. There is a spectrum of platelet activation. The minority of platelets are fully activated, but the majority of platelets circulate with reduced function. Karpatkin[30] reported a marked decrease in larger, younger, and more adherent platelets after CBP.

During the first few hours post-CPB, there is recovery of platelet function and volume, indicating entry of young, larger platelets into the circulation.[31] Recovery of platelet function and normalization of bleeding times occur when there is adequate replacement or recovery of platelet morphology.

Platelet aggregation induced by pulmonary artery catheters, heparin,[32] protamine,[33] and heparin/protamine complex[34] may also cause thrombocytopenia and/or platelet dysfunction. As a rise in intracellular calcium may be the final common pathway mediating platelet granule secretion, a low ionized calcium level may decrease platelet responsiveness to triggering stimuli.[35]

Coagulation Factors

A consistent reduction in the levels of coagulation factors, fibrinogen, plasminogen, and antithrombin III (AT-III) occurs during CPB. The primary cause of the reduction is thought to be dilutional, because the decline (approximately 30%-40%) parallels the decrease in the hematocrit.[11] For unknown reasons, factor V levels decrease more than others. Variations in the reported decrease in coagulation factor levels may be due to differences in priming solutions, flow rates, and pumping techniques.[20] Levels remained low during CPB, although a slight increase was noted for most parameters towards the end of CPB.[11] All levels returned to normal within 48 hours.

Fibrinolysis

Primary fibrinolysis involves the primary activation of circulating plasminogen to plasmin, with resultant increase in plasmin induced lysis of fibrinogen to fibrin (Fig. 2). The lysis of fibrinogen and fibrin generates fibrin degradation products (FDP). The fibrinolytic system alters hemostasis by conversion of plasminogen to plasmin, plasminogen depletion, and subsequent fibrinolytic degradation of fibrinogen and factors V, VIII, and IX.[36]. The resultant degradation products interfere with thrombin activity, fibrin monomer polymerization, and platelet function.[2] Secondary fibrinolysis is the activation of the fibrinolytic system secondary to activation of the coagulation system.

Pathogenesis of fibrinolytic activation during CPB remains unclear. It is also unclear whether adequate heparinization alone can completely suppress fibrin formation on foreign extracorporeal surfaces. Primary fibrinolysis may be stimulated by release of thromboplastic tissue substances into the circulation from disruption of vascular endothelium rich in plasminogen activator substances, ischemia, interface of blood with ECC, physiologic alter-

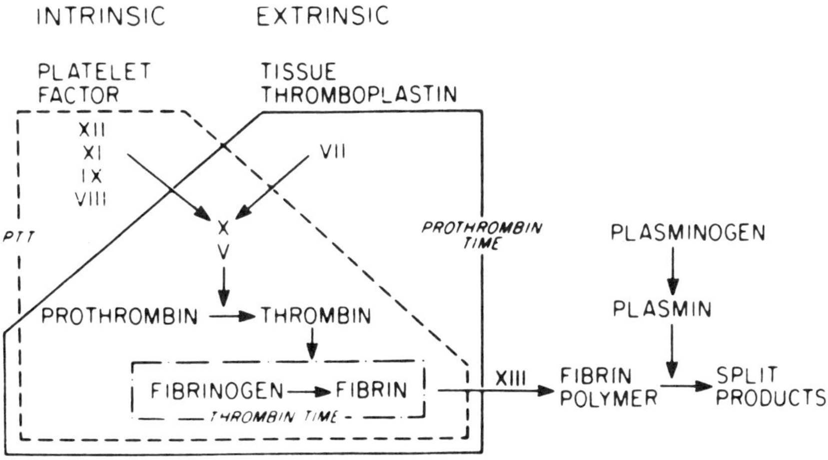

Figure 2. Fibrinolytic system and the effects of plasmin and fibrinogen degradation products on hemostasis.

ations associated with CPB, prekallikrein activation by synthetic surfaces, and hypothermia. Tanaka et al.[37] have suggested that the activation of the intrinsic fibrinolytic system is mainly limited to the beginning of CPB, while enhanced fibrinolytic activity during CPB is predominantly of extrinsic origin by the release of TPA from vascular endothelium. Whatever the exact mechanism, there is an imbalance between the ability to form clots and the strength of the lytic process.

The incidence of primary fibrinolysis during CPB varies from 0%-85% depending on the testing technique. Bick et al.[20,38] found the presence of FDP in all patients with appearance of active plasmin and depletion of fibrinogen and plasmin in 46% of the patients. Conversion of factor XII to XIIa, which activates the intrinsic fibrinolytic system by converting plasminogen to plasmin, was noted in 70% of the patients.

There is controversy regarding incidence and significance of fibrinolysis during CPB. Different assays used to quantitate fibrinolysis may be responsible for the variation.[39] The clinical and laboratory manifestations of systemic hyperfibrinolysis result from the ability of plasmin to degrade established fibrin clots, fibrinogen, and factors V and VIII:C.

Disseminated Intravascular Coagulation

Disseminated intravascular coagulation (DIC) occurs when there is activation of the coagulation system through intrinsic or extrinsic pathways. There is uncontrolled systemic fibrin deposition and coagulation with simultaneous fibrinolysis by intrinsic or extrinsic plasminogen activators. A combination of intravascular thrombosis, with consumption of platelets, fibrin, and coagulation factors, and liberation of fibrin split products occurs with resultant coagulopathy.

As CPB causes depletion of coagulation factors, thrombocytopenia, and elevation of fibrin split products, many early investigators concluded that DIC occurred during CPB.[40,41] These changes that were thought to be reflective of DIC during CPB, may have been based on isolated measurements reflecting fibrinolysis. Decreased AT-III levels, which are indicative of acute or chronic DIC, have been shown in only one study.[42] There appears to be less chance of low grade coagulation and secondary fibrinolysis with wide acceptance of heparin titration during CPB in the 1970s.[11]

The incidence of DIC during CPB appear to be low.[20] Disseminated intravascular coagulation is unlikely to occur with massive heparinization as evidenced by the absence of significant thrombocytopenia, rapid correction of hypofibrinogenemia and hypoplasminogenemia post-CPB, and lack of massive thrombosis after protamine administration. In Bick's experience, only two of several thousand patients have had DIC in association with CPB. Both patients developed DIC pre-CPB, one from cardiac arrest and the other from sepsis. Protamine administration in these patients caused massive vascular thrombosis.

Diagnosis of Postcardiopulmonary Bypass Bleeding: Incidence, Criteria, Classification

The incidence of post-CPB bleeding is variable due to different institutional protocols in the type of CPB circuit, priming solutions, type of oxygenators, intraoperative blood scavenging techniques, use of hypothermia, the duration of CPB, and the definition of excessive bleeding. The Kirklin criteria is a frequently used guideline for excessive bleeding and reoperation.[43]

Diagnosis of excessive bleeding post-CPB is made after protamine reversal of heparin anticoagulation and inspection of the surgical field. Alterations in the coagulation system due to CPB do not predict excessive post-CPB bleeding. As different institutions may have different protocols resulting in varying defects, no one specific approach is best for all institutions.

The causes of postoperative bleeding are loosely divided into "surgical" and "nonsurgical" bleeding. The distinction is often blurred as hemostatic defect in one patient may cause bleeding while not in others. Bleeding at specific sites such as anastomotic sites, cannulation sites, or bleeding vessels is controlled by surgical technique. In various studies, the incidence of such "surgical" bleeding was 33 to 62%.[1] "Nonsurgical" bleeding is manifested as continued, generalized bleeding from multiple sites, such as the intravenous sites, skin edges, sternum, mammary and saphenous harvest beds, without significant clot in the surgical field.

The treatment of post-CPB bleeding places significant demands on blood bank resources. In the 1970s, the average case utilized 6 U/case, with tranfusion of 10 U of blood products being not uncommon.[1] However, with improvements in surgical technique, extracorporeal technology, blood scavenging systems, as well as acceptance of hemodilution and lower hematocrits, a significant number of patients (greater than 30%) receive no blood products in certain centers.[44]

Activated Clotting Time

After administration of protamine, an anticoagulation test (ACT) is performed. The ACT should be ± 10% of the control, when adequate heparin neutralization is achieved. While an elevated ACT may indicate inadequate heparin reversal, a normal ACT does not ensure complete heparin neutralization.[45] Although ACT may be affected by many factors, including severe depletion of intrinsic coagulation factors and severe thrombocytopenia due to insufficient platelet factor III, platelet dysfunction will not elevate ACT. The ACT is relatively insensitive to low heparin levels.

If the ACT remains elevated after initial protamine administration, an additional incremental dose of protamine is given. If there is no improvement in the ACT following additional administration of protamine, then the question of excess protamine, marked platelet abnormalities, fibrinolysis, or coagulation factor deficiency, must be addressed.

Heparin Concentration Assays

Due to the limitations of the ACT, direct measurement of circulating heparin has been developed. Heparin concentration may be measured either by titration methods (protamine or polybrene) or by chromogenic assays. The titration method is by far more commonly available and detects the formation of a clot as its end point. The results are available in 2 minutes unless there is severe anticoagulation. The titration method for heparin level is exceedingly accurate. Teien and Lie[46] have shown that only the polybrene titration method gives accurate results at heparin concentration of 0.05 U/mL plasma compared to four other tests including aPTT and calcium thrombin time. The chromogenic substrate assay of heparin may be performed as an assay of heparin activity or heparin concentration with AT-III added. The assay had a correlation coefficient of 0.85 when the patients had AT-III level greater than 1.00 U/mL versus a correlation coefficient of only 0.36 for patients with AT-III level less than 0.5 U/mL.[47]

However, heparin concentration assays are not functional tests of heparin activity and therefore may not reflect the adequacy of anticoagulation during CPB.[48,49] Their primary use is as a guide in determining protamine dosage and to diagnose unneutralized circulating heparin post-CPB.

Laboratory Tests

A complete laboratory coagulation profile should be performed for excessive post-CPB bleeding (Table III). Tests include: PT, aPTT, complete blood count (CBC) with platelet count, examination of the peripheral smear, fibrinogen and fibrinogen split products, thrombin or reptilase time, and plasmin(ogen) levels.

Adequate protamine reversal of heparin can be assessed by measuring heparin concentration. An increased thrombin time is

Table III
Laboratory Evaluation of Cardiopulmonary Bypass Hemorrhage

Complete blood and platelet count
Blood smear evaluation
Prothrombin time
Activated partial thromboplastin time
Febrin split products tites
Heparin assay (synthetic substrate)
Thrombin time (observe for lysis)
Plasminogen and plasmin assay

also seen with residual heparin. Platelet count and peripheral smear will reveal thrombocytopenia. Prolonged PT or aPTT may indicate a deficiency in the coagulation factors. The clot from reptilase or thrombin time is observed for 5 minutes for evidence of lysis, which along with fibrinogen level and fibrinogen degradation products, will reveal the presence of hyperfibrinolysis. The absence of significant clot lysis without significant elevation in fibrin split products is strong evidence against primary fibrinolysis. Euglobin lysis time is a measure of clot lysis in the euglobin fraction of plasma that contains fibrinogen, plasminogen, and plasminogen activator. Increase in plasminogen activator levels will shorten euglobin lysis time (normal < 80 minutes). Template bleeding time (normal 1-8 minutes) is technically difficult to perform intraoperatively and is probably underutilized postoperatively. The bleeding time is more predictive of postoperative bleeding than platelet count. However, the test is subject to wide variations and lacks correlation with clinically significant bleeding. The utility of tests for platelet aggregation and function is limited by the time required for results.

Laboratory tests of coagulation measure specific coagulation parameters. With hemostatic alterations from CPB, dilution, and platelet dysfunction, the tests results are difficult to interpret. Several studies have demonstrated poor predictability of bleeding by laboratory test. Oh et al.[50] showed prolonged PT and aPTT in pediatric cardiac patients without excessive bleeding. Bachmann et al.[2] have shown an 80% prolongation of PT, even though extrinsic coagulation factors were 70%-80% of normal value, with only 4% clinically significant bleeding,[2] while Tuman et al.[51] have shown only 33% overall accuracy by routine coagulation tests consisting of ACT, platelet count, PT, and aPTT in predicting postoperative hemorrhage. Therefore, an abnormal laboratory test in patients with adequate hemostasis is not an indication for therapy. Despite limitations of laboratory coagulation tests post-CPB, they may serve as a guide to therapy.

Thromboelastography

First introduced in 1948 by Hartert,[52] thromboelastography (TEG) has recently gained recent interest as an intraoperative coagulation monitor for liver transplantation[53] and cardiac surgery.[54] Thromboelastography is a qualitative viscoelastic measure of clot formation from initial procoagulant activation and fibrin formation through fibrin cross linking and clot retraction to eventual clot lysis over time. The test requires 0.35 mL of blood pipetted into a continuously rotating stainless steel crucible maintained at 37°C. A polished metal piston is suspended by a torsion wire 1 mm from the inner wall of the crucible. Fibrin strands form between the piston and the wall of the crucible, and as the clot matures, the rotational motion of the piston is electronically amplified to create the characteristic TEG tracing (Fig. 3).

Characteristic tracings and parameters can be measured. The R value (reaction time: normal 7.5-15 minutes) is the time of blood

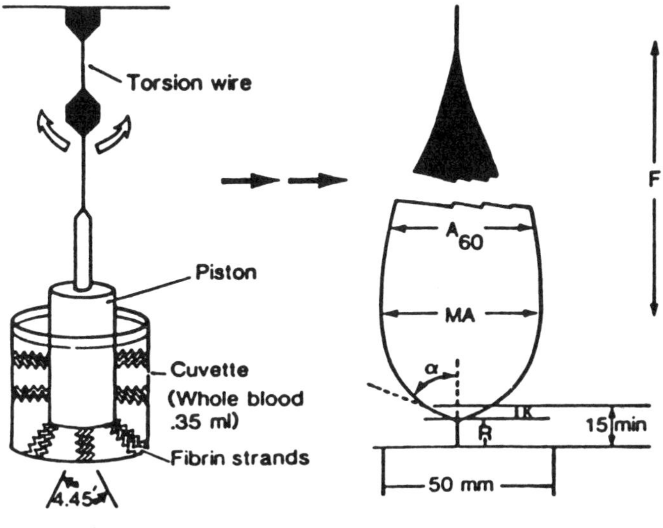

Figure 3. Generation of normal thromboelastogram. R: reaction time. Time from blood placement to 1-mm amplitude, measures the time to initial fibrin formation. K: time from R to amplitude of 20 mm. α Value: Angle of upslope of tracing from R value. Both K and α measures speed of clot formation, fibrin cross-linking, and platelet fibrin interaction. MA: Maximun amplitude represents the maximum clot strenth. A60: Amplitude of tracing 60 minutes after MA, Ratio of A60:MA, and F value: Time from MA to 0 amplitude all represents clot retraction or lysis.

placement to 1-mm amplitude and represents time required for initial fibrin formation. Its prolongation may be due to coagulation factor deficiencies, heparin, or severe hypofibrinogenemia. The K value (coagulation time: normal value 3-6 minutes) is the time from R value until the amplitude of the TEG is 20 mm. The α value (α angle: normal 45-50°) is the angle formed by the upslope of the TEG tracing from the R value. Both K and α values represent the speed of clot formation, fibrin cross-linking, and platelet-fibrin interaction. Thrombocytopenia or hypofibrinogenemia may decrease K and α values (Fig. 4). Maximum amplitude (MA) (MA: normal 50-60 mm) represents maximum clot strength, and depends on platelet number and function, as well as fibrinogen levels. The MA value may be very small with DIC, primary fibrinolysis, and uremia (Fig. 4). A60 (normal value MA: 5mm) is the amplitude of the tracing 60 minutes after MA. Ratio of A60:MA (normal value > 0.85) and the F value (time from MA until 0 amplitude: normal

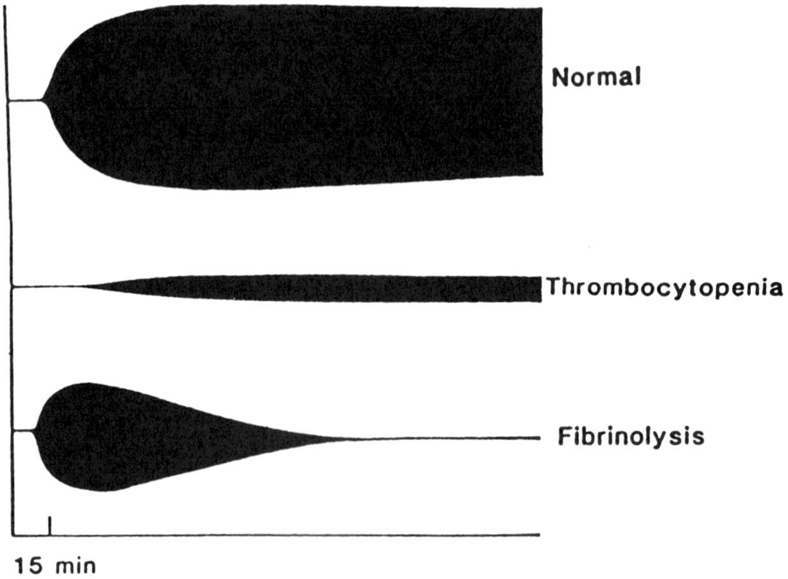

Figure 4. TEG tracings obtained from (top) normal patient; (middle) patient with thrombocytopenia; (bottom) patient with primary fibrinolysis.

value > 300 minutes) along with A60 is a measure of clot retraction or lysis.

Tuman[51] and Speiss[54] have shown TEG monitoring for clinical hemostasis post-CPB to be 80%-100% accurate in predicting postoperative bleeding and found the TEG to be more sensitive and specific than ACT or coagulation profile. Thromboelastography showed 88% overall accuracy with 0% false negative and 15% false-positive, as compared to only 33% overall accuracy with 44% false-negative and 73% false-positive rates for routine coagulation testing consisting of ACT, platelet count, PT, PTT, and fibrinogen. Thromboelastography offers other important advantages compared to the routine coagulation tests, as it is: (1) economical, using a simple reusable machine; (2) easy to use; (3) available in the operating room and allows intraoperative monitoring of coagulation; (4) highly predictive of post surgical bleeding; (5) able to assess heparinization and platelet-protein interaction; (6) able to easily diagnose fibrinolysis, DIC, and hypercoagulable states; (7) allows assessment of coagulation factor, fibrinogen, platelet activity, as well as clot maturation and lysis, all from a single blood sample.

The main disadvantage TEG is the time required to obtain a complete analysis. Initial evaluation of fibrin formation is available within 12-25 minutes given normal R and K values. Platelet function may be assessed from the amplitude of the tracing in another 20 minutes. Evaluation of clot lysis for fibrinolysis requires a variable amount of time.

Thromboelastography data have shown to be loosely correlated with various coagulation tests. Lack of significant correlation exists because while coagulation tests examine isolated coagulation factors, the TEG examines whole blood coagulation, interaction of the protein coagulation cascade, fibrinogen, and platelet surface. However, there are specific changes in the TEG associated with cardiac surgery (Fig. 4). Full heparinization and afibrinogenemia will result in a straight line tracing with infinite value for R and K, with MA value being 0. Near complete heparinization or extremely severe platelet deficiency will result in markedly prolonged R and K values, with MA less than 20 mm. Thrombocytopenia or platelet dysfunction will result in a diminished MA (< 50 mm) with a normal A60:MA value. With severe platelet deficiency, there may be prolonged R and K values, along with markedly diminished MA value. Factor deficiency or moderate anticoagulation therapy will result in prolongation of the R value, and possibly prolongation of the K value, with normal MA and A60 values. Primary fibrinolysis will present nearly normal R and K values, with diminished MA value, and markedly diminished A60:MA value. Secondary fibrinolysis is contrasted by markedly prolonged R and K values, as well as severely diminished MA and A60:MA ratios. Hypercoagulable states can be determined perioperatively by decreased R and K values with increased α and MA values. This may be seen with patients with deep vein thrombosis (DVT) or excessive tranfusion of platelets or coagulation factors.

An exceedingly important advantage of TEG is the ability to test therapeutic interventions in vitro prior to the administration of drugs or blood products. For example, the differentiation of DIC versus fibrinolysis is often difficult as both will yield consumption of protein factors and fibrinogen with production of fibrin degradation products. Small increments of ϵ-aminocaproic acid (EACA) may be added and the TEG repeated. Improvement of the TEG tracing will confirm the diagnosis of fibrinolysis and antifibrinolytic agents may be administered safely. A similar method can be used for protamine titration of unneutralized heparin and deficiencies in platelets and coagulation factors. Thromboelastography guided therapy reduced blood product transfusion by 33% in patients undergoing liver transplantation.[53] For patients on urokinase or streptokinase, TEG may be used to monitor and guide thrombolytic therapy.[55]

Sonoclot

In 1975, von Kaulla[56] described a device that utilizes changes in impedance to assess coagulation. The sonoclot uses 0.4 mL of whole blood or plasma with a vertical plastic vibrating (approximately 200 Hz) probe immersed in a fixed depth. The increasing impedance to the vibration by formed fibrin strands is detected by an electronic circuit that converts it into a output signal proportional to the fluid's viscoelasticity. A typical "signature" tracing consists of the clotting, clot retraction, and clot lysis process (Fig. 5).

The onset time, T1 (normal 3.5 minutes), reflects the inititation of fibrin formation. The primary slope, R1 (normal 2.3 ± 0.5 cm/

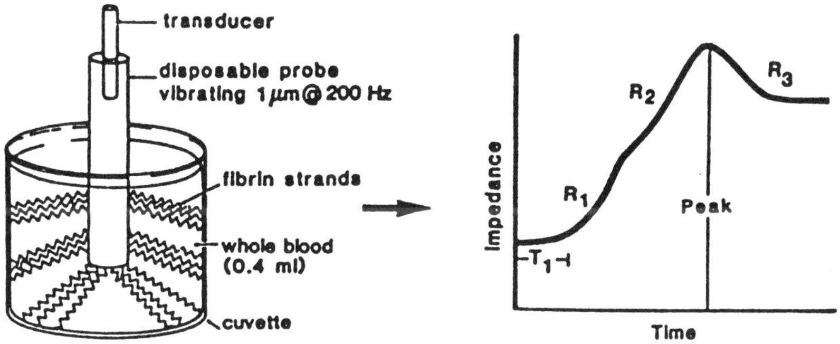

Figure 5. Generation of sonoclot analysis of viscoeleasticity. T1: initiation of fibrin formation. R_1: "primary" slope. Further fibrin formatin and the rate of clot formation. R_2: "secondary" slope Fibrinogenesis and platelet-fibrin interaction. R_3: downward slope. Platelet-induced contraction of completed clot. Peak: maximum fibrin formation and impedance.

min), reflects further fibrin formation and the rate of clot formation. The secondary slope, R2 (normal 3.5 ± 0.6 cm/min), represents further fibrinogenesis and platelet-fibrin interaction. In between R1 and R2, there is often an inflection point that represents the point at which the platelets begin to contract the fibrin strands. PEAK is the peak impedance at which there is maximum fibrin formation. The downward slope, R3, is produced as platelets induce contraction of the completed clot.

Sonoclot tracing is dependent on the number and function of platelets. As platelet number increases, the lag time and the shoulder-peak interval decreases, while the slope of R1 and R2 increases. R2 first appears with platelet count of 30,000, while R3 appears at platelet count of 60,000. Saleem et al.[57] has demonstrated greater effectiveness of the sonoclot in assessment of excessive bleeding post-CPB compared to template bleeding time or platelet aggregation tests.

While the sonoclot tracing is used primarily to assess functional integrity of platelets, it also may be used to aid in the diagnosis of other coagulation deficits. Correlation to specific coagulation tests has not been demonstrated. Sonoclot tracing can detect the presence of heparin, and with celite activation, can monitor heparin therapy. Clot lysis may be determined by measuring the final impedance as a function of time (i.e., severe fibrinolysis results in a final impedance similiar to the impedance at the onset of clot formation). Peck[58] has shown that the soncolot and thrombin generation time (TGT) are practical, rapid and useful tests for the detection and monitoring of hypercoagulable states.

Management and Therapy for Postcardiopulmonary Bleeding: Guidelines and Supportive Therapy

Cardiopulmonary bypass creates tremendous alterations in the coagulation system. After successful hemodynamic separation from CPB, heparin is neutralized and surgical bleeding controlled. The surgical field should be inspected to assess adequate hemostasis. If there is continuous "nonsurgical" bleeding, the cause of coagulopathy is investigated.

Due to the lack of timely and specific laboratory tests, the "shot gun" empirical transfusion of platelets, fresh frozen plasma, and cryoprecipitate is often used. However, this nearsighted approach is to be discouraged, as it places an unnecessary burden on the blood supply and increases the long-term complications of transfusions. Empiric therapy may be required for hemodynamic stability, to control hemorrhage, and to prevent further dilution of coagulation factors. Furthermore, circulatory insufficiency and resultant shock may even cause DIC. Transfusion of platelets is reasonable empiric therapy, as platelet dysfunction appears to be the primary cause of post-CPB bleeding.

During assessment of coagulopathy, factors such as hypothermia and hypertension should be avoided and treated as these factors may increase postoperative bleeding. The institution of positive end-expiratory pressure may tamponade mediastinal oozing. With supportive therapy, the bleeding, if not severe, will often resolve spontaneously with a "tincture of time". If there is persistent bleeding despite normal coagulation profile, immediate reexploration should be performed.

Heparin Rebound

Heparin rebound is the reappearance of free heparin after complete protamine neutralization. The proposed etiologies include: the longer elimination time of heparin compared to protamine, greater body stores of heparin, incomplete rewarming with delayed heparin release from the tissues, exogenous heparin (heparin flush solutions and pump blood), and reentry of free heparin into the circulation via the lymphatics system.[59]

Heparin rebound is reported to occur in 0-100% of patients post-CPB.[60] Most cases of heparin rebound have been reported to occur within 8-9 hours after initial heparin neutralization, but delayed heparin rebound has been reported as late as 18 hours postoperatively.[61] Ellison et al.[60] demonstrated heparin rebound in all patients who received lower doses (0.56 mg protamine per 1 mg total heparin administered) of protamine.[60] Others have reported a much lower incidence of heparin rebound (4.5%) without clinical significance.[62]

Administration of excess protamine at the time of initial heparin neutralization will not prevent heparin rebound and may actually increase bleeding due to the detrimental effects of protamine on platelet function. Zaidan et al.[63] have demonstrated that a slow (> 30 minutes) administration of protamine reduced the initial incidence of early (< 2 hours) heparin rebound.[63] Interestingly, the chloride salt of protamine has been suggested to cause less heparin rebound than the commercially available and more rapidly metabolized sulfate preparation.[64]

Whatever its cause, incidence, or clinical significance, heparin rebound is easily treated by administration of additional protamine in 25-50 mg increments. Indeed, any diagnostic work-up or treatment of post-CPB bleeding should be initiated after elimination of heparin rebound.

Platelets

As discussed in the section on CPB effects on coagulation, the primary hemostatic derangement associated with CPB is platelet dysfunction.[1,2,20,29] The assessment of post-CPB bleeding after documented neutralization of heparin with protamine essentially deals with the adequacy of platelet function. Routine prophylactic platelet transfusion is unjustified due to the risks of transfusion and the documented inefficiency of prophylactic platelet administration.[65]

Simon et al.[66] demonstrated no differences in blood loss, transfusion requirement, or clinical outcome in patients who were given 4 U of platelets prophylactically after protamine administration. Furthermore, thrombocytopenia (platelet count 58,000/mL) and transient platelet dysfunction do not require platelet transfusion in coronary artery bypass surgery and uncomplicated valvular surgery as there is recovery of platelets in number and function post-CPB. In the absence of bleeding, prophylactic transfusion of platelets should be reserved for platelet counts of < 60,000. Because a single unit of platelets will raise the platelet count by 5-10,000, administration of 4-8 U should raise the platelet count to adequate levels.

In cases of bleeding post-CPB, there may be platelet dysfunction despite adequate platelet count[29] and many have advocated transfusion of platelets regardless of platelet count or documentation of abnormal coagulation tests.[20] If there is bleeding with abnormal template bleeding time, TEG, or sonoclot platelets should be transfused. Any transfusion therapy should be monitored to minimize the amount of transfusion. As platelet concentrates contain 40-60 mL of plasma per unit, there is also replenishment of active coagulation factors.[67] Another indication for platelet transfusion is the presence DIC.

Fresh Whole Blood

Fresh whole blood administration is gaining popularity to decrease blood loss post-CPB. Mohr et al.[68] compared the hemostatic effects of tranfusion of 1 U of fresh whole blood and 10 U of platelets. Whole blood group showed an increase in the platelet count equal to 4 U of platelets with normalization of bleeding time. Furthermore, postoperative platelet aggregation to collagen and epinephrine improved after whole blood, but not with platelet concentrates. The 24-hour blood loss was lower in the whole blood group. A recent study in children undergoing open heart surgery showed a significant decrease in postoperative blood loss in patients receiving fresh whole blood.[69] The benefit appears greatest for children less than 2 years of age who have had complex surgery. The difference in blood loss is most probably due to better platelet function in fresh whole blood.

Pharmacologic Platelet Therapy

Because the major effect of CPB on hemostatic function is platelet dysfunction, pharmacological preservation of platelet function have been studied. Iloprost, a potent synthetic analog of prostacyclin, has been used successfully to prevent platelet activation for patients with heparin-induced thrombocytopenia undergoing CPB cardiac surgery.[70] Due to the hypotensive side effects, the routine use of prostacylin is probably unjustified[1]

Desmopressin Acetate

1-Deamino-8-D-arginine vasopressin (DDAVP), a synthetic analog of antidiuretic hormone L-arginine vasopressin, induces release of increase factor VIII:C and von Willebrand's factor (vWF), a large polymeric glycoprotein required for normal platelet adhesion and normal bleeding time. Release from endothelial cells appears to be the major source of vWF, which serves as a bridge for adhesion of platelets to the subendothelium or between platelets.[71] However, DDAVP does not affect platelet count nor platelet aggregation.[72]

Desmopressin may be administered intravenously, intranasally, or subcutaneously. Intravenously, there is an almost immediate release of factor VIII:C and vWF levels that persists for 6 hours. The maximal effect is seen with doses of 0.3-0.4 μg/kg.[73] In both volunteers and hemophiliacs, DDAVP shortens the PTT, even if not prolonged, but does not shorten the PT.[74]

Side effects of DDAVP appear to be minor:[75] transient mild vasodilation, 10%-20% decrease in systolic blood pressure with facial flushing are the most frequent side effect and there appears to be less incidence with slow ($>$ 15 minute) administration. Tachyphylaxis with therapy every 12-24 hours for several days in some patients seems to validate the mechanism of DDAVP release from stored factors. Although DDAVP has potent antidiuretic effect, there have been no reports of its clinical significance. Unlike other natural antidiuretic hormones, DDAVP has very little effect on the V-1 vasopressin receptors on smooth muscle and thus does not produce vasoconstriction or contraction of visceral smooth muscles.[76]

1-Deamino-8-D-arginine vasopressin has been shown to shorten bleeding times in certain forms of hemophilia, von Willebrand's disease, uremia, and other conditions, as well as improving hemostasis in conditions with no known abnormality of factor VIII:C or vWF.[77] Kobrinsky,[77,78] in a series of studies on the effects of DDAVP in surgical patients, demonstrated that DDAVP reverses aspirin-induced prolongation of bleeding time in normal subjects and decreases surgical blood loss during spinal-fusion surgery, even in subjects who were hemostatically competent preoperatively.

In cardiac surgery, Salzman et al.[79] used DDAVP 0.3 μg/kg intravenously post-CPB in 70 patients undergoing various cardiac surgery, excluding routine coronary bypass surgery, and found decreased perioperative blood loss, 1,317 $\pm$ 486 mL compared to 2,210 $\pm$ 1,415 mL in the control group. An unexpected finding of their study was the correlation of preoperative plasma vWF levels with subsequent blood loss. Czer et al.[80] found a decrease in bleeding time from 17 minutes to 12.5 minutes with administration of 20 μg of DDAVP and decreased blood product usage in the treatment group.

Despite enthusiasm generated after initial studies, further studies have questioned the value of DDAVP in cardiac surgery. Brown et al.[81] have demonstrated no difference in perioperative bleeding or transfusion requirement in a study of 20 patients undergoing routine coronary artery bypass. Furthermore, 4 of the 10 patients in the DDAVP group experienced hypotension with administration of the drug. In view of the side effect and the cost of DDAVP administration, they concluded that the prophylactic administration of DDAVP in routine coronary artery bypass surgery is unwarranted. Further studies are required to elucidate those who will benefit from DDAVP therapy. At this time, the only indication for DDAVP in cardiac surgery is efficiency of factor VIII:vWF.

Dipyridamole

Dipyridamole, a pyridopyrimidine compound, inhibits platelet phosphodiesterase activity, increases platelet cyclic adenosine monophosphate concentrations, and decreases calcium mobilization.[82] Clinically, dipyridamole has been used to inhibit venous thrombosis, and improve myocardial and cerebral blood flow. Platelet inhibiting agents may preserve platelet counts during CPB by preventing platelet aggregation on foreign surfaces and at sites of endothelial injury. Although dipyridamole limits platelet activation, aggregation, and granular release, it preserves platelet adhesion and therefore does not inhibit platelet hemostatic functions unlike other antiplatelet agents such as aspirin that may increase postoperative bleeding.[83]

Nuutinen and Mononen[84] found a significantly higher platelet count (129,000 versus 82,0000) post-CPB in the group treated with 40-80 mg of intravenous dipyridamole during CPB without increased postoperative bleeding.[84] Teoh et al.[85] found preservation in platelet count with decreased postoperative bleeding (42%-46%) in patients treated with dipyridamole during CPB. Intravenous administration resulted in higher platelet count and less blood loss than the oral administration. Additional benefit of perioperative dipyridamole is improved early bypass graft patency.[86] A side effect of dipyridamole is a 20%-25% decrease in blood pressure due to vasodilation upon rapid intravenous administration,[87,88] which may be minimized by slow administration over 10 minutes.

Aprotinin

The complement system may be activated by the blood:foreign surface interaction through the Hageman factor or via the alternative pathway by C3b binding on the surface of extracorporeal circuit.[87] The activation of the fibrinolytic and the complement systems may also affect platelets and leukocytes.

Aprotinin is a proteolytic enzyme known to inhibit plasmin and kallikrein. van Oeveren et al.[26] studied the effects of high-dose (plasma concentration > 150 kallikrein inactivator U/mL) aprotinin during CPB in 11 patients and found preservation of platelet number, decreased platelet release product thromboxane B2, and significantly less postoperative bleeding. As aprotinin was not successful in preventing complement activation, plasmin appears to play an important role in the prevention of platelet impairment. Plasmin may remove the bound fibrinogen from the platelets, thereby decreasing the postoperative platelet function.

Platelets were protected by aprotinin, probably at the molecular level, during CPB against pathologic stimuli, but functioned normally on a physiological basis postoperatively. Royston et al.[89] found an eightfold reduction in postoperative blood tranfusion requirement for patients undergoing repeat cardiac surgery with a similiar high-dose aprotinin therapy. The benefits of aprotinin on platelet function occur only when aprotinin is given pre-CPB.

Coagulation Factors

Primarily due to hemodilution, there is a decrease in the levels of coagulation factors during CPB. There is an especially low level of factor V. Rush and Ellis[90] have shown that levels greater than 30% for all coagulation factors, 15% for Factor V, is adequate for normal hemostasis. Therefore, even with lower levels after CPB, bleeding is infrequently due to inadequate coagulation.

Prophylactic therapy with 6 U fresh frozen plasma after CPB for elective coronary artery surgery in 100 patients showed no differences in blood loss or transfusion requirements as body stores and synthesis of coagulation proteins maintain levels above those required for adequate hemostasis.[91]

Indications for transfusion of fresh frozen plasma have been delineated by a multidisciplinary panel conference (Table IV).[92] The indications for administration of FFP include (1) replacement of isolated factor deficiencies; (2) reversal of warfarin effect; (3) massive blood transfusion; (4) antithrombin-III deficiency; (5) treatment of immunodeficiencies; and (6) treatment of thrombotic thrombocytopenic purpura.

Table IV
Indications for Fresh Frozen Plasma

1. Replacement of isolated factor deficiencies
2. Reversal of warfarin effect
3. Massive blood transfusion
4. Antithrombin III deficiency
5. Treatment of thrombotic thrombocytopenic purpura

However, preoperative coagulation defects or excessive dilution by crystalloid, colloids, or packed red blood cells may result in bleeding due to factor deficiencies. Patients receiving thrombolytic therapy in the immediate preoperative period may require FFP and cryoprecipitate (CP) for excessive bleeding.

Cryoprecipitate (CP) contains a concentrated solution of factors VIII:C and vWF, XIII, fibrinogen, and fibronectin. Cryoprecipitate is indicated in the treatment of hemophilia A, von Willebrand's disease (types II and III), and deficiencies in factor XIII or fibrinogen. Excessive use of CP elevates fibrinogen levels and increases risk of thrombosis. There is no indication for CP in the absence of documented laboratory data.

Primary Fibrinolysis

The occurrence and clinical significance of primary fibrinolysis during CPB are controversial. Due to early reports of primary fibrinolysis during CPB, the use of empirical antifibrinolytic therapy was advocated.[93] Bick[20] found evidence of almost universal fibrinolysis during CPB and has postulated that the presence of fibrinolysis and fibrinogen degradation products may cause platelet dysfunction. However, there was no correlation between plasmin levels and platelet adhesion. Marengo-Rowe and Levenson,[94] who found only 8 of 774 patients with platelet counts of less than 40,000 with only 3 out of those 8 experiencing abnormal bleeding, consider fibrinolysis as the most common and important cause of bleeding after cardiac surgery. They have therefore tailored their treatment of post-CPB bleeding with emphasis on antifibrinolytics as first line therapy.

Other studies have failed to show any difference in postoperative bleeding with antifibrinolytic therapy, while McGoon and Gomes[95] have shown an increased postoperative bleeding with empirical use of antifibrinolytic therapy. Although fibrinolytic activity is shown to be increased on initiation of CPB, there is prompt resolution within minutes after cessation of CPB.[96]. As incidence of hypofibrinogenemia or elevated FSP titers post-CPB is low, postoperative bleeding due to fibrinolysis is rare unless there is excessive or persistent plasminogen activation and plasmin generation during or post-CPB.

Antifibrinolytics

ϵ-Aminocaproic acid (EACA), a ϵ-amino-carboxylic acid analog of lysine, binds to the outpouchings of plasminogen at their lysine binding sites and displaces plasminogen from the fibrin surface, thereby interfering with plasminogen's ability to split fibrinogen. Effective EACA levels are achieved with a loading dose of 100-150 mg/kg followed by an infusion of 10-15 mg/kg/h.[97] Tranexamic acid, a cogenor of EACA, is ten times more potent and appears to have a higher therapeutic index.

Risks of EACA therapy include hypokalemia, hypotension, ventricular dysrhythmias, thromboses, and DIC.[98] This agent should only be used in bleeding patients with definitive laboratory evidence of primary fibrinolysis and consultation with a hematologist.[20]

Disseminated Intravascular Coagulation

Disseminated intravascular coagulation (DIC) is a condition of uncontrolled systemic fibrin formation leading to intravascular thrombosis with simultaneous coagulopathy caused by consumption of coagulation components and presence of fibrin degradation products. The differential diagnosis of DIC with secondary fibrinolysis and primary fibrinolysis may be exceedingly difficult.

Disseminated intravascular coagulation due to CPB appears to be rare with the wide acceptance of heparin titration during CPB in the mid-1970s. Earlier reports of DIC may have been due to low grade coagulation from inadequate heparinization. However, DIC may occur during cardiac surgery by the activation of intrinsic or extrinsic coagulation system or fibrinolytic system from shock, transfusion reactions, sepsis, and aortic dissections.

Therapy for DIC requires treatment of the precipitating cause and supportive therapy in terms of hemodynamic support, organ preservation, and transfusion of platelets, FFP, and cryoprecipitates.

Risks of Transfusion Therapy

Risks of transfusion therapy during cardiac surgery have been well documented.[99] The primary risks of tranfusion are transfusion reactions and infectious complications. The risk of hepatitis has been estimated to range from 4% in St. Louis to 18% in Houston.[100] Despite the risks, there are certain situations where the benefits of transfusion outweigh the risks. However, a recent study showed that 22%-26% of all intraoperative transfusions were inappropriate.[101] Those who are transfusing blood products need to understand the indications and appropriately document them.[102]

Conclusion

This chapter has reviewed the etiology, incidence, pathophysiology, diagnosis, and therapy for altered hemostatic system in patients undergoing cardiac surgery with CPB. Although tremendous progress has been made, further research is required to delineate the complex interaction of blood elements with foreign surfaces during CPB. With further progress, cardiac surgery may be performed with less bleeding and safer use of blood products.

REFERENCES

1. Ciavarella D, Snyder EL. Effects of cardiopulmonary bypass on platelet function. In: Dutcher JP, ed. *Modern Transfusion Therapy*. Volume II, Boca Raton, FL: CRC Press Inc.; 1990:3-23.
2. Bachman F, McKenna R, Cole ER, et al. The hemostatic mechanism after open heart surgery. *J Thorac Cardiovasc Surg* 70:76-85, 1975.
3. Torosian M, Michelson EL, Morganroth J, et al. Aspirin and coumadin-related bleeding after coronary-artery bypass graft surgery. *Ann Intern Med* 89:325, 1978.
4. Kennedy RH, McGoon DC, Smith HC, et al. Trends in cardiac surgery in the United States. *N Engl J Med* 312:119, 1985.
5. Freedman J, Lim C, Wright J. Changing patterns of transfusion practice in a tertiary area hospital from 1977-1984. *Can Anaesth Soc J* 33:458-465, 1986.

6. Bick RL. Shanbrom E. A systemic approach to the diagnosis of bleeding disorders. *Med Counterpoint* 6:27, 1972.
7. Ferraris VA, Ferraris SP, Lough FC, et al. Preoperative aspirin ingestion increases blood loss after coronary bypass grafting. *Ann Thorac Surg* 45:71-74, 1988.
8. Campbell FW, Jobes DR, Ellison N. Coagulation management during and after cardiopulmonary bypass. In: Hensley FA Jr, Martin DE, eds. *The Practice of Cardiac Anesthesia*. Boston, MA: Little, Brown, & Co.; 1990:546-582.
9. Kirklin JK, Westaby SW, Blackstone EH, et al. Complement and the damaging effects of cardiopulmonary bypass. *J Thorac Cardiovasc Surg* 86:845-857, 1983.
10. Porter DM, Silver D. Alterations in fibrinolysis and coagulation associated with cardiopulmonary bypass. *J Thorac Cardiovasc Surg* 56:869, 1968.
11. Mammen EF, Koets MH, Washington BC, et al. Hemostasis changes during cardiopulmonary bypass surgery. *Semin Thromb Hemostas* 11:281-292, 1985.
12. Hope AF, Heyns AduP, Lotter MG, et al. Kinetics and sites of sequestration of Indium III-labeled human platelets during cardiopulmonary bypass. *J Throrac Cardiovasc Surg* 81:880, 1981.
13. Aster RH. Thrombocytopenia due to sequestration of platelets. In: Williams WJ, Beutler E, Erslev AJ, et al., eds. *Hematology*. Third ed. New York, NY: McGraw-Hill; 1983:1338-1340.
14. Holmson H, Karpatkin S. Metabolism of platelets. In: Williams WJ, Beutler E, Erslev AJ, et al., eds. *Hematology*. Third ed. New York, NY: McGraw-Hill; 1983:1157-1176.
15. Edmunds LH Jr, Saxena NC, Hillyer P, et al. Relationship between platelet count and cardiotomy suction return. *Ann Thorac Surg* 25:306-10, 1978.
16. Morris KN, Kinross FM, Stirling GR. Hemolysis of blood in the pericardium: the major source of plasma hemoglobin during total body perfusion. *J Thorac Cardiovasc Surg* 49:250, 1965.
17. van Oeveren W, Kazatchkine MD, Descamps-Latscha B, et al. Deleterious effects of cardiopulmonary bypass: a prospective study of bubble versus membrane oxygenation. *J Thorac Cardiovasc Surg* 89:888-889, 1985.
18. Peterson KA, Dewanjee MK, Kaye MP. Fate of indium m-labeled platelets during cardiopulmonary bypass performed with membrane and bubble oxygenation. *J Thorac Cardiovasc Surg* 84:39-43, 1982.
19. Solis RT, Kennedy PS, Beall Jr AC, et al. Cardiopulmonary bypass. Microembolization and platelet aggregation. *Circulation* 52d:103-108, 1975.
20. Bick RL. Hemostasis defects associated with cardiac surgery, prosthetic devices, and other extracorporeal circuits. *Semin Thromb Hemostas* 11:249-280, 1985.

21. Heyns A duP. Kinetics and in vivo redistribution of 111 Indium-labeled platelets after intravenous protamine sulfate. *Thromb Haemost* 44:65, 1980.
22. Baier RE, Dutton RC. Initial events in interaction of blood with a foreign surface. *J Biomed Mater Res* 3:1919, 1969.
23. Wenger RK, Lukasiewicz H, Mikuta BS, et al. Loss of platelet fibrinogen receptors during clinical cardiopulmonary bypass. *J Thorac Cardiovasc Surg* 97:235-239, 1989.
24. Addonozio VP Jr, Macarak J, Nicolaou KC, et al. Effects of prostacyclin and albumin on platelet loss during in vitro stimulation of extracorporeal circulation. *Blood* 53:1033-42, 1989.
25. Wachtfogel Y, Kucich U, Greenplate JK, et al. Human neutrophil degranulation during extracorporeal circulation. *Blood* 69:324-330, 1987.
26. van Oeveren W, Jansen NJG, Bidstrup BP, et al. Effects of aprotinin on hemostatic mechanisms during cardiopulmonary bypass. *Ann Thorac Surg* 44:640-645, 1987.
27. Zilla P, Fasol R, Groscurth P, et al. Blood platelets in cardiopulmonary bypass operations. *J Thorac Cardiovasc Surg* 97:379-388, 1989.
28. Zilla P, Groscurth P, Rhyner K, et al. Surface morphology of human platelets during in vitro aggregation. *Scand J Haematol* 33:440-447, 1984.
29. Harker LA, Malpass TW, Branson HE, et al. Mechanism of abnormal bleeding in patients undergoing cardiopulmonary bypass: acquired transient platelet dysfunction with selective α-granule release. *Blood* 56:824-834, 1980.
30. Karpatkin S. Heterogenicity of human platelets. II. Functional evidence suggestive of young and old platelets. *J Clin Invest* 47:1083-1087, 1969.
31. Mohr R, Golan M, Martinowitz U, et al. Effect of cardiac operations in platelets. *J Thorac Cardiovasc Surg* 92:434-442, 1986.
32. Ellison NE, Edmunds Jr LH, Colman RW. Platelet aggregation following heparin and protamine administration. *Anesthesiology* 48:65-68, 1978.
33. Jacques LB. A study of the protamine salmine. *Br J Pharmacol* 4:135, 1949.
34. Wallace HW, Brooks H, Stein TP, et al. The contribution of anticoagulants to platelet dysfunction with extracorporeal circulation. *J Thorac Cardiovasc Surg* 72:735-741, 1976.
35. Steer ML, Slazman EW. Intracellular regulatory processes in platelets. In: Colman RW, Hirsh J, Marder VJ, eds. *Hemostasis and Thrombosis*. Philadelphia, PA: JB Lippincott Company; 1982:485-495.
36. Bick RL. Syndromes associated with hyperfibrino(geno)lysis. In: Bick RL, ed. *Disseminated Intravascular Coagulation*. Boca Rota, FL: CRC Press; 1983:105.
37. Tanaka K, Takao M, Yuasa H, et al. Alterations in coagulation and fibrinolysis associated with cardiopulmonary bypass during open heart surgery. *J Cardiothorac Anesth* 3:181-189, 1989.

38. Bick RL, Frazier BL, Saunders CL, et al. Alterations of hemostasis during cardiopulmonary bypass: the potential role of factor XII activation in inducing primary fibrino(geno)lysis. *Blood* 64:926, 1984.
39. Marengo-Rowe AJ, Lambert CJ, Levenson JE, et al. The evaluation of hemorrhage in cardiac patients who have undergone extracorporeal circulation. *Transfusion* 19:426-433, 1979.
40. Blomback M, Noren I, Senning AK. Coagulation disturbances during extracorporeal circulation and the postoperative period. *Acta Chir Scand* 127:433, 1964.
41. Trimble AS, Herst R, Grady M, et al. Blood loss in open heart surgery. *Arch Surg* 93:323, 1966.
42. Muller N, Popov-Cenic S, Buttner W, et al. Studies of fibrinolytic and coagulation factors during open heart surgery II. Postoperative bleeding tendencies and changes in the coagulation system. *Thromb Res* 7:589, 1975.
43. Kirklin JW, Barratt-Boyes BG. Postoperative care. In: *Cardiac Surgery*. New York, NY: Wiley & Sons; 1986:139-176.
44. Milam JD. Blood transfusion in heart surgery. *Surg Clin North Am* 63:1127, 1983.
45. Gravelee G, Goldsmith J, Low J, et al. Heparin sensitivity comparison of the ACT, SCT, and aPTT. *Anesthesiology* 71:A4, 1989.
46. Teien AN, Lie M. Heparin assay in plasma: a comparison of five clotting methods. *Thromb Res* 7:777-788, 1975.
47. Holm HA, Abildgaard U, Larsen ML, et al. Monitoring heparin therapy: should heparin assays reflect the patient's antithrombin concentration. *Thromb Res* 46:669-675, 1987.
48. Culliford AT, Gitel SN, Starr N, et al. Lack of correlation between activated clotting time and plasma heparin during cardiopulmonary bypass. *Ann Surg* 193:105, 1981.
49. Haddon WS, Gravelee GP, Bean VE, et al. The activated clotting time independently determines adequate anticoagulation during hypothermic cardiopulmonary bypass. *Anesthesiology* 67:3A, 1987.
50. Oh TH, Bell C, Hughes C. Prolonged PT and PTT despite adequate heparin neutralization following cardiopulmonary bypass in children. *Anesthesiology* 67:A22, 1987.
51. Tuman KJ, Speiss BD, McCarthy RJ, et al. Comparison of viscoelastic measures of coagulation after CPB. *Anesth Analg* 69:69-75, 1989.
52. Hartert H. Blutgerinnung studien mit der thromboelastographie, einen neuen untersuchingsverfahren. *Klin Wochenschr* 26:577-583, 1948.
53. Kang YG, Martin DJ, Marquez J, et al. Intraoperative changes in blood coagulation and thromboelastographic monitoring in liver transplantation. *Anesth Analg* 64:888-896, 1985.
54. Speiss BD, Tuman KJ, McCarthy RJ, et al. Thromboeleastography as an indicator of post-cardiopulmonary coagulopathies. *J Clin Monit* 3:25-30, 1987.
55. Summaria L, Sandesara J, Yang G, et al. In vitro comparison of fibrinolytic activity of plasminogen activators using a thromboelasto-

graphic method: in-vivo evaluation of the B-chain streptokinase complex in the dog model using pretitered doses. *Thromb Haemost* 56:1147-1163, 1986.
56. von Kaulla KN, Ostendorf P, Von Kaulla E. The impedence machine: a new bedside coagulation recording device. *J Med* 6:73-87, 1975.
57. Saleem A, Blifeld C, Saleh SA, et al. Viscoelastic measurement of clot formation: a new test of platelet function. *Ann Clin Lab Sci* 13:115-124, 1983.
58. Peck SD. Evaluation of the in vitro detection of the hypercoagulable state using the thrombin generation test and plasma clot impedence test. *Thromb Haemost* 42:764-777, 1979.
59. Schreiner R. Discussion of: Our experience in regional heparinization by Nakamoto S, Holmes JH. *Trans Am Soc Artif Organs* 4:36, 1958.
60. Ellison N, Beatty CP, Blake DR, et al. Heparin rebound, studies in patients and volunteers. *J Thorac Cardiovasc Surg* 67:723-729, 1974.
61. Estas JW. Kinetics of the anticoagulant effect of heparin. *J Am Med Assoc* 212:1492-1495, 1970.
62. Esposito RA, Culliford AT, Colvin SB, et al. The role of activated clotting time in heparin administration and neutralization for cardiopulmonary bypass. *J Thorac Cardiovasc Surg* 85:174-185, 1983.
63. Zaidan JR, Johnson S, Brynes R, et al. Rate of protamine administration: its effect on heparin reversal and antithrombin recovery after cornonary artery surgery. *Anesth Analg* 65:377-380, 1986.
64. Frick DG, Brogli H. The mechanism of heparin rebound after extracorporeal circulation for open cardiac surgery. *Surgery* 59:721, 1966.
65. Concensus Conference: platelet transfusion therapy. *J Am Med Assoc* 257:1777-1780, 1987.
66. Simon TL, Bechara FA, Murphy W. Controlled trial of routine administration of platelet concentrates in cardiopulmonary bypass surgery. *Ann Thorac Surg* 37:359-364, 1982.
67. Ciavarella D, Lavallo E, Reiss RF. Coagulation factor activity in platelet concentrates stored up to 7 days: an in vitro and in vivo study. *Clin Lab Haematol* 8:233, 1986.
68. Mohr R, Martinowitz U, Lavee J, et al. The hemostatic effect of transfusion fresh whole blood versus platelet concentrates after cardiac operations. *J Thorac Cardiovasc Surg* 96:530-534, 1988.
69. Lavee J, Martinowitz U, Mohr R, et al. The effects of transfusion of fresh whole blood versus platelet concentrates after cardiac operations. A scanning microscope study of platelet aggregation on extracellular matrix. *J Thorac Cardiovasc Surg* 97:204-212, 1989.
70. Kappa JR, Horn MK III, Fisher CA, et al. Efficacy of iloprost (ZK36374) versus aspirin in preventing heparin induced platelet activation during open cardiac surgery. *J Thorac Cardiovasc Surg* 94:405-413, 1987.
71. Coller BS. von Willebrand's disease. In: Ratnoff OD, Forbes CD, eds. *Disorders of Hemostasis*. Orlando, FL: Grune & Stratton; 1984:241-269.

72. D'Angelo A, Capitano A, Smith JB, et al. Effect of desamino-D-arginine vasopressin on plasma levels of platelets and endothelial cell release products. *Thromb Haemost* 49:64-65, 1983.
73. Mannucci PM. Desmopressin for treatment disorders of hemostasis. In: Coller BS, ed. *Progress in Hemostasis and Thrombosis*. Orlando, FL: Grune & Stratton; 1986:19-45.
74. Cash JD, Gader AMA, DaCosta J. The release of plasminogen activator and factor VIII by LVP, AVP, DDAVP, ATIII, and OT in man. *Br J Haematol* 27:363-364, 1974.
75. Ware JA. Desmopressin acetate in hemorrhagic conditions, with emphasis on use after cardiopulmonary bypass. In: Ellison N, Jobes DR, eds. *Effective Hemostasis in Cardiac Surgery*. Philadelphia, PA: W.B. Saunders; 1988:137-154.
76. Richardson DW, Robinson AG. Desmopressin. *Ann Int Med* 103:228-239, 1985.
77. Kobrinsky NL, Israels ED, Gerrard JM, et al. Shortening of bleeding time by 1-deamino-8-D-arginine vasopressin in various bleeding disorders. *Lancet* 1:1145-1148, 1984.
78. Kobrinsky NL, Israels ED, Letts M, et al. DDAVP shortens the bleeding time and decreases operative blood loss in hemostatically normal subjects undergoing spinal-fusion surgery. *Blood* 66:323A, 1985.
79. Salzman EW, Weinstein MJ, Weintraub RM, et al. Treatment of desmopressin acetate to reduce blood loss after cardiac surgery. A double-blind randomized trial. *N Engl J Med* 314:1402-1406, 1986.
80. Czer LS, Bateman TH, Gray RJ, et al. Treatment of severe platelet dysfunction and hemorrhage after cardiopulmonary bypass: Reduction in blood product usage with desmopressin. *J Am Coll Cardiol* 9:1139-1147, 1987.
81. Brown MR, Swygert TH, Whitten CW, et al. Desmopressin acetate following cardiopulmonary bypass: Evaluation of coagulation parameters. *J Cardiothorac Anesth* 3:726-729, 1989.
82. Best LC, McGuire MB, Jones PB, et al. Mode of action of dipyridamole on human platelets. *Thromb Res* 16:367-377, 1979.
83. Emmons PR, Harrison MJG, Honour AJ, et al. Effect of dipyridamole on human platelet behavior. *Lancet* 2:603-606, 1965.
84. Nuutinen LS, Mononen P. Dipyridamole and thrombocyte count in open-heart surgery. *J Thorac Cardiovasc Surg* 70:707-711, 1975.
85. Teoh KH, Christakis GT, Weisel RD, et al. Dipyridamole preserved platelets and reduced blood loss after cardiopulmonary bypass. *J Thorac Cardiovasc Surg* 96:332-341, 1988.
86. Chesebro JH, Clements JP, Fuster V, et al. A platelet inhibitor drug trial in coronary artery bypass operations: benefit of perioperative dipyridamole and aspirin therapy on early postoperative vein graft patency. *N Engl J Med* 307:73-78, 1982.
87. Kadatz R. Die pharmakologischen eigenschaften der neuen coronarerweitervden substanz 2,6 bis(diaethanoamino)-4,8,-dipiperidino-pyrimido (5,4-d)pyrimidin. *Artzneinmittel-Forsch* 9:39, 1959.

88. Fishelson Z, Pangburn MK, Muller-Eberhard HJ. Characterization of the initial C3 convertase of the alternative pathway of human complement. *J Immunol* 132: 1430, 1984.
89. Royston D, Bidstrup BP, Taylor KM, et al. Effect of aprotinin on need for blood transfusion after repeat open-heart surgery. *Lancet* 1:1289-1292, 1987.
90. Rush B and Ellis H: The treatment of patients with factor V deficiency. *Thromb Diasth Haemorrh* 14:74-82, 1965.
91. Roy RC, Stafford MA, Hudspeth AS, et al. Failure of prophylaxis with fresh frozen plasma after cardiopulmonary bypass. *Anesthesiology* 69:254-257, 1988.
92. Tullis JL, Alving B, Bove JR, et al. Fresh frozen plasma: indications and risks. *J Am Med Assoc* 253:551-553, 1985.
93. Kevy SV, Glickman RM, Bernhard WF, et al. The pathogenesis and control of the hemorrhagic defect in open-heart surgery. *Surg Gynecol Obstet* 123: 313, 1966.
94. Marengo-Rowe AJ, Levenson JE. Fibrinolysis: a frequent cause of bleeding. In: Ellison N, Jobes DR, eds. *Effective Hemostasis in Cardiac Surgery*. Philadelphia, PA: W.B. Saunders Co.; 1988:41-55.
95. McGoon MM, Gomes D. Bleeding patterns after open heart surgery. *J Thorac Cardiovasc Surg* 60:87, 1970.
96. Gans H, Lillehei CW, Krivit W. Problems in hemostasis during open-heart surgery I. On the release of plasminogen activator. *Ann Surg* 154:915-924, 1961.
97. Verstraete M. Clinical application of inhibitors of fibrinolysis. *Drugs* 29:236-261, 1985.
98. Naeye RL. thrombotic state after a hemorrhagic state: a possible complication of therapy with epsion-aminocaproic acid. *Blood* 19:694, 1962.
99. Ushijima K, Lee S, Oka Y. Transfusion therapy in cardiac surgery. In: Dutcher JP, ed. *Modern Transfusion Therapy*. Boca Raton, FL: CRC Press Inc.; 1990:135-156.
100. Buimovici-Klein E, Sonnnabend JA, Lange M, et al. Tranfusion-associated hepatitis and AIDS: what is the risk? *N Engl J Med* 317:242-245, 1987.
101. Stehling L, Esposito B. An analysis of the appropriateness of intraoperative transfusion. *Anesth Analg* 68:Sl-S321, 1989.
102. Rabkin B, Rabkin MS. Individual and institutional liability for transfusion-acquired diseases. An update. *J Am Med Assoc* 256:2242-2243, 1986.

Chapter 9

Renal Failure Following Open Heart Surgery

Pierre A. Casthely, MD,
B. Chandrasekaran, MD,
and Thil Yoganathan, MD

Acute renal failure (ARF) is a syndrome characterized by the sudden deterioration of renal function with accumulation of metabolic waste products in the body fluid. Nonoliguric, oliguric, and anuric represent a spectrum of insult to the kidney; with nonoliguria considered as minor insult, oliguria moderate insult, and anuria severe insult. Acute renal failure is usually associated with oliguria (urine output less than 400 mL/day) or anuria (urine output of less than 50 mL/day) although 25% of patients with acute renal failure will not be oliguric.[1] Many theories have been proposed to explain the oliguria of acute renal failure. They include tubular theories, back leak, obstruction, and vascular theories. However, no single theory will be sufficient to explain all aspects of acute renal failure because different mechanisms may be active at different times during the course of the syndrome.[2,3] Because improved methods for treating acute tubular necrosis have failed to improve the mor-

From Casthely PA, Bregman D, (eds): *Cardiopulmonary Bypass: Physiology, Related Complications, and Pharmacology.* Mount Kisco, NY, Futura Publishing Company, Inc., © 1991.

tality rate over the past 20 years prevention should be the goal. The mortality rate of acute renal failure is approximately 60% but this varies from 20% to 30% for patients with nonoliguric renal failure up to 90% in patients critically ill who develop renal failure.[4]

The incidence of renal failure following open heart surgery ranges from 1.5% to 2.5%.[5,6] Oliguria may result from prerenal causes, parenchymal renal damage, or postrenal obstruction. Predisposing factors include advanced age, diabetes, preexisting impairment of renal function, prolonged cardiopulmonary bypass, and low cardiac output state.[7,8] Large doses of loop diuretics, aud aminoglycosides can precipitate ARF in the postoperative period. Direct renal parenchymal damage may occur from hemoglobinopathies or intravenous contrast. Low cardiac output state is the most common cause of renal failure in the postoperative open heart patient. Controversy still exists over protective advantages of pulsatile or nonpulsatile flow on renal function during cardiopulmonary bypass, because both produce almost identical renal blood flow rates.

Appropriate diagnostic measures include fluid challenge, urine osmolality, urine to plasma osmolality ratio, urine to plasma urea nitrogen ratio, urine to plasma creatinine ratio, urine sodium excretion, urine sodium concentration, renal failure index, fractional excretion of sodium, ultrasound and scanning of the kidney, monitoring of cardiac output and intravascular pressures, and bladder catheterization. To discriminate between prerenal and renal causes of ARF fractional excretion of sodium is the best test with an accuracy of 90% (Table I).

Prevention of renal failure in patients undergoing open heart surgery is mainly based on maintenance of adequate perioperative cardiac output.[9,10] Low doses of dopamine have been found to improve renal function after cardiopulmonary bypass.[10] Diuretics, particularly furosemide, are commonly used to treat oliguria if cardiac output and filling pressures are adequate, because they can help maintain renal cortical blood flow during cardiopulmonary bypass[11,12] and may have a synergistic effect with dopamine.[13] Mannitol and furosemide have been used to increase urine output in the patient with renal failure, but there is no clear evidence that they decrease the morbidity and mortality associated with ARF in humans.[12] They do have an advantage by converting oliguric renal

Table I
Diagnostic Indices for Prerenal Azotemia (PA) and Acute Tubular Necrosis (ATN)

Measure*	PA	ATN
Uosm	> 500 mOsm	< 350 mOsm
U:Posm	> 1.2	< 1.2
U:Pun	> 10	< 13
U:Pcr	> 40	< 20
Una	< 20 mEq/L	> 40 mEq/L
RFI	< 1	> 1
Fexc Na	< 1	> 1

Uosm = urine osmolality; U:Posm = urine to plasma osmolality ratio; U:Pun = urine to plasma urea nitrogen ratio; U:Pcr = urine to plasma creatine ratio; Una = urine sodium concentration. RFI (renal failure index) = Una/U:Pcr; Fexc Na (fractional sodium excretion) = U:Pna/U:Pcr. (Modified from Miller TR, Anderson RJ, Linas SL, et al.: Urinary diagnostic indices in acute renal failure. A prospective study. *Ann Intern Med* 89:47, 1978).

failure (RF) to nonoliguric RF that has a shorter and more benign course.

Acute renal failure results in several metabolic derangements: hyperkalemia, acidosis, hypocalcemia. The physiologic effects of potassium accumulation are worsened by the development of acidosis and the appearance of lethal arrhythmias, particularly ventricular fibrillation. Hypocalcemia, hypoglycemia, and hypermagnesemia may precipitate seizures in ARF.[13,14]

In the setting of low cardiac output, compensatory vasoconstriction may occur and result in prerenal azotemia. Initial treatment for prerenal azotemia includes volume expansion, afterload reduction, and augmentation of cardiac output to preserve renal blood flow and prevent progression to renal failure. The treatment of renal failure is based on avoiding hypervolemia, bleeding, encephalopathy, and electrolyte imbalances such as hyperkalemia. Fluid intake should be adjusted to replace only insensible losses and total output. Emergency treatment of hyperkalemia includes administration of sodium bicarbonate, calcium chloride, dextrose and insulin, kayexalate enemas. and dialysis (Table II). The use of large doses of $NaHCO_3$ should be used cautiously because it can cause hypernatremia, pulmonary edema, and hypertension.

Table II
Emergency Treatment of Hyperkalemia

Mechanism	*Treatment*	*Limitations*
Antagonism of K^+ effect on cell membranes.	Calcium chloride, 1 g IV slowly.	Usually exacerbate digitalis toxicity.
Shift of K^+ from extracellular to intracellular space.	Sodium bicarbonate, 50–100 mEq IV slowly. Mechanical ventilation. IV infusion of insulin 5 u, dextrose 50 g over 20 minutes.	May induce pulmonary edema, hypotension. Short-lived (30–40 min)
Removal of K^+ from body.	Kayexalate 0.5 g/kg per rectum (sodium polystyrene sulfonate). Emergency peritoneal dialysis. Emergency hemodialysis.	Exchanges for sodium, may induce pulmonary edema. Inefficient K^+ removal, respiratory compromise. Hypotension, hemorrhage.

Method of Dialysis

Different methods of blood purification are available in acute uremia. They include hemodialysis, hemofiltration, peritoneal dialysis, and a combination of hemofiltration and hemodialysis (hemodiafiltration). Each method can be used either intermittently or continuously (Table III).

There are no randomized clinical studies comparing one method with another. The only nonrandomized interinstitutional studies that have been performed have compared hemodialysis with intermittent peritoneal dialysis in patients with acute renal failure. They have all shown similar mortality.[15] No comparison of mortality has been done for slow continuous hemofiltration, but the mortality rate does not seem to be high. This procedure is reserved for those patients who physiologically are too unstable to tolerate conventional dialytic management.

Hemodialysis is indicated to treat fluid overload, encephalopathy, severe azotemia, and electrolyte imbalance (Fig. 1). Vascular access for acute hemodialysis is established either through percuta-

Table III
Methods of Dialysis

	Hemodialysis	*Peritoneal Dialysis*	*Hemofiltration*	*Hemodiafiltration*
Intermittent	Most clinical experience "gold standard"	Results equal to intermittent hemodialysis	Anecdotal experience only. Technically complicated	No clinical reports. Very complicated
Continuous	Anecdotal experience. Technically complicated	CAPD needs catheter to be in place at least for 10–14 days to avoid hernia and leaks.	Rapidly accumulating experience. Technically simple	No clinical reports. Very complicated

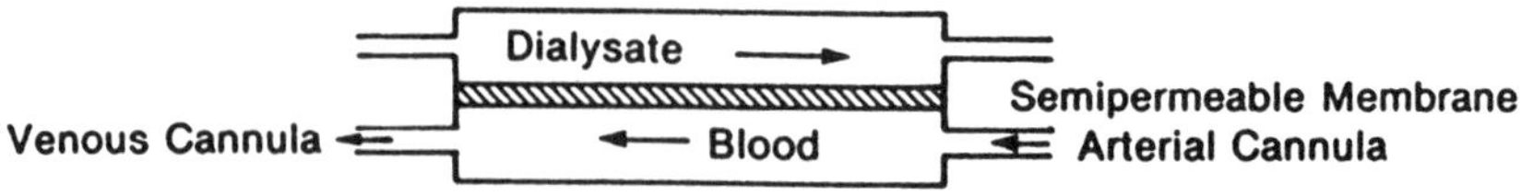

Figure 1. Schematic diagram of hemodialysis. The dialysate is circulated past the blood flowing in the opposite direction (countercurrent flow) on the other side of a thin semipermeable membrane.

neous cannulation of the femoral or subclavian veins. The dialysis solution is usually adjusted based on electrolytes considerations for individual patients (potassium, sodium, calcium).

Dextrose is added to the dialysate to prevent inducing a negative nitrogen balance secondary to gluconeogenesis[16] and other side effects of dialysis.[17] Very high dextrose levels, over 1,000 mg/dL, should probably be avoided because postdialysis hypoglycemia and convulsions have been described with such solutions. A dialysate dextrose concentration close to 700 mg/dL may be optimal to inhibit gluconeogenesis. It supplies calories, causes only moderate elevation of blood sugar (50 mg/dL) at the end of dialysis, and minimizes the disequilibrium syndrome.[16,18]

Bicarbonate or acetate are the two buffer bases in the dialysate.[19] When acetate is metabolized through the Krebs cycle, hydrogen ions are consumed as it is metabolized to acetylcoenzyme A. Severe metabolic acidosis may result from the removal of bicarbonate by dialysis and the failure to regenerate bicarbonate from acetate secondary to incomplete metabolism.

Bicarbonate and acetate have different effects on the cardiovascular system. Both ions, when infused, cause vasodilatation, but this is most pronounced with acetate. Previous clinical studies have shown that more mannitol and albumin infusions were necessary to maintain blood pressure during acetate dialysis than during bicarbonate dialysis.[20,21] In most patients, the choice between buffer base is probably arbitrary, but it seems prudent to use bicarbonate in the most desperately ill patients. In selected patients with abnormally high bicarbonate levels, lower than normal acetate or bicarbonate dialysate should be used.[22] Chloride simply makes up the difference between cations and anions in dialysate.

Hemodialysis solution contains acetate that is metabolized to form bicarbonate. This bicarbonate is intended to correct the high anion gap acidosis found in renal failure patients. The advantage of using acetate solutions over initially using $NaHCO_3$ is that acetate solutions remain stable for a greater time than bicarbonate, thus they are used in most commercially available solutions. The major disadvantage is that acetate produces vasodilatation that may further compromise the hemodynamic status of the patient. Eleven out of thirteen of our postoperative open heart patients, who required hemodialysis, tolerated it very poorly. They were all mechanically ventilated and recovering from low output syndrome in the postoperative period. Most of them became hypotensive, acidotic, and four of them had experienced cardiac arrest during hemodialysis.

Anticoagulation

The anticoagulant of choice during dialysis remains heparin. However, the administration of a bolus of heparin as used in chronic dialysis patients should be avoided. Clotting times should not be allowed to rise more than 25% above baseline. Most patients can be anticoagulated with this schedule, which uses 1,500 to 2,000 U of heparin per therapy, and still have only a 2% to 5% incidence of dialyzer clotting. This approach will minimize bleeding even in those high-risk patients.[23]

In patients at an extremely high risk for bleeding, one can occasionally use dialysis with no anticoagulation. Cellulose acetate dialyzer may be most suitable, although no controlled studies are available.

Regional heparinization, involving simultaneous infusion of heparin into the arterial line and protamine into the venous line, is inferior to the methods described above. There is a high risk of rebound anticoagulation after dialysis has ceased because heparin is metabolized more slowly than protamine. Several other methods of anticoagulation have been described. They include citrate,[24] prostacyclins,[25] ticlopidine, gabexate mesilate, and the new heparinoids.[24-27] There is little clinical experience with these anticoagulants.

Complications

Standard hemodialysis, although beneficial in the chronic maintenance of renal failure patients, is associated with numerous detrimental physiologic changes that may be poorly tolerated in an already hemodynamically unstable patient. Severe fluid shifts may occur with overzealous hemodialysis and up to 1 L of fluid can be removed per hour of hemodialysis.[28] Hypotension, especially in hypovolemic patients and in those renal failure patients with autonomic dysfunction, may be fatal, because few physiologic compensatory methods are available to the patient on hemodialysis. Most interventions, with fluids or colloids such albumin, are not intrinsically controlled by the dialysis system.

The pathogenesis of these effects is multifactorial, and poorly understood (Table IV). Acute decreases in plasma osmolality contribute significantly to dialysis hypotension.[29-31] A decrease in plasma osmolality decreases extracellular fluid volume because water moves from the extracellular to the intracellular space resulting in cell dysfunction. This dysfunction enhances the release of prostaglandins causing vasodilatation, and decreases vasopressin and vasoactive amine release in stress.[32] Although vasoactive amines are small molecules and easily dialyzable, most patients show no fall in epinephrine and norepinephrine blood levels during dialysis.[33,34] The infusion of acetate during dialysis has been shown to cause a fall in blood pressure, but only if dialysate sodium is low.

A number of pharmacologic interventions can decrease dialysis hypotension (Table IV). The use of hyperosmolar agents such as mannitol, sodium, or glucose, as mentioned above, prevents or

Table IV
Pathogenesis of Dialysis Induced Hypotension

Pathogenic factors →	*Mediators*	*Pathophysiology*
Ultrafiltration	↓ Vasopressin	↓ Cardiac output
+	+	
Fall osmolality →	↑ Prostaglandin release →	↓ Peripheral Resistance
+	+	
Acetate infusion	Complement activation	Hypotension
+	+	
Bioincompatibility	Neutropenia	
	+	
	Hypoxemia	

ameliorates dialysis hypotension.[35] Oxygen was shown to decrease dialysis hypotension in one controlled study.[36] Bicarbonate dialysate may also facilitate blood pressure stability, particularly if low-sodium dialysate has to be used.[37] Infusions of vasoactive amines or hyperoncotic albumin are empirical treatment method.[38]

Dialysis-disequilibrium syndrome is a well recognized central nervous system (CNS) complication of rapid correction of uremia by hemodialysis. The intracellular/extravascular concentration gradients of the solutes urea and sodium are rapidly modified. The extracellular levels are effectively lowered, but prior to the equilibration of intracellular/extravascular a marked disequilibration may result. The increased intracellular osmolality attracts H_2O that may lead to cerebral edema and resultant CNS symptoms.

Hypoxemia, a devastating challenge to critically ill patients, has routinely been associated with hemodialysis.[39,40] Several explanations have been described. Blood passing through the extracorporeal hemodialysis membranes may initiate complement activation with a resultant leukocyte margination in the lung.[41-45] This leads to inadequate ventilation and subsequent hypoxia.[44,45] All currently available dialysis membranes are bioincompatible and induce complement activation, neutropenia, and thrombocytopenia.[41,42] The cellophane and cuprophane membranes seem to be more bioincompatible than cellulose acetate, polyacrylonitrile, and polycarbonate membranes.[43,44] There has been suggestion of much less complement activation from the Amicon filter. Romaldini demonstrated a decline in alveolar ventilation, respiratory quotient, and PaO_2 with an unchanged alveolar-arterial O_2 tension difference.[39] If an acetate bath is utilized for dialysis, CO_2 is lost through the dialyzer membrane; this reduces the respiratory quotient (CO_2 excreted by lungs/O_2 consumption). This can be attenuated by using a bicarbonate diasylate but the practical consideration as mentioned must be remembered.

Normally hypoxemia during hemodialysis can be easily managed with supplemental O_2. The postoperative open heart patient may not be able to tolerate even mild decreased pO_2. Furthermore, if the patient is extubated, additional O_2 by face mask/nasal cannula may be insufficient to prevent this hypoxemia. The intubated patient with seriously compromised pulmonary function may require positive end-expiratory pressure (PEEP) to increase its PO_2 while increasing the fractional inspired oxygen tension. This will decrease the risk of oxygen toxicity and prevent further damage to the lungs.

Peritoneal Dialysis

Peritoneal dialysis (PD) has been used as a renal replacement therapy for many years by making use of a natural semipermeable membrane namely peritoneal membrane (Fig. 2). However, until 1968 when Tenchoff introduced the silicone rubber in-dwelling catheter, PD was not used that widely because this made repeated access to the peritoneal easy. In 1976, Papovich and Moncrief described what is known today as chronic ambulatory peritoneal dialysis and since then PD has become a standard renal replacement therapy. There are four different types of PD:

(1) Chronic ambulatory peritoneal dialysis (CAPD). This is usually done as three or four exchanges of PD fluid per day, 1 to 2 liters each time, enabling dialysis to be a 24-hour process. Because of the increased intra-abdominal pressure and other related problems, this is usually not used for acute renal failure.
(2) Intermittent peritoneal dialysis (IPD). A mechanical device is used to do the exchanges, usually on a hourly basis. Depending on the blood chemistries value this can be used from every other day to every day. However, because the exact amount of fluid removed is difficult to determine, this may not be advisable in the acutely sick patient, such as the postoperative open heart patient.

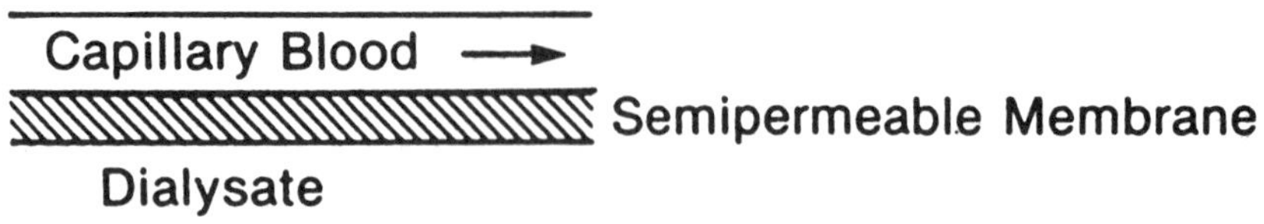

Figure 2. Schematic diagram of peritoneal dialysis. Nonflowing dialysate is separated from capillary blood by the peritoneal lining, which is a complex semipermeable, biologic membrane.

(3) Continuous cyclic peritoneal dialysis (CCPD). This is similar to CAPD. Here, however, a cycler (mechanically devised) is used at night to do the three or four exchanges. Hence it is used only for chronic renal failure.
(4) Manual peritoneal dialysis (MPD). This most commonly used for acute renal failure. Because you can manually alter the PD fluid volume, and also can add and delete medications to the dialysate at any given time and measure the fluid volume removed accurately this modality is more appropriate for the postoperative open heart patients with acute renal failure.

Choice of Buffer Anion

Both lactate and acetate have been used in commercial peritoneal dialysis solutions.[45] Although lactate is a racemic mixture of natural and unnatural isomers, metabolism of both forms seems to equal peritoneal dialysis absorption rates at low blood levels. The L (+) isomer may be absorbed slightly more rapidly.[46]

Acetate and lactate solutions yield similar peritoneal transport results in acute studies.[45] However, recent reports suggest losses of ultra-filtration and rapid glucose absorption with repeated or continuous acetate exposure.[47,48] There appears to be a high association of acetate use with sclerosing peritonitis but a causative role is unproven.[49,50]

Factors Influencing Peritoneal Dialysis Efficiency

There is indirect evidence to suggest that peritoneal capillary blood is the major sources of solutes and water removed during peritoneal dialysis.[51] Vasoconstrictors administered systemically or intraperitoneally can reduce peritoneal clearances.[52] They cause a decrease in the number of peritoneal capillaries perfused and in peritoneal capillary blood flow.

The intraperitoneal administration of vasodilators increases peritoneal clearances,[2,53] increases peritoneal capillary blood flow as well as the number of capillaries perfused. Vasodilation and/or direct effects of vasodilator agents may increase capillary permeability. Peritoneal clearance increases with vasodilators support the contention that blood flow, the number of capillaries perfused and vascular permeability influence peritoneal dialysis efficiency.[52]

Reduced peritoneal clearances have been reported in patients with severe systemic vascular diseases, presumably involving the peritoneal microcirculation. Reduced peritoneal clearances have been reported in patients with systemic lupus erythematosus, malignant hypertension, and widespread diabetic vascular disease.[54,55] Reduced clearances are not universal to all diabetics but may reflect the degree of capillary basement membrane thickening and vascular disease in the peritoneal microcirculation.

Other physical factors influencing peritoneal dialysis include dialysate flow, temperature,[56] pH,[57] protein content of dialysis solution,[58] osmolality,[59] buffer anion, and PCO_2.[60]

Complications

Some of the common complications of PD are outlines in Table V.

(1) Peritonitis. Most commonly it is due to staph species. By carefully monitoring the dialysis effluent and checking the PD fluid cell count this can be treated quickly and successfully. Gram-negative and fungal peritonitis rarely occur and usually require removal of the catheter.
(2) Electrolytes. Hypernatremia and hypokalemia may occur. Hypokalemia can be avoided by adding potassium to PD fluid. Hypernatremia is indicative of water loss and may need appropriate replacement.
(3) Hyperglycemia occurs especially in diabetics and when high dextrose concentration dialysate is used for fluid removal purposes. This may need either intraperitoneal or parenteral insulin therapy.
(4) Protein loss could be a problem especially in patients with peritonitis.

Table V
Complications of Peritoneal Dialysis

Mechanical	Hemorrhage Puncture of intraabdominal organ Leakage Inadequate drainage Dissection of fluid into tissue spaces Wound/bowel suture problems Intraperitoneal catheter loss
Metabolic	Hypoglycemia or hyperglycemia Electrolyte abnormalities Fluid imbalance Acid-base problems Protein/amino acid loss
Cardiovascular/pulmonary	Pulmonary edema Hypotension Hypertension Arrhythmia/cardiac arrest Atelectasis Pneumonia Hydrothorax
Infectious complications	Abscess at puncture site Bacterial peritonitis Fungal peritonitis Sterile peritonitis

(5) Mechanical problems such as catheter leak, drainage problem, hemorrhage, pain, hernias, reflex esophagitis secondary to increased intra-abdominal pressure.
(6) Alkalosis can occur very rarely.
(7) Pneumonia and atelectasis can occur due to increased intra-abdominal pressure and elevated diaphragm that can compromise the respiration especially if the patient is already extubated. Hydrothorax occurs in up to 10% of the patients.

Heparin

Routine addition of heparin is no longer practiced. In the patient with an intact peritoneum, only small amounts of heparin are reportedly absorbed from the dialysate.[74,75] However, if high concentrations are used, significant absorption can occur, resulting in severe anticoagulation and bleeding (personal observation). It is customary to add heparin to the dialysis fluid if the patient has peritonitis to prevent obstruction of the catheter by fibrin.

Antibiotics

Prophylactic antibiotics are of no value in preventing peritonitis.[76,77] In fact, the incidence of infections with more highly resistant organisms may increase. Addition of antibiotics to peritoneal dialysis solution is recommended only for therapy and not for prophylaxis.

Several pharmacologic agents have been added to the dialysate to improve clearance or ultrafiltration rates. They include prostaglandins, prostaglandin precursors, dopamine, glucagon, isoproterenol, tolazoline, nitroprusside, and dipyridamole.[79,82]

Continuous Artery Venous Hemofiltration

Continuous arteriovenous hemofiltration (CAVH), first proposed in 1974, was modified to its present form in 1977.[61-63] Continuous arteriovenous hemofiltration works as a standard dialysis method, and has been increasingly used as the optimal modality of emergency fluid removal in the critically ill patient with renal failure. The system is pressure dependent and utilizes the patient's arteriovenous pressure gradient as the driving force through a Diafilter (Fig. 3). Continuous arteriovenous hemofiltration has many advantages over conventional hemodialysis or peritoneal dialysis, including ease of vascular access, maintenance of hemodynamic stability, low cost, and a reduced side-effect profile.

Vascular access for CAVH does not require shunt implantation or surgical modification of vessels. The standard method of vascular cannulation involves insertion of 14 gauge hemodialysis catheters in the femoral artery and vein utilizing the Seldinger technique. This bedside procedure produces the greatest flow rate when compared with fistula or shunt access.

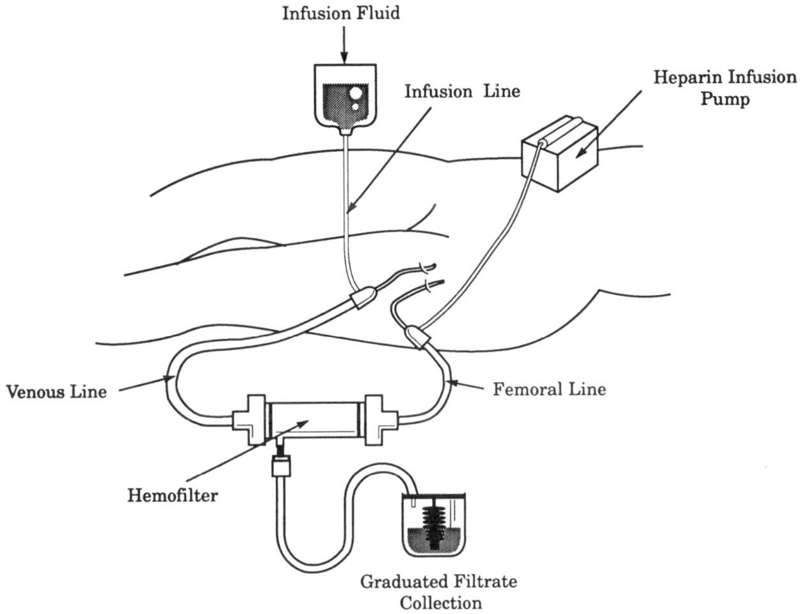

Figure 3. Schematic diagram of continuous arteriovenous hemofiltration.

Continuous arteriovenous hemofiltration flow rate, unlike hemodialysis flow, is linearly variable with the patient's blood pressure. Theoretically CAVH may be used in any patient with a systolic blood pressure > 40 mm Hg with the limiting factor being clotting of the filter secondary to low blood flow. If a significant fall in circulating volume occurs, the resultant decrease in blood pressure will slow CAVH flow. This early compensation in flow filtration rate will assure that only small changes in blood pressure occur. This negative feedback mechanism has been demonstrated in several studies to provide hemodynamic stability to critically ill patients while on CAVH dialysis.[64,65] This is in distinct contrast to hemodialysis, which is poorly tolerated in many patients with multisystem failure. Hemodialysis may be difficult when systolic blood pressure is below 90 mm Hg, because it causes rapid fluid shifts with precipitous falls in blood pressure in hypovolemic patients.

Continuous arteriovenous hemofiltration removes fluids, electrolytes, and small and medium size molecules with a molecular weight less than 50,000 kd. The ultrafiltrate formed contains potassium, sodium, phosphate, urea, and creatinine in concentrations that were within 0.7 mmol/L of serum values.[66] With CAVH, blood urea nitrogen is maintained below 90 mL/L with daily filtration of 14.2 ± 4.6 L.[67] Replacement fluid composed of sodium chloride, 50% magnesium sulfate, and sodium bicarbonate is used in a varying percentage replacement to achieve the desired fluid balance. This allows aggressive hyperalimentation to be added to therapy without the usual problems concerning fluid balance in an anuric patient.

The close correlation between ultrafiltrate and plasma concentrations of sodium, potassium, phosphate, urea, creatinine negate the need for analysis of ultrafiltrate concentration. The notable exception of this ratio is the concentration of calcium. This is probably because only ionized calcium is filtered. The concentration of water soluble antibiotics is also imbalanced with free filtration.[68] To achieve therapeutic levels several dosing adjustments may be required with monitoring of serum antibiotic levels.

Factors That Affect Ultrafiltration Rate

Continuous arteriovenous hemofiltration, although a simple system, requires many technical considerations for the system to run efficiently. Any factor that affects blood flow through the system ultimately affects ultrafiltration rates (UFR) and solute clearance. Variables to be considered include the balance between hydrostatic and oncotic forces, the location of arterial and venous access, the length and diameter of the arterial and venous cannulae and tubing, and the arterial/venous hemofilter pressure gradient.

For CAVH to be effective, there must be a filter transmembrane pressure gradient and a balance between hydrostatic and oncotic forces that favors ultrafiltration. Hydrostatic pressure is positive on the blood side and negative on the ultrafiltration side. It favors movement of water across the filter membrane, and as the hydrostatic pressure becomes greater, the ultrafiltration rate also becomes greater. On the other hand, oncotic pressure tends to retain plasma water and solutes on the blood side of the filter membrane. Consequently, increased oncotic pressure yields a slower ultrafiltration rate. As these two forces (hydrostatic and oncotic pressure) become equal, the transmembrane gradient necessary for ultrafiltration to occur ceases. Hence, an ideal balance must be achieved if adequate volume and solute removal are to occur.

The hydrostatic pressure across the filter membrane is reflected in the arterial blood pressure delivered to the filter membrane. The location of the arterial/venous access, the length, the width of the vascular cannulae and tubing, the arterial/venous pressure gradient across the filter, and the height of the ultrafiltration column are all factors that may be manipulated in an attempt to preserve the mean arterial pressure delivered to the filter. As the blood traverses the hemofilter, plasma matter is removed and hemoconcentration occurs. Oncotic pressure eventually becomes equal to hydrostatic pressure, and ultrafiltration ceases. Although fluid may be delivered to the patient through the arterial limb of the system, blood products and protein solutions should only be given on the venous side. If given arterially, they increase oncotic pressure and decrease ultrafiltration rates. The primary factors opposing ultrafiltration are oncotic pressure, blood viscosity, and increased venous back pressure across the filter.

Blood pressure, blood flow, and vascular access are related. Large-bore arterial/venous access provides the least resistance to blood flow and best preserves hydrostatic pressure. For any given arterial pressure, blood flow increases as central rather than peripheral vascular access is used. According to Pouiselle's law, the pressure drop or resistance across a vascular catheter is proportional to the length and inversely proportional to the radius of the catheter. Blood pressure thus is best preserved by using short, large-bore catheters. We prefer femoral artery-venous access or axillary artery-venous access in our institution.

The major advantage of femoral access is ease of insertion. The disadvantages include interference with patient mobilization and turning, difficulty in maintaining an uncontaminated site, and increased risk of atherosclerotic complications, specifically, intimal tears, and plaque emboli. Axillary access allows for better patient mobilization. Atherosclerosis of upper extremity vessels is less common than lower extremity vessels and, thus, flow complications may be less, despite the fact that the axillary artery has a smaller lumen than the femoral artery.

The most difficult technical problem encountered when using CAVH in the absence of a blood pump is increased venous back pressure across the filter. This problem results in decreased blood flow and predisposition to filter clotting. It occurs most commonly in patients with severe respiratory compromise who have extremely elevated intrathoracic and right heart pressures.

Variables such as filter surface area, priming volume, membrane permeability, and membrane biocompatibility are unique to each hemofilter system, and they influence ultrafiltration rates.

Although infrequent, complications of CAVH include access complications (infection, thrombosis, hemorrhage, and aneurysm formation), excessive anticoagulation, system disconnections, and errors in fluid and electrolyte balance. These complications are all predictable and can be easily prevented.

Hemodialysis Versus Continuous Arteriovenous Hemofiltration

Several mechanisms differentiate CAVH from traditional diffusion dialysis. The first important distinction is the driving force behind the two systems. Continuous arteriovenous hemofiltration is powered by the patient's blood pressure. Solute removal, which occurs by convective transfer, is dependent on the volume of plasma water filtered. On the other hand, a blood pump is necessary for hemodialysis. Solute removal, which occurs by diffusive transport, is dependent on the solute gradient between the blood and the dialysate bath.

Another major difference between the two systems is the direction of water and solute movement as they are removed from the vascular space. With CAVH, as plasma water and solutes are removed, they are quickly replaced by interstitial and cellular constituents. The osmolality of the vascular space remains virtually unchanged. Conversely, with diffusion dialysis, solutes are preferentially removed from the vascular space. Cells become hypertonic compared to the extracellular fluid, thus producing a disequilibrium state. Water consequently moves into the cells and decreases vascular volume. This mechanism, in part, may be responsible for the hemodynamic instability brought by hemodialysis.[69]

Filter membranes used with CAVH are different than those used in hemodialysis. Continuous arteriovenous hemofiltration uses synthetic membranes that are more fragile, porous and more biocompatible than those used in hemodialysis. Hypoxia also occurs with most hemodialysis membranes. Leukocyte and total hemolytic complement values were preserved with CAVH membranes while there was a decrease in leukocyte and platelet counts with certain hemodialysis membranes.[70,71]

Difference in filter membrane material also affects solute removal. Removal of middle molecular weight solutes is greater with CAVH than with hemodialysis.

Management of renal failure in the postoperative open heart patient is very complex. Long cardiopulmonary bypass, low cardiac output with massive utilization of vasoactive drugs (levophed), and borderline renal function in the preoperative period predispose to this untoward event. Use of $NaHCO_3$, $CaCl_2$, kayexalate, and glucose and insulin all have their limitations; sodium bicarbonate produces hypotension and may induce pulmonary edema; $CaCl_2$ usually exacerbates digitalis toxicity.

The main advantage of hemodialysis is its efficiency between 10 and 20 times that of peritoneal dialysis and slow continuous hemofiltration. Treatment times can, therefore, be kept short, and the patient is free to be mobilized and undergo other therapeutic or diagnostic procedures. The main disadvantages are the cardiovascular effects, particularly hypotension, that occur in 10% to 50% of treatments and the intermittent cell edema that to some degree seems to occur with each treatment. A relative disadvantage is the need for anticoagulation during treatment.

The main advantages of peritoneal dialysis are that no anticoagulation is needed and there is minimal effect on the cardiovascular function of the patient. The mechanical cleaning of the abdominal cavity may be an advantage in a patient with a soiled peritoneal cavity. The main disadvantages are its low efficiency, the requirement for an intact peritoneum, and the risk of peritonitis.

The main advantages of slow continuous hemofiltration are the absence of cardiovascular effects, at least early during the treatment, and the ease with which clearance can be manipulated through the use of negative pressure. The main disadvantages include its relatively low efficiency, the need for continuous anticoagulation in most patients, and possible cardiovascular complications occurring later in treatment. Most patients beginning dialysis show the greatest cardiovascular instability during the first several treatments. Early in the treatment it is better to use peritoneal dialysis or CAVH. Later, patients tend to become more stable, and intermittent hemodialysis seems more suitable.

REFERENCES

1. Anderson RJ, Linas SL, Berns AS, et al. Nonoliguric acute renal failure. *N Engl J Med* 296:1134, 1977.
2. Gabow PA, Anderson RJ, Schrier RW. Acute renal failure. *Cardiovasc Med* 2:1161, 1977.
3. Schrier RW. Acute renal failure. *Kidney Int* 15:205, 1979.
4. Abbott WM, Abel RM, Beck CH Jr, et al. Renal failure after ruptured aneurysm. *Arch Surg* 110:1110, 1975.
5. Gailiunas P Jr, Chawla R, Lazarus JM, et al. Acute renal failure following cardiac operations. *J Thorac Cardiovasc Surg* 79:241-243, 1980.
6. Hilberman M, Myers BD, Carrie BJ, et al. Acute renal failure following cardiac surgery. *J Thorac Cardiovasc Surg* 77:880-888, 1979.
7. Abel RM, Buckley MJ, Austen WG, et al. Etiology, incidence, and prognosis of renal failure following cardiac operations. *J Thorac Cardiovasc Surg* 71:323, 1976.
8. Hilberman M, Myers BD, Carrie BJ, et al. Acute renal failure following cardiac surgery. *J Thorac Cardiovasc Surg* 77:881, 1979.
9. Kron IL, Joob AW, Van Meter C. Acute renal failure in the cardiovascular surgical patient. *Ann Thorac Surg* 39:590-598, 1985.
10. Davis RF, Lappas DG, Kirklin JK, et al. Acute oliguria after cardiopulmonary bypass: renal functional improvement with low dose dopamine infusion. *Crit Care Med* 10:852-856, 1982.
11. Engelman RM, Gouge TH, Smith SJ, et al. The effect of diuretics on renal hemodynamics during cardiopulmonary bypass. *J Surg Res* 16:268-276, 1974.
12. Lawson DH, Macadam RF, Singh H, et al. Effect of furosemide and antibiotic induced renal damage in rats. *J Infect Dis* 126:593-600, 1972.
13. Lindner A, Cutler RE, Goodman WG. Synergism of dopamine plus furosemide in preventing acute renal failure in the dog. *Kidney Int* 16:158-166, 1979.
14. Reese GN, Appel SH. Neurologic complications of renal failure. *Semin Nephrol* 1:137-150, 1981.
15. Kleinknecht D, Junger P, Chanard J, et al. Uremic and non-uremic complications in acute renal failure: evaluation of early and frequent dialysis on prognosis. *Kidney Int* 1:190, 1972.
16. Wathen R, Keshaviah P, Hommeyer P, et al. Role of dialysate glucose in preventing gluconeogenesis during hemodialysis. *Trans Am Soc Artif Intern Organs* 23:393, 1977.

17. Leski M, Niethammer T, Wyss T. Glucose-enriched dialysate and tolerance to maintenance hemodialysis. *Nephron* 24:271, 1979.
18. Rodrigo F, Shideman J, McHugh R, et al. Osmolality changes during hemodialysis. Natural history, clinical correlations, and influence of dialysate glucose and intravenous mannitol. *Ann Intern Med* 86:554, 1977.
19. Kjellstrand CM, Pru C, Borges H. Acetate versus bicarbonate dialysis: a review of biochemical and clinical side effects. *Controv Nephrol* 3:92, 1981.
20. Barcenas CG, Olivero J, Ayus J. Bicarbonate dialysis is hemodynamically superior to acetate dialysis (abstracts). *Am Soc Nephrol* 14:11A, 1979.
21. Raja RM, Henriquez M, Kramer MS, et al. Improved dialysis tolerance using Redy sorbent system with bicarbonate dialysate in critically ill patients. *Dial Transplant* 8:241, 1979.
22. Ayus JC, Olivero JJ, Adrogue HJ. Alkalemia associated with renal failure. *Arch Intern Med* 140:513, 1980.
23. Swartz RD, Port FK. Preventing hemorrhage in high-risk hemodialysis: regional versus low-dose heparin. *Kidney Int* 16:513: 1979.
24. Pinnich RV, Wiegmann TB, Diederich DA. Regional citrate anticoagulation for hemodialysis in the patient at high risk for bleeding. *N Engl J Med* 308:258, 1983.
25. Turney JH, Williams LC, Fewell MR, et al. Use of prostacyclin in regular dialysis therapy. *Proc Eur Dial Trans Assoc* 17:318, 1980.
26. Turney JH, Williams LC, Fewell MR, et al. Platelet protection and heparin sparing with prostacyclin during regular dialysis therapy. *Lancet* 2:291, 1980.
27. Woods HF, Ash G, Weston MJ, et al. Prostacyclin can replace heparin in haemodialysis in dogs. *Lancet* 2:1075, 1978.
28. Reese GN, Appel SH. Neurologic complications of renal failure. *Semin Nephrol* 1:137-150, 1981.
29. Kjellstrand CM. Controversies and issues for future renal substitute therapy: sodium, acetate and bicarbonate. *Jpn J Artif Organs* 12:732, 1983.
30. Kjellstrand CM, Rosa AA, Shideman JR. Hypotension during hemodialysis: osmolality fall is an important pathogenetic factor. *ASAIO J* 3:11, 1980.
31. Kjellstrand CM, Evans RL, Petersen RJ, et al. The "unphysiology" of dialysis: a major cause of dialysis side effects? *Kidney Int* 7:S30, 1975.
32. Leithner C, Sinzinger H, Stummvoll HK, et al. Enhanced 6-OXO-PGF_{1a} levels in plasma during hemodialysis. *Prostaglandins Med* 5:425, 1980.
33. Korchik WP, DeMaster EG, Brown DC. Plasma norepinephrine and hemodialysis. *Kidney Int* 12:484, 1977.
34. Korchik WP, Brown DC, DeMaster EG. Hemodialysis induced hypotension. *Int J Artif Organs* 1:5, 1978.
35. Chen WT, Ing TS, Daugirdas JT, et al. Hydrostatic ultrafiltration during hemodialysis using decreasing sodium dialysate. *Artif Organs* 4:187, 1980.

36. Maierhofer W, Maymon HL, Woods MP, et al. Hypoxemia during hemodialysis: effects of hourly changes in bath composition. *Am Soc Nephrol* 14:46A, 1981.
37. Wehle B, Asaba H, Castenfors J, et al. The influence of dialysis fluid composition on the blood pressure response during dialysis. *Clin Nephrol* 12:62, 1978.
38. Marty AT. Hyperonocotic albumin therapy. *Surg Gynecol Obstet* 139:105, 1974.
39. Romaldini H, Rodriguez-Roisin R, Lopez FA, et al. The mechanisms of arterial hypoxemia during hemodialysis. *Am Rev Respir Dis* 129:780-784, 1984.
40. Maierhofer W, Maynon HL, Woods MP. Hypoxemia during hemodialysis: effects of hourly changes in both compositions. *Am Soc Nephrol* 14:46A, 1981.
41. Lynch RE, Bosl RH, Streifel AJ, et al. Dialysis thrombocytopenia: parallel plate vs hollow fiber dialyzer. *Trans Am Soc Aftif Inter Organs* 24:704, 1978.
42. MacGrigor RR. Granulocyte adherence changes induced by hemodialysis, endotoxin, epinephrine, and glucocorticoids. *Ann Intern Med* 86:35, 1977.
43. Hakim RM, Breillatt J, Lazarus JM, et al. Complement activation and hypersensitivity reactions to dialysis membranes. *N Engl J Med* 311:878, 1984.
44. Hakim RM, Fearon DT, Lazarus JM, et al. Biocompatibility of dialysis membranes: effects of chronic complement activation. *Kidney Int* 26:194, 1984.
45. Rubin J, Nolph KD, Argahnia D, et al. Comparison of the effects of lactate and acetate on clinical peritoneal clearances. *Clin Nephrol* 12:145, 1979.
46. Rubin J, Adair C, Johnson B, et al. Stereo specific lactate absorption during peritoneal dialysis. *Nephron* 31:224, 1982.
47. Rubin J, Kirchner K, Bower J. Evaluation of stagnant fluid films during simulated peritoneal dialysis: in-vitro and in-vivo studies. *Clin Exp Dial Aphersis* 5:285, 1981.
48. Slingeneyer A, Canaud B, Mion C. Permanent loss of ultrafiltration capacity of the peritoneum in long-term peritoneal dialysis: An epidemiological study. *Nephron* 33:133, 1983.
49. Gahndi VC, Humayun JM, Ing TS, et al. Sclerotic thickening of the peritoneal membrane in maintenance peritoneal dialysis patients. *Arch Intern Med* 140:1201, 1980.
50. Gahndi VC, Ing TS, Daugirdas JT, et al. Failure of peritoneal dialysis due to peritoneal sclerosis (letter). *Am J Artif Organs* 6:97, 1983.
51. Nolph KD, Sorkin MI. The peritoneal dialysis system. In: Nolph KD, ed. *Peritoneal Dialysis*. The Hague: Maftinus Nijhoff; 1981.
52. Nolph KD, Ghods AJ, Brown P, et al. Factors affecting peritoneal dialysis efficiency. *Dial Transpl* 652, 1977.

53. Nolph KD, Ghods AJ, Brown PA, et al. Effects of intraperitoneal nitroprusside on peritoneal clearances with variations in dose, frequency of administration, and dwell times. *Nephron* 24:114, 1979.
54. Nolph KD, Stoltz M, Maher JF. Altered peritoneal permeability in patients with systemic vasculatis. *Ann Intern Med* 78:891, 1973.
55. Nolph KD, Miller L, Husted FC, et al. Effects of intraperitoneal isoproterenol on reduced peritoneal clearances in patients with systemic vascular disease. *J Int Urol Nephrol* 8:161, 1976.
56. Gross M, McDonald HP Jr. Effects of dialysate temperature and flow rate on peritoneal clearance. *J Am Med Assoc* 202:215, 1967.
57. Knochel JP, Mason AD. Effects of alkalinization on peritoneal diffusion of uric acid. *Am J Physiol* 210:1160, 1966.
58. Cole DEC, Lirenman DS. Role of albumin enriched peritoneal dialysate in acute copper poisoning. *J Pediatr* 92:955, 1978.
59. DeSanto NG,Capodicassa G,Capasso G,et al. Development of means to augment peritoneal urea clearances: the synergistic effects of combining high dialysate temperature and high: dialysate flow rates with dextro and nitroprusside. *Artif Organs* 5:409, 1981.
60. Nolph KD, Popovich RP, Ghods AJ,et al. Determinants of low clearances of small solutes during peritoneal dialysis. *Kidney Int* 13:117, 1978.
61. Silverstein ME, Ford CA, Lysaght MT, et al. Treatment of severe fluid overload by ultrafiltration. *N Engl J Med* 291:747-751, 1974.
62. Kaplan AA, Longnecker RE, Folker VW. Continuous arterio-venous hemofiltration. a report of six months experience. *8Ann Intern Med* 100:358-367, 1984.
63. Maguire WC, Anderson RJ. Continuous arteriovenous hemofiltration in the intensive care unit. *J Crit Care* 1:54-56, 1986.
64. Lauer A, Saccaggi A, Rosco C, et al. Continuous hemofiltration in the critically ill patient. *Ann Intern Med* 99:454-460, 1983.
65. Olbricht C, Mueller C, Schurek HJ, et al. Treatment of acute renal failure in patients with multiple organ failure by continuous spontaneous hemofiltration. *Trans Am Soc Artif Intern Organs* 28:33-37, 1982.
66. Prough DS, Adams L. Physiologic effects of dialysis and ultrafiltration. *ASA Refresher Courses Anesthesiol* 14:185-198, 1986.
67. Maher JF, Schreiner GE. Hazards and complications of dialysis. *N Engl J Med* 273:370-377, 1965.
68. Lawson DH, Macadam RF, Singh H, et al. Effect of furosemide and antibiotic induced renal damage in rats. *J Infect Di* 126:593-600, 1972.
69. Schuenermann B, Borghardt J, Falda Z, etal. Reactions of blood pressure and body spaces to hemofiltration treatment. *Trans Am Soc Artif Intern Organs* 24:687, 1978.
70. Jacob AI, Gravellas G, Zarco R, et al. Leukopenia hypoxia and complement function with different hemodialysis membranes. *Kidney Int* 18:505, 1980.
71. Bohler J, Kramer P, Goltze O, et al. Leukocyte counts and complement activation during pump-driven and arteriovenous haemofiltration. *Contrib Nephrol* 36:15, 1983.

Chapter 10

Neurological Complications Following Open Heart Surgery

Andrew Karlin, MD

Neurological and psychological complications of heart surgery and cardiopulmonary bypass (CPB) have been reported for more than 35 years.[1,2] Their reported incidence varies from 0% to 100% depending upon the criteria used and the frequency and timing of postoperative examinations.[3,4]

Most post-CPB neurological and psychological deficits appear to be due to focal damage caused by hypoperfusion or embolic events,[5] although other etiologies are common (Table I). That is,

Table I
Etiologies of Neurological Complications of Cardiopulmonary Bypass

Emboli
Hypoperfusion
Hypoxia
Cerebrovascular disease
Metabolic encephalopathy

From Casthely PA, Bregman D, (eds): *Cardiopulmonary Bypass: Physiology, Related Complications, and Pharmacology.* Mount Kisco, NY, Futura Publishing Company, Inc., © 1991.

Table II
Neurological Complications Following Cardiopulmonary Bypass[6]

Complication	*Incidence (%)*
Cognitive changes	30 –79
Psychiatric dysfunction	1.0–57
Abnormal reflexes	0 –40
Opthalmological abnormalities	17 –25
Depressed level of consciousness (Delayed emergence)	3.2–13
Peripheral nerve damage	2.6–13
Fatal cerebral damage	0.3– 2
Spinal cord injury	0.1– 2

except for peripheral nerve injuries and some instances of psychiatric abnormalities, these are intraoperative strokes: sudden onset central nervous system deficits lasting more than 24 hours. It is the specific manifestations of the stroke that will be discussed now, however. The nature and incidence of manifestations have been summarized in one review[6] and are presented below in Table II.

Although there is some uncertainty in comparing diagnoses in different reports, and patients often have more than one deficit, this table is a good starting point for discussion.

Cognitive Changes

"Cognition" is measured by neuropsychological tests that measure abilities such as memory, learning, and response speed. These tests are termed "psychometric." In general, investigators have shown postoperative scores deteriorating from preoperative scores, and usually, the more extensive the testing and the shorter the interval between operation and retest the more dramatic the deterioration. Also, scores tend to increase with continued retesting, although it is not clear if the increased score is due to the patient's familiarity with the test or to improved neuropsychiatric status.

Other factors cloud the results of psychometric testing. First, these tests study certain abilities, but a low score may not reflect any noticeable deficit. In the Newcastle Study for example, 123 of 235 patients whose scores had deteriorated were asymptomatic.[7] Second, in another report the patients complaining of deficits were more likely to have a depressed mood than a decreased test score.[8] These reports highlight the question of the connection between neuropsychological scores and clinical neurological deficits. The evidence conflicts, with some reporting a correlation[9–11] and others not.[12,13]

Whatever the basis of deteriorated test performance, it resolves within 6 months, according to most reports.

Psychiatric Dysfunction

The wide range of reported incidence of psychiatric dysfunction after cardiac surgery, 1.0% to 57%, is due to the wide range of definitions of psychiatric dysfunction in various reports as well as to the depth of the preoperative examination.[14] The reports of higher incidence usually include postoperative delirium along with thought, mood, and behavior disorders.

There are probably many factors contributing to postbypass psychosis and delirium. Preoperative psychiatric illness[15] and personality type may play a role.[16] Several investigators have found associations between postoperative delirium and preoperative organic brain disease and physical state.[17–19] Two studies have shown a lower incidence of delirium in coronary artery bypass surgery than in valve surgery,[20,21] implying that intraoperative focal neurological damage from emboli may play a role in postoperative delirium.[9,22] On the other hand, delirium after cardiac surgery usually occurs after 2 days of lucidity,[23] therefore, perhaps sleep deprivation and the ICU environment are responsible for inducing delirium in some patients.[15,16]

Abnormal Reflexes

One large study found that about 39% of post-CPB patients demonstrated primitive and abnormal reflexes. The authors felt that these findings might reflect mild cerebral injury, especially because there was a correlation with both stroke and depressed level of consciousness.[7] It is difficult to interpret the significance of abnormal reflexes in an otherwise normal patient.

Ophthalmological Abnormalities

Visual problems are not uncommon, if carefully sought. Their source are often emboli in vessels of the retina,[24,25] optic nerve,[26] and cerebral cortex.[27] The prognosis for these injuries is usually good.

Stroke and Spinal Cord Injury

The reported incidence of stroke varies with the nature of both the study and of the surgery. Prospective studies report a rate of about 5%,[7,28] whereas retrospective studies report a rate of less than 1%.[29,30] Valve procedures seem to put the patient at higher risk than coronary artery bypass graft surgery,[11,31] although not all studies confirm this.

Spinal cord injury appears to be an unusual complication of CPB. One series of patients undergoing valve surgery reported postoperative spinal injury in one patient of one hundred,[11] whereas another reported injury in 1 of 1,427 patients.[30] In addition to CPB, intra-aortic balloon counterpulsation may cause spinal cord infarction.[32–34]

Delayed Emergence and Fatal Cerebral Damage

Delayed emergence from anesthesia unrelated to sedative drugs is reported with a widely varying incidence, 3.2% to 13%. A Cleveland Clinic report of over 12,000 bypass procedures found that postoperative nonmetabolic coma was rare and that the prognosis was poor, with a mortality of 85%. Only 1 of 34 comatose patients had functional neurological recovery. In this report, coma was caused by global ischemia in 20% of patients, hemispheric infarction with herniation in 15%, and multiple cerebral infarcts in 9%. The etiology of the remaining 56% was unknown.[35] Another study looking at 214 patients who died after CPB found a triad of focal hemorrhage, acute neuronal necrosis, and emboli; however, the time in the postoperative course and the cause of death were not given.[36]

Peripheral Nerve Damage

The Newcastle study reported peripheral nerve damage in 12% of their patients,[7] however, one of the authors later noted that "many of the problems would not have been detected without systematic and detailed postoperative neurological assessment."[6] In general, upper extremity nerve injuries are more common than lower extremity or phrenic nerve injuries. Of the upper extremity nerves, the most common site of injury is the brachial plexus.[37,38] Intercostal nerve damage is also not uncommon. The mechanism of brachial plexus and intercostal nerve injury is not certain, but sternal retraction causing stretching of the nerves,[39] or trauma by a first rib fractured during sternal retraction[40] or by a needle during internal jugular vein catherization,[41] have all been proposed.

The phrenic nerve may also be injured during CPB and surgery, presumably by local hypothermia induced for myocardial preservation and by trauma during excision of the internal mammary artery.

The etiology of other peripheral neuropathies is even less clear, although both trauma and position-induced stretch and compression injuries are likely causes.

Risk Factors

Some risk factors for neurological injury cannot be changed. The patient's age is significant in many studies.[22,42–47] A history of neurologic disease may also put the patient at higher risk.[9,11,43]

The nature of the surgery itself may also be a risk factor. Valve surgery may be a higher risk than coronary bypass surgery;[47] mitral valve surgery may be a higher risk than aortic valve surgery;[11] and multiple valve surgery may be a higher risk than single-valve surgery.[10,11]

Ironically, two factors subject to a high level of control are also subject to the most controversy: (1) pump flows and mean arterial pressures, and (2) carbon dioxide tension. Arguments both for low pressures, from 30 to 50 mm Hg,[48] and for high pressures above 50 mm Hg[49] have been presented recently. Flow rate is also the subject of some debate, but both of the above papers recommend a flow of at least 1.5 L/min/m^2. Some institutions, however, still adhere to higher flows, 2.0–2.4 L/min/m^2, which were established for CPB in the 1950s.[50]

The importance of carbon dioxide in controlling cerebral blood flow is well known,[51] and CO_2 tension is easily controlled during CPB. The measurement of carbon dioxide and pH, however, have been much debated recently. Essentially, one school of thought argues that pH and blood gas values should be temperature corrected, termed "pH stat,"[52] while the other argues that they should not be temperature corrected, termed "α-stat".[53] At the present time, both methods are widely used and there are no clear data supporting one method over the other.

Lastly, the one risk factor that seems widely accepted is the duration of CPB,[9–12,22,36,43,44] with 2 hours generally reported as the threshold for increased neurologic damage.

Mechanisms of Injury and Their Modification

Emboli, both large and microscopic, are commonly considered the major cause of neurological deficit. Macroemboli can come from heart valves[22] and atheromata.[54] Large air emboli are uncommon,[55] which is somewhat surprising when all the possible sources are considered. Air may enter the system from the reservoir if the blood level is allowed to fall; if the tubing or pump direction is reversed; if there is unexpected resumption of ventricular contractions; if the heart chambers are inadequately vented of air; if deep suction is used in the pulmonary artery; and from the oxygenator if it is not airtight.

Embolization of small particles of plastic and antifoaming agents as well as thrombus, aggregated platelets, and small air bubbles into the arterial line has been noted for many years.[25,56] The clinical efficacy of arterial line filters, even Dacron wool, in reducing these microemboli has also long been noted.[36] In one study in dogs, for example, it was shown that the intra-bypass release of brain enzymes was greatly decreased when a 40 μm filter was placed in the arterial line.[57] Furthermore, their use seems virtually free of complications.[58] Interestingly, smaller pore filters may yield no additional benefit. Two studies from different groups, one using a 25-μm nylon filter,[59] and the other a 20-μm nylon filter,[60] showed the same or poorer neurologic outcome compared to 40-μm polyester filter.

A second strategy for reducing embolic neurological damage is based on oxygenator design. A membrane oxygenator may cause far fewer emboli than a bubble oxygenator.[61]

The last approach to protecting the brain from ischemia due to emboli and hypoperfusion has been to reduce its demand for oxygen ($CMRO_2$). Hypothermia appears to the most commonly used means of reducing $CMRO_2$ during CPB.[62] Cooling the brain causes a slowing of biochemical processes, thus both the energy needed to maintain cellular integrity, 40%–50% of the total $CMRO_2$, and the energy needed to maintain electrical activity, 50%–60% of the total $CMRO_2$, are decreased. The decrease in energy used is expressed as the Q_{10}, which is the ratio of CMROs after a cooling of 10 °C has occurred. When electrical activity is present in the brain, the Q_{10} between 28 °C and 18 °C is about 5.[63] But when cerebral electrical activity has been suppressed prior to inducing hypothermia, say by barbiturates, the Q_{10} is less, 2.1–2.4.[63]

With these facts as a background, the role of barbiturates and other drugs that suppress cerebral electrical activity may be better understood. In 1982, a large study looked for a cerebral protective effect of barbiturates during coronary artery bypass grafts placed during normothermic CPB.[46] No protective effect was found, but this is a relatively low-risk procedure. In 1986 a similar study was performed on patients undergoing open heart surgery (which is a higher risk procedure) during normothermic CPB, and a protective effect was found.[31]

In this last study, the barbiturates were titrated to isoelectric electroencephalogram (EEG) tracings. However, no one has yet shown that administering barbiturates in doses that do not achieve EEG isoelectricity is protective, nor has anyone shown that administering barbiturates during hypothermic CPB yields more protection than hypothermia alone. It should be pointed out that in the above study the use of barbiturates in doses sufficient to cause isoelectricity, an average dose of 39.5 mg/kg, caused clinically significant difficulties when coming off bypass.

The general problem of cerebral protection from ischemia has led to the investigation of other drugs, but their use during CPB is speculative. Nimodipine, a calcium blocker,[64,65] excitatory amino acid inhibitors,[66,67] and phenytoin,[68] all fall into this category.

Other mechanisms have been reported but are not well explained. Both intra-aortic balloon pumps and massive doses of vasopressors significantly correlate with postoperative encephalopathy, although brain isoemzymes, a marker of organic damage, did not correlate with the degree of encephalopathy.

Diagnosis and Treatment

A full discussion of diagnosis of all the complications associated with CPB is beyond the scope of this chapter. However, some points should be made. Determining the etiology of the deficit, mental or psychiatric versus organic, requires:

(1) A review of the patient's psychiatric and medical history. This must include mental disease, drug and alcohol use, and cerebrovascular disease. All perioperative drugs and their time of administration should be noted.
(2) A physical examination. Although gross neurological abnormalities may help form a diagnosis, primitive, abnormal, or asymmetric reflexes can occur immediately after general anesthesia in patients who will show no neurological deficits after full emergence. Also, global derangements, such as hypoglycemia, may produce focal signs.
(3) Laboratory studies. Serum sodium, potassium, chloride, blood urea nitrogen, calcium, and magnesium concentrations should be normal. An arterial blood gas is also needed.
(4) A consultation with a neurologist or neurosurgeon. The patient can require special diagnostic procedures with which the neurologist or neurosurgeon is probably

more familiar than either the cardiac surgeon or anesthesiologist.

If the patient has a new mental or psychological disorder postoperatively, hyper- and hypoglycemia, drug and alcohol withdrawal, and lidocaine toxicity should be considered in the differential diagnosis. Fever, sepsis, and uremia can also cause neuropsychiatric dysfunction, but these usually do not occur in the immediate postoperative period. If the above investigations are all normal, a psychiatrist should be consulted. If, however, a focal deficit is found, emergency computed tomography (CT) will help diagnose an ischemic, hemorrhagic, or other etiology. An ischemic stroke may not appear on CT for some time after the event. Doppler flow studies and angiography can help both make the diagnosis and locate the lesion. Ordinarily, if a thrombotic embolism appears to have caused a stroke, a patient receives anticoagulants; however, this can be impossible in the immediate postoperative period.

If physical examination reveals global deficits, the three most likely causes are prolonged drug effects, encephalopathy, and coma.[69] Of the anesthetic drugs commonly used during cardiac surgery, narcotics, benzodiazepines, and muscle relaxants are probably the most likely to have prolonged effects. Postoperative encephalopathy has many causes. Some common causes more specific to the cardiac surgery patient are ischemia, hypoxia, hypo- and hypercalcemia, and hypothermia. Other causes that may occur later in the postoperative course are sepsis, uremia, hyperosmolar syndrome, and endocrine diseases that may be a consequence of or exacerbated by CPB.

Coma implies absence of recovery from anesthesia. If prolonged drug effects, encephalopathies, and focal lesions having global effects are ruled out of the diagnosis, then supportive medical management should be given. As mentioned above, the prognosis is poor.

Conclusion

Neurological deficits after CPB are common, but are usually mild and often so subtle that they are found only after careful pre- and postoperative examinations. Serious deficits are uncommon, but have a poor prognosis. To date, no drug has been shown to increase or surpass the cerebral protection of hypothermia.

REFERENCES

1. Fox HM, Rizzo ND, Gifford S. Psychological observations of patients undergoing mitral surgery. *Psychosom Med* 16:186; 1954.
2. Torres F, Frank GS, Cohen M, et al. Neurological and electroencephalographic studies in open-heart surgery. *Neurology* 9:174; 1959.
3. Sachdev NS, Carter CC, Swank RL, et al. Relationship between post-cardiotomy delirium, clinical neurological changes and EEG abnormalities. *J Thorac Cardiovasc Surg* 54:557; 1967.
4. Frank KA, Heller SS, Kornfeld SS, et al. Long term effects of open-heart surgery on intellectual functioning. *J Thorac Cardiovasc Surg* 64:811; 1972.
5. Taylor KM. Brain damage during open-heart surgery. *Thorax* 37:873; 1982.
6. Shaw PJ. Neurological complications of cardiovascular surgery: II. Procedures involving the heart and thoracic aorta. *Int Anesth Clin* 24:159; 1986.
7. Shaw PJ, Bates D, Cartlidge NEF, et al. Early neurological complications of coronary artery bypass surgery. *Br Med J* 291:1384; 1985.
8. Newman S, Klinger L, Venn G, et al. Subjective reports of cognition in relation to assessing cognitive performance following coronary artery bypass surgery. *J Psychosom Res* 33:227; 1989.
9. Tufo HM, Ostfeld AM, Shekelle R. Central nervous system dysfunction following open-heart surgery. *J Am Med Assoc* 212:1333; 1970.
10. Aberg T, Kihlgren M. Effect of open-heart surgery on intellectual function. *Scand J Thorac Cardiovasc Surg* 15(Suppl):1; 1974.
11. Sotaniemi KA. Brain damage and neurological outcome after open-heart surgery. *J Neurol Neurosurg Psychiatry* 43:127; 1980.
12. Lee WH, Miller W, Rowe J, et al. Effects of extracorporeal circulation on personality and cerebration. *Ann Thorac Surg* 7:562; 1969.
13. Juolasmaa A, Outakoski J, Hirvenoja R, et al. Effect of open-heart surgery on intellectual performance. *J Clin Neuropsychol* 3:181; 1981.
14. Adrian J, Crankshaw DP, Tiller JW, et al. Affective, cognitive and subjective changes in patients undergoing cardiac surgery—a preliminary report. *Anaesth Intensive Care* 16:144; 1988.
15. Sveinsson IS. Post-operative psychosis after heart surgery. *J Thorac Cardiovasc Surg* 70:117; 1975.
16. Kornfeld DS, Heller SS, Frank KAO, et al. Personality and psychological factors in post-cardiotomy delirium. *Arch Gen Psychiatry* 31:249; 1974.
17. Blachly PH, Starr A. Post-cardiotomy delirium. *Am J of Psychiatry* 121:371; 1964.

18. Edgerton N, Kay JH. Psychological disturbances associated with open-heart surgery. *Clev Clin Q* 48:205; 1981.
19. Rubinstein D, Thomas JK. Psychiatric findings in cardiotomy patients. *Am J Psychiatry* 126:108; 1969.
20. Rabiner CJ, Wilner AE, Fishman J. Psychiatric complications following coronary bypass surgery. *J Nerv Ment Dis* 160:342; 1975.
21. Wilner AE, Rabiner CJ, Wisoff GB, et al. Analogical reasoning and post-operative outcome. *Arch Gen Psychiatry* 33:255; 1976.
22. Gilman S. Cerebral disorders after open-heart operations. *N Engl J Med* 272:489; 1965.
23. Yate PM, Holt GM. Psychological responses to anaesthesia. In: Taylor HT, and Major E, eds., *Hazards and Complications of Anaesthesia.* London; Churchill Livingstone; 1986:50.
24. Williams IM. Intravascular changes in the retina during open-heart surgery. *Lancet* ii:688, 1971.
25. Williams IM. Retinal vascular occlusions in open-heart surgery. *Br J Ophthalmol* 59:81; 1975.
26. Sweeny PJ, Breuer AC, Selhorst JB, et al. Ischemic optic neuropathy: a complication of cardiopulmonary bypass surgery. *Neurology* 32:560; 1982.
27. Ross Russell RW, Bharucha N. The recognition and prevention of border zone cerebral ischemia during cardiac surgery. *J Med* 47:303; 1978.
28. Breuer AC, Furlan AJ, Hanson MR. Central nervous system complications of coronary artery bypass graft surgery: prospective analysis of 421 patients. *Stroke* 14:682; 1983.
29. Lee MC, Geiger J, Nicoloff D, et al. Cerebrovascular complications associated with coronary artery bypass (CAB) procedure. *Stroke* 10:107; 1979.
30. Gonzales-Scarano F, Hurtig HI. Neurological complications of coronary artery bypass grafting: case control study. *Neurology (NY)* 31:1032; 1981.
31. Nussmeier NA, Arlund C, Slogoff S. Neuropsychiatric complications after cardiopulmonary bypass. *Anesthesiology* 64:165; 1986.
32. Cleveland JC, Lefemine AA, Mardoff I, et al. The role of intra-aortic balloon counterpulsation in patients undergoing cardiac operations. *Ann Thorac Surg* 20:652, 1975.
33. Rose DM, Jacobwitz, IJ, Acinapura AJ, et al. Paraplegia following percutaneous insertion of an intra-aortic balloon. *J Thorac Cardiovasc Surg* 87:788; 1984.
34. Harris RE, Reimer KA, Crain BJ, et al. Spinal cord infarction following intra-aortic balloon support. *Ann Thorac Surg* 42:206; 1986.
35. Furlan AJ, Breuer AC. Central nervous system complications of open-heart surgery. *Stroke* 15:912; 1984.
36. Aguilar MJ, Gerbode F, Hill JD. Neuropathologic complications of cardiac surgery. *J Thorac Cardiovasc Surg* 61:676; 1971.
37. Morin JE, Long R, Elleher MG, et al. Upper extremity neuropathies following median sternotomy. *Ann Thorac Surg* 34:181; 1982.

38. Lederman RJ, Breuer AC, Hanson MR, et al. Peripheral nervous system complications of coronary artery bypass graft surgery. *Ann Neurol* 12:297; 1982.
39. Kirsh MM, Magee KR, Gago O, et al. Brachial plexus injury following median sternotomy incision. *Ann Thorac Surg* 11:315; 1971.
40. Vander Salm TJ, Cereda JM, Cutler BS. Brachial plexus injury following median sternotomy. *J Thorac Cardiovasc Surg* 80:447; 1980.
41. Hanson MR, Breuer AC, Furlan AJ, et al. Mechanism and frequency of brachial plexus injury in open-heart surgery: a prospective analysis. *Ann Thorac Surg* 36:675; 1983.
42. Javid H, Tufo HM, Najafi H, et al. Neurological abnormalities following open-heart surgery. *J Thorac Cardiovasc Surg* 58:502; 1968.
43. Branthwaite MA. Neurological damage related to open-heart surgery. *Thorax* 27:748; 1972.
44. Savageau JA, Stanton BA, Jenkins CD, et al. Neuro-psychological dysfunction following elective cardiac operation: I. Early assessment. *J Thorac Cardiovasc Surg* 84:585; 1982.
45. Savageau JA, Stanton BA, Jenkins CD, et al. Neuro-psychological dysfunction following elective cardiac operation: II. A six month reassessment. *J Thorac Cardiovasc Surg* 84:585; 1982.
46. Slogoff S, Girgis KZ, Keats AS. Etiologic factors in neuro-psychiatric complications associated with cardiopulmonary bypass. *Anesth Analg* 61:903; 1982.
47. Kolkka R, Hilberman M. Neurologic dysfunction following cardiac operation with low-flow, low pressure cardiopulmonary bypass. *J Thorac Cardiovasc Surg* 79:432; 1980.
48. Reeves JG, Govier A, Croughwell N. Low pressure during cardiopulmonary bypass is preferable. In: Fyman P, Gotta AW, eds., *Controversies in Cardiovascular Anesthesia.* Boston, MA: Kluwer Academic Publishers; 1988:90.
49. Shevde K, Mylavarapu S. High pump flows are desirable during cardiopulmonary bypass. In: Fyman P, Gotta AW, eds., *Controversies in Cardiovascular Anesthesia.* Boston, MA: Kluwer Academic Publishers; 1988:53.
50. Kirklin JW, Dushane JW, Patrick RT, et al. Intracardiac surgery with the aid of a mechanical pump-oxygenator system (Gibbon-type): report of eight cases. *Proc Mayo Clin* 30:201; 1955.
51. Michenfelder JD. Cerebral blood flow and metabolism. In: Cucchiara RF, Michenfelder JD, eds., *Clinical Neuroanesthesia.* New York, NY: Churchill Livingstone; 1990:120.
52. Camporesi EM, Moon RE. Blood gas values should be corrected for body temperature during hypothermia. In: Fyman P, Gotta AW, eds., *Controversies in Cardiovascular Anesthesia.* Boston, MA: Kluwer Academic Publishers; 1988:30.
53. Goldiner PL, Oka Y, Svadjian E. Blood gases should not be temperature corrected during hypothermia. In: Fyman P, Gotta AW, eds., *Controversies in Cardiovascular Anesthesia.* Boston, MA: Kluwer Academic Publishers; 1988:55.

54. McKibbon DW, Bulkley BH, Green WR, et al. Fatal cerebral atheromatous embolization after cardiopulmonary bypass. *J Thorac Cardiovasc Surg* 71:741; 1976.
55. Stoney WS, Alford WC, Burrus GR, et al. Air embolism and other accidents using pump oxygenators. *Ann Thorac Surg* 29:336; 1979.
56. Pearson DT, Carter RF, Hammo MB, et al. Gaseous microemboli during open-heart surgery. In: Longmore DB, ed. *Towards Safer Cardiac Surgery.* Lancaster, PA: MTP Press; 1981:90.
57. Taylor KM, Devlin BJ, Mittra SM, et al. Assessment of cerebral experimental model. *Scand J Thorac Cardiovasc Surg* 14:197; 1980.
58. Miller, Jr., DW, Binford JM, Hessel EA. Results of a survey of the professional activities of 811 cardiopulmonary perfusionists. *J Thorac Cardiovasc Surg* 83:385; 1982.
59. Wilner AE, Caramente LL, Garvey JW, et al. The relationship between arterial filtration during open-heart surgery and mental abstraction ability. *Proc Am Acad Cardiovasc Perf* 4:56; 1983.
60. Aris A, Solanes H, Camara ML, et al. Arterial line filtration during cardiopulmonary bypass. *J Thorac Cardiovasc Surg* 91:526; 1986.
61. Smith PLC. Interventions to reduce cerebral injury during cardiac surgery—introduction and the effect of oxygenator type. *Perfusion* 4:139; 1989.
62. Gisvold SE, Steen PA. Drug therapy in brain ischemia. *Br J Anaesth* 57:96; 1985.
63. Steen PA, Newberg LA, Milde JH. Hypothermia and barbiturates: individual and combined effects on canine cerebral oxygen consumption. *Anesthesiology* 58:527; 1983.
64. Steen PA, Newberg LA, Milde JH. Nimodipine improves cerebral blood flow and neurologic recovery after complete ischemia in the dog. *J Cereb Blood Flow Metab* 3:38; 1983.
65. Steen PA, Newberg LA, Milde JH. Cerebral blood flow and neurologic outcome when nimodipine is given after complete cerebral ischemia in the dog. *J Cereb Blood Flow Metab* 4:82; 1984.
66. Duverger D, Benavides J, Cudennec A, et al. A glutamate antagonist reduces infarction size following focal cerebral ischemia independently of vascular and metabolic changes. *J Cereb Blood Flow Metab* 7[Suppl]:S144; 1987.
67. Swan JH, Evans MC, Meldrum BS. Ischemic brain damage: protection by 2-chloroadenosine, a modulator of excitatory neurotransmission. *J Cereb Blood Flow Metab* 7[Suppl]:S146; 1987.
68. Artru AA, Michenfelder JD. Cerebral protective, metabolic, and vascular effects of phenytoin. *Stroke* 11:377; 1980.
69. Denlinger JK. Prolonged emergence and failure to regain consciousness. In: Orkin FK, Cooperman LH, eds. *Complications of Anesthesiology.* Philadelphia, PA: JB Lippincott; 1983:368.

Chapter 11

Respiratory Complications Following Open Heart Surgery

Michael J. Given, MD
and M. Anees Khan, MD

Pulmonary complications after open heart surgery are sometimes serious and may be life-threatening. Pulmonary complications seen most frequently include tracheobronchitis, atelectasis (segmental and lobar), pneumonia, and respiratory insufficiency. These complications may occur in normal patients and in many patients who are at high risk due to an underlying pulmonary or systemic disease. A vast majority of patients require little ventilatory support after cardiac surgery and are weaned from mechanical ventilation within 24 hours. There is a small percentage of patients who require prolonged ventilatory support. When possible, it is important to identify those patients who are at risk of developing pulmonary complications.[1] This may be achieved by obtaining a thorough history and physical examination and a preoperative evaluation of pulmonary function.

From Casthely PA, Bregman D, (eds): *Cardiopulmonary Bypass: Physiology, Related Complications, and Pharmacology.* Mount Kisco, NY, Futura Publishing Company, Inc., © 1991.

Preoperative Assessment

History and Physical Examination

History of past or present medical illnesses and the presence or absence of physical findings of disease are helpful in predicting the possibility of pulmonary complications. In terms of mortality, preoperative studies may help to separate the operable from inoperable patient. By taking into account the predisposing factors which are responsible for postoperative pulmonary complications, we are better able to identify potential problem areas and initiate treatment early.

Operative mortality increases in the presence of respiratory tract infection.[2] Recent fever and cough productive of purulent sputum should alert the physician that an infectious process is likely and any surgical procedure should be postponed until the respiratory infection has been properly treated.

Wheezing may indicate reversible obstructive airways disease and appropriate bronchodilator therapy should be initiated prior to surgery.

Cigarette smoking increases respiratory morbidity after cardiac surgery.[3-5] The mechanism whereby current cigarette smoking contributes to postoperative morbidity is speculative. Cigarette smoke is known to induce secretion of mucus, stimulate goblet cell hyperplasia, alter ciliary function, and cause small airways dysfunction. Cessation of smoking is encouraged prior to surgery, however the short term abstinence from smoking is not efficacious in decreasing the incidence of pulmonary problems.[6,7] After many weeks of abstinence from smoking, there is improvement in ciliary activity[8] and small airway function[9] and a reduction in the amount of mucous hypersecretion and sputum produced.[10] The combination of mucous hypersecretion and airway inflammation secondary to cigarette smoke and an impaired cough reflex secondary to incisional site pain and the use of analgesics lead to airway obstruction and atelectasis.

Morbid obesity is associated with an increased risk of complications.[11] Obesity imposes high metabolic postoperative demands on its subject. This is reflected by an increase in oxygen consumption and carbon dioxide production both at rest and during exercise.[12]

The major respiratory complications of obesity include: increased demand for ventilation; elevated work of breathing; respiratory muscle inefficiency; decreased lung and chest wall compliance; diminished functional residual capacity (FRC) and expiratory reserve volume (ERV); and high closing volume (CV) to FRC ratio that is associated with closure of peripheral lung units, ventilation-perfusion abnormalities, and hypoxemia, especially in the supine position.[12]

Obesity is associated with an increased risk of postoperative pneumonia. Patients who weighed more than 250 pounds have a significantly higher rate of pneumonia than patients who weighed less than 250 pounds.[13] These patients are susceptible to basilar atelectasis, progressive hypoxemia, and resultant infection.[14]

Nutritional assessment is an important component of every patient's preoperative evaluation.[15,16] Malnutrition is associated with impairment of respiratory muscle function, ventilatory response to hypoxia, and lung water homeostasis. Malnourished patients tend to have inspiratory and diaphragmatic muscle wasting and frequently require prolonged ventilatory support after cardiac surgery.

Pulmonary Function Tests and Arterial Blood Gas Analysis

Preoperative assessment of pulmonary function is a useful means of identifying patients who are at risk of developing postoperative pulmonary complications.

Gaensler and associates[17] used spirometry to assess the operative mortality and morbidity after surgery for pulmonary tuberculosis. The maximal breathing capacity (MBC) was identified as the single best predictor of mortality. Preoperative maximal breathing capacity of less than 50% was associated with increased morbidity and mortality.[17]

Lockwood[18] used multiple spirometric tests to separate patients into four risk categories: very low risk, low risk, high risk, and very high risk. Patients with very low risk had essentially normal pulmonary function. Patients with very high risk had severe limitation in pulmonary function ($FEV_1 < 1.2$ liters or $FEV_1\% <$ 35% predicted; maximal voluntary ventilation < 28 L/min; vital capacity (VC) < 1.85). He found it difficult to separate the two middle groups, the low-risk and high-risk patients.

Several other investigators agree that the low-risk patient will have $FEV_1 > 50\%$ predicted, MBC > 50% predicted, VC > 60% predicted, residual volume (RV) < 40% of the total lung capacity (TLC), and an arterial $PO_2 > 50$ mm Hg.[2,19,20]

Arterial blood gas analysis is frequently performed prior to surgery. Preoperative hypercapnia ($PaCO_2 > 45$ mm Hg) may indicate severe lung dysfunction with minimal pulmonary reserve and is a relative contradiction to surgery.

Preoperative arterial hypoxemia ($PaO_2 < 50$ mm Hg) with widening of the alveolar-arterial oxygen tension gradient in a patient without cardiogenic shock may be a factor for increased risk of postoperative pulmonary complications. Emergency coronary bypass for cardiogenic shock has been associated with high perioperative mortality.[21,22] These patients have a high rate of pulmonary complications. Preoperative pulmonary evaluation is usually not possible in this situation. Patients at high risk of developing pulmonary complications are not identified and preoperative medical management is not initiated.

Pathophysiologic Changes in Lung Function After Surgery

Pulmonary function deteriorates after open heart surgery. The changes in pulmonary function depend upon several factors that occur in the perioperative period. These include the location of the incision, length of anesthesia, timing of the procedure, mental status of the patient, and postoperative medications. Coronary revascularization procedures are done through a median sternotomy incision in a vast majority of cases because of the excellent exposure obtained and the reduced morbidity as compared to lateral thoracotomy.[23] Some authors believe that pulmonary function is better preserved using median sternotomy rather than anterior or lateral thoracotomy.

Postoperatively, there are significant changes in static lung volumes, gas exchange, and pattern of ventilation. The interventions likely to cause alteration in pulmonary function include: median sternotomy incision; use of extracorporeal circulation; deflating of the lungs during the ischemic period; and the dissection of the internal mammary artery (IMA) from the chest wall.

Static Lung Volumes

Patients undergoing open heart surgery develop a pulmonary restrictive pattern early in the postoperative period.[24] Lung volumes decline and a proportional reduction in expiratory flow rates is observed.[25] At discharge, with the exception of residual volume, all lung volumes may be reduced by as much as 19%-33% of preoperative values. The peak expiratory flow rate (PEFR), the only bedside test that could be measured immediately after extubation, is as low as 35% of the preoperative value. Residual lung volume is unchanged in the postoperative period. The dead space to tidal volume ratio is increased, signifying ventilation of unperfused portions of the lung and airways.[26]

Dissection of the internal mammary artery adversely affects the PEFR after surgery.[27] This may be the result of muscle weakness and chest wall pain and stiffness by IMA dissection and retractor pressure to the cartilages and ribs.

Lung volumes usually return to preoperative level within 3 months, however a mild pulmonary restrictive pattern may persist for many more months. Patients who develop wound infections may have depressed lung volumes for a greater length of time. All expiratory flow rates return to preoperative level by 3 months except for forced vital capacity (FVC) and forced expiratory volume at 1 second (FEV_1) that remain reduced.

The mechanisms causing the reduction in lung function are not well understood. Although pain and reduced chest wall compliance are the principle causative factors, total relief of pain with opiate analgesics and epidural anesthesia results in only partial restoration of vital capacity and FRC. Postoperative diaphragm dysfunction may be at least partly responsible for the low lung volumes, however, further studies are necessary to resolve this issue.[28]

Gas Exchange

Postoperatively, ventilation-perfusion mismatch develops secondary to airway narrowing and closure. The result is hypoxemia and a widening of the alveolar-arterial oxygen tension gradient.[29] Generally, there is no radiographic evidence of gross pulmonary collapse to explain the degree of intrapulmonary shunting.

The diffusion capacity (DLCO) is adversely affected by open heart surgery.[27] Postoperative values are significantly lower than predicted preoperative values. The DLCO will return to baseline at 3 months and may be greater than the preoperative value in patients who stop smoking.

Pattern of Ventilation

While breathing spontaneously or with ventilatory support when periodic hyperinflation is stopped, pulmonary compliance declines an average of 33%.[30] Reduction in lung volumes after surgery is known to cause a reduction in lung compliance.[31]

An increase in respiratory rate does not in itself cause a reduction in lung compliance until the rate is greater than 48 breaths per minute.[32] The respiratory rate rarely reaches this level without medical intervention.

Ferris and Pollard[33] showed that, after a series of deep breaths, shallow breathing resulted in a reduction in lung compliance by 26%-40%. Two or more deep breaths to the limit of inspiration after a period of shallow breathing, resulted in an increase in lung compliance to near normal level. In the postoperative patient, the frequency of sighing, deep breathing, and coughing is reduced.[34] This is, in part, due to postoperative incisional site pain, the use of analgesics, and the prolonged effects of anesthetic agents. Therefore, the postoperative open heart patient must be encouraged to breath deeply and cough frequently.

Early Pulmonary Dysfunction

Postperfusion Lung Injury

Fine structural changes are known to occur in the lung following cardiopulmonary bypass surgery. The alterations in the structure of the alveoli are similar to those seen with hemorrhagic shock, severe soft tissue trauma, and endotoxemia.[35] Microscopically, there is swelling of endothelial cells, membranous pneumocytes, and the mitochondria of granular pneumocytes. There is interstitial edema; interstitial hemorrhage, and engorgement of the pulmonary vascular bed.[36]

During extracorporeal circulation, there is sequestration of polymorphoneucleocytes (PMNS) within the alveolar vasculature. The PMNS degranulate into the pulmonary circulation leading to interstitial and alveolar injury. Further injury occurs with obstruction of pulmonary microvasculature by microaggregates of fragmented PMNS and microaggregates from stored blood.[37]

With the rapid advances in cardiac surgery and perfusion, the incidence of postperfusion lung injury following cardiopulmonary bypass has declined.[38]

Cardiogenic Pulmonary Edema

Cardiogenic pulmonary edema is another important cause of early pulmonary dysfunction in the postoperative cardiac patient.[39] The possibility exists that all patients undergoing cardiopulmonary bypass and open intracardiac surgery develop some degree of subclinical pulmonary edema.[35] Pulmonary edema may be the result of increased microvascular pressure, possibly due to poor left ventricular function, or to increased permeability of the pulmonary vessels to protein and solute. There is a progressive decline in pulmonary capillary perfusion as interstitial lung water accumulates. Hypoxia develops as ventilation-perfusion mismatch worsens. Fluid initially accumulates within the interstitium and then fills the lymphatic vessels. Alveolar edema is a late occurrence. Pulmonary edema causes the lungs to become stiff, lung compliance falls, and the work of breathing is increased.

Noncardiogenic Pulmonary Edema

Noncardiogenic pulmonary edema is virtually indistinguishable clinically from cardiogenic pulmonary edema. Clinical features common to both include: tachypnea, rales on auscultation, widespread radiographic infiltrates, and arterial hypoxemia.[40] Noncardiogenic pulmonary edema differs from cardiogenic pulmonary edema in that mean left atrial and pulmonary wedge pressures are low or normal and the protein content of pulmonary edema fluid is dramatically higher than that of cardiogenic pulmonary edema.[40]

Noncardiogenic pulmonary edema and peripheral vascular collapse following cardiopulmonary bypass is a rare event. Several causes have been implicated. These include drug reaction, endotoxin shock, allergic anaphylaxis, and nonimmunologic reaction mediated by complement or histamine.[41-43] Severe anaphylactoid reaction to protamine administration after cardiopulmonary bypass may be a causative factor in the development of noncardiogenic pulmonary edema.[41]

Atelectasis and Pneumonia

Despite advances in modern medicine, lower respiratory tract infections rank as the third most common cause of nosocomial infection behind urinary tract and wound infections.[13] Pneumonias account for approximately 15% of all hospital-acquired infections, and 50% of these pneumonias occur in surgical patients.[44]

The causes of acute atelectasis include: space occupying lesions of the chest (pneumothorax, pleural effusion, etc.) causing compression atelectasis; total obstruction of an airway causing absorption of the distal alveolar air (absorption atelectasis) and microatelectasis (the closure of nonradiographically evident small distal airways). Macroatelectasis involves collapse of a segment, lobe, or lung, usually apparent radiographically.

There are several mechanisms believed to be responsible for postoperative atelectasis: (1) impaired mucociliary clearance and retained secretions; (2) loss of sigh mechanism; (3) impaired cough reflex; (4) diminished lung volumes; and (5) diaphragm dysfunction.[11]

Retained secretions are no longer believed to be the sole mechanism responsible for postoperative atelectasis. Atelectasis is seen in patients without increased secretions and in patients with otherwise normal lungs. Retained secretions may lead to cessation of ventilation distal to the occluded airway, while perfusion persists. A true shunt develops causing a widened alveolar-arterial oxygen tension difference.

Collapse is more common in the dependent regions of the lung. The airways and alveoli are relatively poorly expanded in the dependent zones and secretions tend to collect here due to gravitational force.

The rate at which the lung behind an occluded airway will collapse is believed to be a function of the nature of the gas trapped. Because of its high concentration of nitrogen (nitrogen has low solubility and the absorptive process is slow), air requires the most time for complete resorption. High concentrations of oxygen, perioperatively, promote more rapid resorption and earlier collapse of the airways.

Postoperatively, patients with severe incisional pain are treated with opiate analgesics. This leads to a reduction in the frequency of sighing secondary to the respiratory depressive effects of the analgesics. The loss of the sigh mechanism and the reduction of tidal volume have been shown to produce airway closure and atelectasis.

Several factors are responsible for the retention of secretions and airway obstruction. These include narcotic-induced suppression of the cough reflex, prolonged postoperative immobilization, splinting from pain or constricting bandages, pulmonary congestion, dehydration, and weakness of respiratory muscles.

Airway closure secondary to the reduction of lung volumes postoperatively appears to be an important factor in the genesis of atelectasis.[45,46] The CV responsible for airway closure usually occurs within the ERV. Postoperatively, however, there is a decline in the ERV, and even in the presence of a normal CV, the CV may exceed the ERV. The closing volume may now be above the end-tidal point, causing airways to close during tidal breathing (Fig. 1).[46]

Some patients with preoperative abnormalities in lung volumes, such as reduced ERV and increased closing volume, are at an increased risk of postoperative atelectasis. Obesity is associated with reduction in ERV and RV. Smokers have an increased closing volume above the ERV and within tidal breathing. Elderly patients

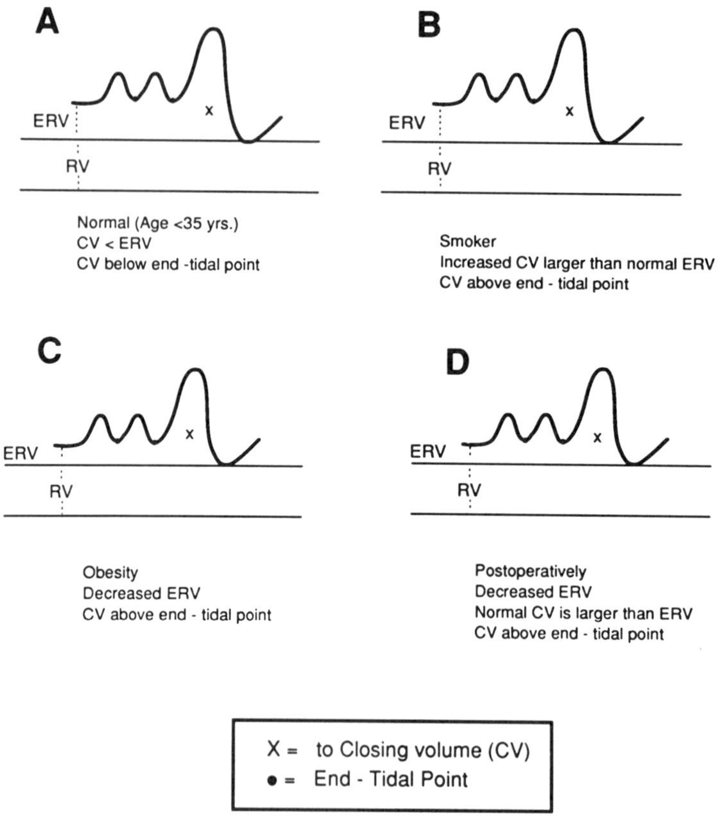

Figure 1. Relationship between expiratory reserve volume (ERV) and closing volume (CV) in (A) normals; (B) smokers; (C) obesity; (D) postoperatively.

also have an increased CV and frequently experience airway closure during tidal breathing.[47]

Patients with chronic airways obstruction have reduced ERV and increased CV.[46] These patients are at increased risk of atelectasis postoperatively because the reduced ERV secondary to chronic obstructive pulmonary disease (COPD) is now further reduced by surgery. Airway closure will now occur above the end-tidal point.

Pneumonia

Pneumonia refers to inflammation of the lung parenchyma associated with alveolar filling by exudate. The usual criteria for the diagnosis of nosocomial pneumonia include the presence of fever, leukocytosis, purulent tracheobronchial secretions, new or progressing infiltrates on chest radiograph, and the presence of pathogenic bacteria in respiratory secretions.[48-53] Resolution may occur or suppuration may result in necrosis of tissue, causing lung abscess.

Conditions that predispose a patient to develop pneumonia include: impaired cough reflex, aspiration of oral/gastric secretions, dehydration, impaired mucociliary clearance, prolonged postoperative immobilization, supplemental oxygen, low serum albumin, and microatelectasis and macroatelectasis.[5,13,50,51]

The upper airways are normally inhabited by a multitude of organisms, yet few bacteria exist below the level of the larynx in normal man. Within 24 hours of intubation, the trachea is colonized with bacteria commonly found in the upper airway. Gram-negative and anaerobic organisms will colonize the airway shortly thereafter. Colonization does not necessarily lead to pneumonia, and many patients without major risk factors never develop clinical illness despite colonization. Cultures of sputum obtained from intubated patients are usually positive for a variety of organisms and such results must be interpreted with caution.

Pneumonitis often supervenes if airway collapse persists for more than 2 or 3 days. Almost all patients with pneumonitis develop an infiltrate on chest roentgenogram. Physical signs may antedate the roentgenographic signs. These include the onset of fever, tachycardia, tachypnea, purulent sputum production, presence of moist rales on auscultation of the chest, bronchial breathing, and dullness to percussion note.

In patients with abnormal chest radiographs, it is important to distinguish pneumonia from noninfectious pulmonary conditions such as pulmonary emboli, congestive heart failure, pleural effusion, and atelectasis. Bacteriologic studies of expectorated sputum or endobronchial secretions are of limited value. Frequently these specimens are contaminated by oropharyngeal and tracheal flora during passage through upper airways.[48,54] Postoperative pulmonary infections are likely to involve a great array of bacteria including gram-negative, anaerobic bacteria, and staphylococcal aureus. There is a multitude of likely pathogens with variable antimicrobial susceptibility patterns, and all attempts should be made to obtain uncontaminated sputum specimens. It may be necessary to resort to the use of deep suction catheters, protective brush catheter via flexible fiberoptic bronchoscopy, or transtracheal aspiration.[55] The specimen should be properly collected and processed before antibiotic therapy is initiated. Empiric therapy may be necessary in seriously ill patients. Broad spectrum coverage is appropriate and should include an aminoglycoside or third-generation cephalosporin in combination with a penicillinase-resistant penicillin or clindamycin. If methicillin-resistant staphylococcal aureus is suspected, vancomycin should be started. Prophylactic antimicrobial therapy prior to surgery used to reduce septic complications at the operative site does not appear to reduce the incidence of postoperative pneumonia, but may help select out more resistant pathogens.

Bronchospasm

Severe bronchospasm after cardiopulmonary bypass surgery is an unusual event.[56] Bronchospasm may be detected when the first attempts to inflate the lungs are accompanied by expiratory wheezing, high inflation pressures, and difficulty in deflation of the lungs. Possible etiologies for bronchospasm are listed in Table I. Bronchodilators and corticosteroids are the mainstay of therapy.

Mechanical Ventilation

Mechanical ventilation is usually maintained for 12-24 hours postoperatively. In most cases, weaning from a ventilator occurs

Table I
Causes of Bronchospasm After Cardiopulmonary Bypass Surgery[56–58]

1.	Exacerbation of preoperative bronchospastic disease
2.	Allergic reaction
3.	Activation of complement anaphylatoxins during cardiopulmonary bypass
4.	Ventricular failure
5.	Cold urticaria syndrome
6.	Drug-induced histamine release
7.	β-Adrenergic blockade induced bronchospasm

without difficulty within 24 hours. Careful observation is vital during this period of potential cardiopulmonary instability prior to the initiation of the weaning process.

The oral route of intubation is preferred to nasotracheal intubation in adult patients undergoing open heart surgery. A larger diameter tube may be placed, allowing for improved suctioning capability and providing a means through which bronchoscopy may be performed in the event such a procedure is necessary.[59] A smaller diameter tube is used with nasotracheal intubation and suctioning is more difficult because of the small caliber of the tube and the possibility of kinking. Because major episodes of epistaxis may occur with nasotracheal intubation,[60] the procedure should be avoided in patients undergoing cardiac surgery where anticoagulation is routinely undertaken.

Mechanical ventilation should minimize respiratory muscle fatigue while providing optimal gas exchange in the postoperative period. Proper selection of tidal volume (Vt), respiratory rate, inspiratory and expiratory times, and inspired concentration of oxygen are crucial.

The tidal volume is generally set at 10-15 mL/kg,[61] but usually not greater than 1,200 mL. This volume should provide small airway patency, prevent atelectasis, as well as provide adequate gas exchange.

In the normal adult patient, the respiratory rate is usually set at 12-16 breaths per minute and adjusted to maintain a PCO_2 of 36-44 mm Hg.

Inspired oxygen should be provided in order to maintain an adequate PO_2 without the deleterious effects of oxygen.[62] In the critically ill patient, periods of hypoxemia may lead to disastrous consequences such as an intractable cardiac arrhythmia, extension of myocardial infarction,[63] and death.

There are three clinical goals that can be accomplished with proper oxygen therapy: (1) Treat hypoxemia; when arterial hypoxemia is the result of decreased alveolar oxygen tensions, an increased inspired oxygen concentration will dramatically improve the hypoxemia. (2) Decrease the work of breathing; hypoxemia is associated with increased ventilatory work load. Enriched inspired oxygen concentration will result in a decrease in the minute ventilation to normal, thus a reduction in the work load of breathing. (3) Decrease myocardial work; the cardiovascular system is a primary mechanism for compensation of hypoxemia. Elimination of hypoxemia with increased inspired oxygen concentration will reduce the demand for increased myocardial work. Positive end-expiratory pressure (PEEP) may be used to reduce the inspired fraction of oxygen to nonhyperoxic levels.

Airway Management

The need for maintaining a patent airway and appropriate removal of tracheobronchial secretions in mechanically ventilated patients cannot be overemphasized. This can be effectively accomplished by careful assessment of patient needs and appropriate application of respiratory therapy. Prophylactic respiratory therapy is important in postoperative patient with hypoventilation, reduced vital capacity, splinting, and altered mental status secondary to the prolonged effects of anesthetic agents.

The goals of aerosol therapy include the humidification of inspired gases, an aid to bronchial hygiene, and a means of delivering medication.

In the intubated patient, where the upper airway is bypassed, the application of aerosol therapy ensures proper humidification of inspired gases. Airways are kept moist and free from desiccated secretions with the use of aerosol therapy. Expectoration is promoted and mucous blanket continuity is maintained with aerosol therapy. It is also possible to deliver medication to the tracheobronchial tree and lung parenchyma via aerosol route.

Chest physical therapy involves a series of manipulative techniques used to prevent the accumulation and improve the mobilization of secretions from the tracheobronchial tree.[64,65] The basic techniques of chest physical therapy are postural drainage, chest percussion, vibration, and cough instruction. Chest physical therapy is frequently used in conjunction with aerosol or intermittent positive pressure breathing (IPPB) therapy.[66] Chest physical therapy is often not tolerated by postoperative cardiac patients.[67] Chest percussion can aggravate incisional site pain beyond a tolerable level.

Suctioning of secretions is an important step in proper airway management. Sterility of suction catheters is essential. The suction catheter should be long enough to pass the tip of the endotracheal tube and it should be made of material that reduces trauma to the tracheal mucosa.

The frequency of suctioning must be individualized. Patients with copious secretions will require more frequent suctioning. There are several complications of airway suctioning worth noting. These include hypoxemia,[68] hypotension, and cardiac dysrhythmia.[69]

Airway suctioning is an important cause of hypoxemia in the intubated patient. Hypoxemia will result in heart rate abnormalities, most frequently sinus tachycardia, and less frequently bradycardia, electromechanical dissociation and ventricular tachycardia. Hypotension may be the result of vagal stimulation or decreased venous return to the heart secondary to excessive coughing episodes. Airway suctioning must stop and ventilation reestablished in the patient who shows significant change in heart rate or rhythm.

These complications are best avoided by limiting the suctioning process to 10 seconds or less and with the use of supplemental oxyen via nasal canula, venturi mask, or ventilatory support.[70]

Respiratory Monitoring During Mechanical Ventilation

Patients requiring mechanical ventilation may develop complications suddenly, either as a result of their underlying disease or as a direct result of ventilator therapy. Close monitoring of these patients will provide early detection of changes in condition and provide an early opportunity to initiate life-saving measures.[71]

Arterial blood gas analysis (ABG) is an integral part of the assessment of respiratory function in intubated patients. Serial ABGs are used to monitor progress routinely in postoperative open heart patients.

Pulse Oximetry

Pulse oximetry has gained enormous popularity in the field of noninvasive continuous monitoring of intensive care patients. Oximeters determine oxygen saturation by either absorption or reflection spectrophotometry. Pulse oximeters do not measure saturation or desaturation directly, but rather observe the pulse-added change in relative absorption at only two wavelengths. Only two wavelengths of light are required to calculate O_2 saturation, because blood is usually composed of only two major light absorbers, HbO_2 and RHb (reduced Hb).[72]

Pulse oximeters correlate significantly with PaO_2 when the saturation of arterial blood with oxygen (SaO_2) is high. Pulse oximetry also appears to be a sensitive indicator of the presence of relative hypoxemia (saturation of < 95% correlated with PaO_2 < 70 mm Hg with a sensitivity of 100%).[73]

The accuracy of oximeters varies among makes and models. On average, oximeters measure saturation with 95% confidence limits of ± 4% when SaO_2 is > 70%.[74] Accuracy of pulse oximeters deteriorates at lower saturation values.[75]

Many factors appear to influence the accuracy of pulse oximetry. These include: poor peripheral perfusion, fingernail polish, presence of carboxyhemoglobin or methemoglobin, hypothermia, intravascular dyes, and mechanical ventilation artifact.[76,77] Theoretically, skin pigmentation should not significantly affect the accuracy of pulse oximetry because only pulse-added change in absorption is considered.[78] However, a recent study has shown that a significant difference in PaO_2 exists between black and white patients at identical saturation values. In the black patient, pulse oximetry targets of 90%, 92%, and 94% were unreliable in predicting a clinically satisfactory level of oxygenation, while in white patients a SaO_2 target value of 92% appeared optimal and correlated with a PaO_2 value of > 60 mm Hg in 92% of the readings.[79]

The role of pulse oximetry in clinical decision making is not well defined.[80] Pulse oximetry has been used as an immediate visual feedback device for pursed lip breathing in patients with COPD.[81] It is also used in the titration of supplemental oxygen with mechanically ventilated patients.[79]

Pulse oximetry has few complications associated with its use. Rare instances of finger burns and necrosis have been reported usually through overheating of a damaged probe or long-term continuous use.[82]

Noninvasive Monitoring of Carbon Dioxide

End-Tidal Carbon Dioxide Monitoring (Capnometry)

Carbon dioxide tension at end expiration can be measured using mass spectroscopy or infrared analysis. The procedure is most easily accomplished in intubated patients, however, sampling from the hypopharynx can be performed in the nonintubated patient.[83] In patients with minimal ventilation-perfusion mismatch, end-tidal PCO_2 closely approximates $PaCO_2$ (within 4 mm Hg).[78] In patients with increased physiologic dead space, i.e., COPD, pulmonary embolism, end-tidal PCO_2 underestimates $PaCO_2$.

Capnography is most useful for the detection of apnea or hypoventilation because end-tidal CO_2 is measured with each breath and changes in ventilatory status may be detected immediately.

Transcutaneous Carbon Dioxide Monitoring

Transcutaneous carbon dioxide partial pressure ($PtcCO_2$) can be measured with the use of an infrared sensor or pH electrode.[84] In hemodynamically stable infants and adults, $PtcCO_2$ reliably follows the trend of $PaCO_2$.[78] However, $PtcCO_2$ is usually from 4 to 25 mm Hg higher than the corresponding $PaCO_2$.[85] Transcutaneous carbon dioxide monitors are slow to respond to changes in $PaCO_2$, often taking as long as 4 minutes for full response. Therefore, $PtcCO_2$ monitoring is not useful in situations where abrupt decompensation is possible. The $PtcCO_2$-$PaCO_2$ gradient increases disproportionately in conditions of low cardiac output or hypotension.[86]

Weaning From Mechanical Ventilation

Following cardiac surgery, there is generally a period of routine ventilatory support. During this time, a careful assessment of the neurologic, hemodynamic, pulmonary, and metabolic status should take place. When the patient is medically stable, weaning from mechanical ventilation is considered. Patients who require prolonged ventilator support often experience intraoperative problems with oxygen transport, carbon dioxide clearance, or congestive heart failure. A number of factors may be responsible for an unsuccessful weaning outcome including excessive ventilatory requirements, hypoventilation secondary to decreased respiratory center output or respiratory muscle fatigue, impaired pulmonary gas exchange, and psychological problems.[87]

The patient's rate, pattern, and symmetry of respiration provide important information about the current clinical status of the patient. Normal respiration should be virtually effortless and symmetric with a rate of 14 to 20 breaths per minute. Tachypnea is an observed response in acidemia, hypoxemia, and hypercapnia. Bradypnea is often the result of central nervous system dysfunction, drug effect, or an agonal event, rarely the result of a primary pulmonary pathologic process. The use of accessory muscles of respiration, intercostal retraction, and nasal flaring indicate labored breathing. Paradoxical motion of the chest wall and abdomen may represent diaphragm or intercostal muscle paralysis. Auscultation of the chcst is a critical part of the physical examination. Auscultation is performed on the naked chest, comparing symmetry side-to-side and top-to-bottom. The diagnosis of pulmonary edema, pneumonia, pleural effusion, and atelectasis can be made early with the use of a stethoscope.

Pump Failure

Respiratory muscle pump failure is probably the most common cause of failure to wean from mechanical ventilation.[80] Pump failure during the weaning process is likely to be secondary to a multitude of factors including poor respiratory muscle strength, phrenic nerve dysfunction, respiratory center dysfunction, and increased respiratory muscle load.

Dynamic hyperinflation or stacking is an important cause of respiratory muscle dysfunction during the weaning process.[88] There is a reduction in the force of contraction with shortened inspiratory muscles at high lung volumes. The flattened diaphragm is less efficient in generating a pressure gradient and the altered muscle fiber orientation at high lung volume leads to a reduction in chest wall expansion.

Poor nutritional status can cause impairment of respiratory muscle function and a reduction in ventilatory drive. In critically ill patients with inadequate caloric intake, energy sources are derived from protein breakdown and gluconeogenesis. Inspiratory and expiratory respiratory muscles, primarily the diaphragm and intercostals, are susceptible to this catabolic effect.[16] Malnutrition reduces diaphragmatic muscle mass resulting in a weaker muscle with reduced contractile capability. Respiratory muscle function can be impaired in inadequately nourished patients by unavailability of energy substrate. Approximately 50% of the energy used by the diaphragm is derived from carbohydrate oxidation that is derived from stored glycogen.[89] Glycogen stores are depleted early in the inadequately nourished patient, thus protein must be utilized as an energy source.

Ventilatory response to hypoxia may be reduced by as much as 42% in malnourished patients.[90] Reducing the protein deficit with amino acid supplementation will restore the depressed ventilatory drive to near normal level.

Electrolyte abnormalities such as hypophosphatemia, hypokalemia, hypocalcemia, or hypomagnesemia may adversely affect respiratory muscle function.[91-93]

Most patients who fail a weaning trial have an elevated respiratory drive,[94] however, patients with respiratory center dysfunction may display hypoventilation while weaning. In the postoperative patient, the likely causes of respiratory center dysfunction include the prolonged effects of anesthetic agents, sedatives, sleep deprivation, cerebrovascular accidents, and metabolic alkalosis.

Left hemidiaphragm dysfunction is seen in a number of patients after coronary artery bypass surgery.[95] An important cause of impairment to diaphragm activity is phrenic nerve paralysis secondary to the saline slush used for topical cold cardioplegia. The incidence of cold injury to the phrenic nerve after open heart surgery is unknown. Recent studies suggest that the cause of left hemidiaphragm elevation may be due to factors other than phrenic nerve injury.[95,96] These include direct lung injury from the use of retractors during surgery and atelectasis secondary to breathing at low lung volumes with a reduction in the frequency of sighing.

Many postoperative patients have increased ventilatory requirements and require prolonged ventilatory support before weaning can be attempted. Patients with elevated CO_2 production, elevated respiratory drive, and increased dead-space ventilation require greater minute ventilation and may display ventilatory difficulty during weaning trials.

Patients receiving excesive caloric intake in the form of carbohydrates have increased CO_2 production. These patients may develop hypercanpic respiratory failure if appropriate minute ventilation is not maintained.[97]

Patients with severe lung disease have increased dead-space to tidal volume ratio (Vd/Vt) and require a greater than normal minute ventilation to prevent the development of hypercapnia. Unsuccessful weaning is likely to occur in patients with Vd/Vt > 0.6 due to the high minute ventilation necessary for carbon dioxide elimination.

Criteria for Weaning

The appropriate time to discontinue mechanical ventilation is often based on clinical judgement and experience, however, several guidelines have been established to reduce the risk of unsuccessful weaning trials (Table II).[98-104]

Table II
Various Criteria for Weaning

(1) Vital capacity of > 10–15 mL/kg body weight
(2) Maximum inspiratory force < −20 cm H_2O
(3) Tidal volume > 5 mL/kg body weight
(4) Minute ventilation < 10 L/min
(5) Maximum voluntary ventilation more than twice minute ventilation
(6) PaO_2 > 60 mm Hg with FiO_2 < 35%
(7) Alveolar-arterial oxygen tension gradient < 350 mm Hg with FiO_2 equal to 100%
(8) Vd/Vt < 0.6
(9) Respiratory rate < 30 breaths/min

The vital capacity is normally 65-70 mL/kg. Safar and Kunkel[103] state that if the adult patient's vital capacity is less than 1 L, weaning should be terminated due to the increased risk of progressive atelectasis.

Maximum inspiratory force (P_{max}) is a measure of respiratory muscle strength. Most patients who have maximum inspiratory force of -20 cm H_2O or less are successfully extubated, while those patients with Pimax > -20 cm H_2O are unable to maintain adequate ventilation without ventilatory support.[100]

Tidal volume should exceed 5 mL/kg body weight.[101] Breathing at lower lung volumes is associated with airway closure, a reduction in lung compliance, and progressive respiratory failure.

Patients with a minute ventilation less than 10 liters per minute and the ability to double the minute ventilation with a maximal voluntary effort are generally weaned successfully. Postextubation maximal voluntary ventilation values are usually greater than those measured while intubated. This may be due to the greater airway resistance imposed by the endotracheal tube.

The alveolar-arterial oxygen tension gradient (A-a gradient) is frequently used as a measure of gas exchange efficiency. Changes in minute ventilation will have little affect on the A-a gradient. Thus, when hypoxemia is due solely to hypoventilation, the A-a gradient will be normal. Abnormalities in gas exchange will be detected by a widening of the A-a gradient.

Calculation of A-a Gradient

$$(A\text{-}a)Do_2 = PAo_2 - Pao_2$$

where: PAo_2 = alveolar o_2 tension
Pao_2 = arterial o_2 tension (measured)

$$PAo_2 = (PB - PH_2O) \times FiO_2 - \frac{PaCO_2}{R}$$

where: PB = barometric pressue
PH_2O = Water vapor pressure
FiO_2 = inspired oxygen concentration
R = respiratory quotient (0.8)
$PaCO_2$ = arterial CO_2 tension (measured)

The normal A-a gradient in a young patient, breathing room air at sea level, is 12 mm Hg. The normal A-a gradient is up to 30 mm Hg in the elderly patient.[105]

High alveolar-arterial oxygen tension gradient (> 350 mm Hg) while on high inspired fraction of oxygen (100%) indicates severe lung disease with poor gas exchange ability. These patients will require prolonged mechanical ventilation and any attempt at weaning should be discouraged (Table III).

Weaning from mechanical ventilatory support should be done in stages. The choice of weaning techniques varies among physicians. There are advantages and disadvantages to each technique. Some patients are able to tolerate abrupt withdrawal of ventilatory support, while others require step-wise withdrawal of ventilatory support. The use of synchronized intermittent mandatory ventilation (SIMV) and pressure support ventilation (psv) as weaning techniques are popular among many physicians.[104,106] Tracheal-tube trials are seldom used in the postoperative open-heart patient.

Synchronized intermittent mandatory ventilation has advantages over other means of weaning (assist-control, T-tube trial).[107] Groegan et al.[108] found oxygen delivery, systemic blood pressure, left ventricular stroke work, and cardiac output to be better with SIMV than with assist-control ventilation.[108]

Pressure support ventilation (PSV) augments a spontaneous breath with a fixed amount of positive pressure.[106] The patient is able to control his respiratory rate, inspiratory time, and inspiratory flow rate. The physician sets the level of positive pressure to provide an average tidal volume of 300 mL. Pressure support ventilation may be used for weaning by gradually reducing the level of positive pressure according to the tolerance of the patient. Extubation can be considered when a PSV level of 5 cmH_2O is

Table III
Contraindications to Weaning

(1) Residual neuromuscular blockade
(2) Neurological complications or a depressed state of consciousness
(3) Low cardiac output syndrome
(4) Malignant ventricular arrhythmias
(5) Excessive postoperative bleeding (150 mL/h)
(6) Absence of gag reflex

achieved. To date, there are no studies showing superiority of PSV over other modes of weaning.

Complications Associated with Mechanical Ventilation

Mechanical ventilation is associated with numerous complications, some of which may be fatal. Complications range from relatively minor, such as nasal necrosis with the use of a nosotracheal tube,[60] to severe and often life-threatening, such as nosocomial pneumonia or pulmonary barotrauma (Table IV).[109-112]

Pulmonary Barotrauma

Barotrauma refers to alveolar gas leak to extraparenchymal structures usually due to excessive volumes with alveolar overdis-

Table IV
Complications of Mechanical Ventilation

(1) Nasal necrosis
(2) Laryngeal complications
  a. sore throat, hoarseness
  b. glottic edema
  c. vocal cord ulceration and paralysis
  d. tracheal ulceration and stenosis
(3) Endotracheal tube malfunction
  a. main-stem intubation
  b. suboptimal cuff inflation and cuff leakage
(4) Pulmonary barotrauma
  a. subcutaneous emphysema
  b. interstitial emphysema
  c. pneumothorax and tension pneumothorax
  d. pneumomediastinum
  e. pneumoperitoneum
(5) Diminished cardiac output and hypotension
(6) Gastrointestinal malfunction
(7) Renal and hepatic malfunction
(8) Alveolar hyperventilation with respiratory alkalosis
(9) Alveolar hypoventilation with respiratory acidosis
(10) Mechanical ventilator failure

tension and/or high airway pressures. Barotrauma may result when very large tidal volumes are used in ventilated patients.

If the visceral pleura is interrupted, air may leak through the alveolar wall into the interstitium and track along the pulmonary vascular structures. The air may then track up or down the mediastinum, into the pleural space, or into the facial planes of the neck resulting in pneumomediastinum, pneumothorax, and subcutaneous emphysema, respectively. Pneumothorax is the most dangerous type of barotrauma in mechanically ventilated patients where tension pneumothorax may develop rapidly. Air in the pleural space causes compression of the lung with hypoxemia, and the possibility of total circulatory collapse.

Diminished Cardiac Output

All modes of positive pressure ventilation cause an increase in mean intrathoracic pressure and a reduction in venous return to the heart.[113-115] Initiation of PEEP leads to a further reduction in right ventricular preload. The primary effect of PEEP is to increase end-expiratory lung volume, hence a reduction in venous return to the heart. Positive pressure ventilation also causes an increase both in pulmonary vascular resistance and in right ventricular afterload.[116] Increased lung volumes result in alveolar distention and stretching of the alveolar septa. Pulmonary capillaries are compressed and pulmonary vascular resistance rises. Regional alveolar hypoxemia ($PaO_2 < 60$ mm Hg) may cause pulmonary vascular resistance to rise further as a result of an increase in pulmonary vasomotor tone. Cardiac output falls as right ventricular preload drops and pulmonary vascular resistance rises. Intravenous fluids will increase the venous return to the heart. However, pulmonary vascular resistance may remain high in the mechanically ventilated patient. Overzealous fluid administration will cause the right ventricle to dilate, pushing the interventricular septum into the left ventricle. Left ventricular compliance and cardiac output will be reduced.[117]

Gastrointestinal Malfunction

Gastric and intestinal distension may occur in patients requiring mechanical ventilation. Air may leak around the endotracheal tube cuff and overcome the lower esophageal sphincter, to enter the stomach. This problem may be alleviated by the passage of a nasogastric tube.

Gastrointestinal bleeding is frequently seen in patients requiring mechanical ventilation for more than 3 days. Acute ulceration of gastric and bowel mucosa is the likely cause of gastrointestinal bleeding in mechanically ventilated patients.[118] Prophylactic use of histamine (H_2) receptor antagonists and antacids has greatly reduced the incidence of gastrointestinal bleeding.[119,120]

Respiratory Alkalosis

Alveolar hyperventilation may be the result of pain, agitation, anxiety, dyspnea, and inappropriate ventilator settings.[121] The resultant respiratory alkalosis may predispose to cardiac dysrhythmia, impair cerebral perfusion, and slow the weaning process. Sedation with proper ventilation adjustment of respiratory rate, tidal volume, and inspiratory flow will generally resolve the unintentional respiratory alkalosis.

Impaired Renal Function

Reduction of renal blood flow and deterioration of renal function may occur with positive pressure ventilation.[122] In general, positive airway pressure results in decreased urine output, sodium retention, and water retention.[123]

Atelectasis and Pneumonia

Atelectasis and pneumonia are common complications of mechanical ventilation. This subject has been discussed earlier in this chapter.

Postextubation Respiratory Care

Many pulmonary complications may be avoided with proper use of postextubation airway management. Aerosol therapy, chest physiotherapy, IPPB, incentive spirometry, and breathing exercises are frequently used. Aerosol therapy and chest physiotherapy have been discussed earlier in this chapter. The use and effectiveness of IPPB, incentive spirometry, and deep breathing exercises requires further elaboration.

Intermittent Positive Pressure Breathing

The use of postoperative IPPB therapy in general has been under criticism for several decades. For IPPB therapy to be effective, it must increase alveolar distending pressure.[124] With the use of IPPB therapy, tidal volume is increased in patients unable to breath deeply in the postoperative period.

Intermittent positive pressure breathing therapy is administered via a pressure cycled ventilator. The treatments are usually given three to four times a day, lasting approximately 15 minutes per treatment. Most patients require 20-40 cmH_2O pressure to have adequate lung expansion. Intermittent positive pressure breathing may be used to deliver air, therapeutic gases, and aerosolized bronchodilators.[125]

Intermittent positive pressure breathing therapy is accompanied by many potential risks. Therefore, IPPB is justified only if the patient's ability to inspire adequately is limited.[126] Intermittent positive pressure breathing therapy has been used in the treatment of acute hypoventilation in an attempt to avoid intubation. Some patients with chronic hypoventilation and carbon dioxide retention feel better after IPPB therapy. Intermittent positive pressure breathing with aerosolized bronchodilators has been used in the treatment of atelectasis. It has also been useful for the clearance of secretions in patients who fail to expectorate adequately.

The major disadvantagese of IPPB therapy include: hyperinflation with air trapping, barotrauma, reduction in venous return to the heart, increased intracranial pressure, gastric distension, increased airway resistance, and nosocomial infection.

Intermittent positive pressure breathing is contraindicated in patients with pneumothorax, subcutaneous or mediastinal emphysema, bullous lung disease, cardiovascular insufficiency, and tracheoesophageal fistulas.[127]

Incentive Spirometry

Breathing at low lung volumes, without sighs, results in gradual alveolar collapse within 1 hour.[128] Alveolar collapse is avoided in the normal adult with sigh breaths occurring approximately six to nine times per hour. In the postoperative patient, when the frequency of sighing is greatly reduced, hourly maximal inspiratory maneuvers should provide an ideal prophylactic measure for alveolar collapse.

Incentive spirometry appears to have several advantages over IPPB as a prophylactic regimen. Incentive spirometry is equally effective, with fewer complications, and requires less personnel time (less costly).[129]

Incentive spirometry is effective only if the patient is cooperative and motivated. The initial inspiratory goal should be at least twice the patients measured tidal volume. The procedure should be repeated every hour while awake. Most patients require some coaching and encouragement in the use of incentive spirometry.

Breathing Exercises

Breathing exercises are beneficial in preventing postoperative pulmonary complications.[66] The beneficial effects are most noteworthy in patients with high risk of developing pulmonary complications (current smokers, FVC < 80% predicted, FEV_1 < 75% of FVC, and patients over 60 years of age). It has been suggested that breathing exercises may be more effective in preventing postoperative pulmonary complications than postural drainage and percussion in open-heart surgical patients.[66] As is the case with incentive spirometry, patients require coaching and encouragement in the use of breathing exercises and coughing.

REFERENCES

1. Olsen GN, Fishman AP. *Pre- and Postoperative Evaluation and Management of the Thoracic Surgical Patient.* New York, NY: McGraw-Hill Book Co.; 1988:2413-2431.
2. Mittman C. Assessment of operative risk in thoracic surgery. *Am Rev Resp Dis* 84:197-207; 1961.
3. Robicsek F, Daugherty HK, Mullen DC, et al. The effect of continued cigarette smoking on the patency of synthetic vascular grafts in Leriche Syndrome. *J Thorac Cardiovasc Surg* 70:107-112; 1975.
4. Braun SR, Birnbaum ML, Chopra PS. Pre- and postoperative pulmonary function abnormalities in coronary artery revascularization surgery. *Chest* 73:316-320; 1978.
5. Wightman JAK. Prospective survey of the incidence of postoperative pulmonary complications. *Br J Surg* 55:85-91; 1968.
6. Warner MA, Offord KP, Warner ME, et al. Role of preoperative cessation of smoking and other factors in postoperative pulmonary complications: a blinded prospective study of coronary artery bypass patients. *Mayo Clin Proc* 64:609-616; 1989.
7. Warner MA, Divertie MB, Tinker JH. Preoperative cessation of smoking and pulmonary complications in coronary artery bypass patients. *Anesthesiology* 60:380-383; 1984.
8. Camner P, Philipson K. Some studies of tracheobronchial clearance in man. *Chest* 63(Suppl):23s; 1973.
9. Buist AS, Sexton GJ, Nagy JM. The effect of smoking cessation and modification on lung function. *Am Rev Resp Dis* 114:115-122; 1976.
10. Mitchell C, Garrahy P, Penke P. Postoperative respiratory morbidity: identification and risk factors. *Aust NZ J Surg* 52:203-209; 1982.
11. Tisi GM. Preoperative evaluation of pulmonary function. *Am Rev Resp Dis* 119:293-308; 1979.
12. Luce JM. Respiratory complications of obesity. *Chest* 78:626-631; 1980.
13. Garibaldi RA, Britt MR, Coleman ML, et al. Risk factors for postoperative pneumonia. *Am J Med* 70:677-680; 1981.
14. Laver MB, Bendixen HH. Atelectasis in the surgical patient: recent conceptual advances. *Prog Surg* 5:1-7; 1966.
15. Memsic L, Silberman AW, Silberman H. Respiratory failure and malnutrition. *J Resp Dis* 11:693-699; 1990.
16. Pingleton SH, Harmon GS. Nutritional management in acute respiratory failure. *J Am Med Assoc* 257:3094-3098; 1987.
17. Gaensler EA, Cugell DW, Lingren I, et al. The role of pulmonary insufficiency in mortality and invalidism following surgery for pulmonary tuberulosis. *J Thorac Surg* 29:163-187; 1955.
18. Lockwood P. The principles of predicting risk of post-thoracotomy-function-related complications in bronchogenic carcinoma. *Respiration* 30:329-344; 1973.

19. Fee HJ, Holmes EC, Gewirtz HS, et al. Role of pulmonary vascular resistance measurements in preoperative evaluation of candidates for pulmonary resection. *J Thorac Cardiovasc Surg* 75:519-524; 1978.
20. Krietersson S, Lindell SE, Svanberg L. Prediction of pulmonary function loss due to pneumonectomy using 133Xe- radiospirometry. *Chest* 62:694-698; 1972.
21. Ratshire RA, Rackley CE, Russell RO. Hemodynamic evaluation of left ventricular function in shock complicating myocardial infarction. *Circulation* 55:127-139; 1972.
22. Guyton RA, Arcidi JM, Langford DA, et al. Emergency coronary bypass for cardiogenic shock. *Circulation* 76:V22-27; 1987.
23. Julian OC, Lopez-Belio M, Dye WS, et al. The median sternotomy incision in intracardiac surgery with extra- corporeal circulation. A general evaluation of its use in heart surgery. *Surgery* 42:753-761; 1957.
24. Bryant LR. Lung perfusion scanning for estimation of postoperative pulmonary function. *Arch Surg* 104:52-55; 1972.
25. Edwards FH, Cohen AJ, Bellamy RF, et al. Risk assessment in urgent/emergent coronary artery surgery. *Chest* 97:1125-1129; 1990.
26. Ghia J, Anderson N. Pulmonary function and cardiopulmonary bypass. *J Am Med Assoc* 212:593-597; 1970.
27. Shapira N, Zabatino SM, Ahmed S, et al. Determinants of pulmonary function in patients undergoing coronary bypass operations. *Ann Thorac Surg* 50:268-273; 1990.
28. Jedrzejowicz AM, Brophy C, Moxham J, et al. Assessment of diaphragm weakness. *Am Rev Resp Dis* 137:877-883; 1988.
29. Rea HH, Harris EA, Seelye ER, et al. The effects of cardiopulmonary bypass upon pulmonary gas exchange. *J Thorac Cardiovasc Surg* 75:104-120; 1978.
30. Mead J, Collier C. Relation of volume history of lungs to respiratory mechanics in dogs. *J Appl Physiol* 14:669-675; 1959.
31. Ellison LT, Duke JF, Ellison RG. Pulmonary compliance following open-heart surgery and its relationship to ventilation and gas exchange. *Circulation* 35:I-217-225; 1967.
32. Albright CD, Bondurant S. Some effects of respiratory frequency on pulmonary mechanics. *J Clin Invest* 44:1362-1370; 1965.
33. Ferris BG, Pollard DS. Effect of deep and quiet breathing on pulmonary compliance in man. *J Clin Invest* 39:143-149; 1960.
34. Egbert LD, Bendixen HH. Effect of morphine on breathing pattern: a possible factor in atelectasis. *J Am Med Assoc* 188:485-488; 1964.
35. Parker DJ, Karp RB, Kirklin JW, et al. Lung water and alveolar and capillary volumes after intracardiac surgery. *Circulation* 45(Suppl I):139-146; 1972.
36. Asada S, Yamaguchi M. Fine structural change in the lung following cardiopulmonary bypass. *Chest* 59:478-483; 1971.
37. Ratliff NB, Young GW, Hackel DB, et al. Pulmonary injury secondary to extracorporeal circulation. *J Thorac Cardiovasc Surg* 65:425-432; 1973.

38. Byrick RJ, Noble WH. Postperfusion lung syndrome. *J Thorac Cardiovasc Surg* 76:685-693; 1978.
39. Fedullo AJ, Swinburne AJ, Wahl GW, et al. APACHE II score and mortality in respiratory failure due to cardiogenic pulmonary edema. *Crit Care Med* 16:1218-1221; 1988.
40. Culliford AT, Thomas S, Spencer FC. Fulminating noncardiogenic pulmonary edema. *J Thorac Cardiovasc Surg* 80:868-875; 1980.
41. Olinger GN, Becker RM, Bonchek LI. Noncardiogenic pulmonary edema and peripheral vascular collapse following cardiopulmonary bypass: rare protamine reaction? *Ann Thorac Surg* 29:20-25; 1980.
42. Curreri PW, Manwaring D. Mechanisms of acute pulmonary dysfunction induced by fibrinogen degradation product D. *Surgery* 84:45-54; 1978.
43. Millen JE, Glauser FL, Smeltzer D, et al. The role of leukocytes in ethchlorvynol-induced pulmonary edema. *Chest* 73:75-78; 1978.
44. Eickhoff TC. Pulmonary infections in surgical patients. *Surg Clin North Am* 60:175-183; 1980.
45. Buist AS, Ross BB. Quantitative analysis of the alveolar plateau in the diagnosis of early airway obstruction. *Am Rev Resp Dis* 108:1078-1087; 1973.
46. Craig DB, Wahba WM, Don HR, et al. Closing volume and its relationship to gas exchange in the seated and supine position. *J Appl Physiol* 31:717-721; 1971.
47. McCarthy DS, 5pencer R, Green R, et al. Measurement of closing volume as a single and sensitive test for early detection of small airway disease. *Am J Med* 52:747-753; 1972.
48. Johanson WG, Pierce AK, Sanford JP, et al. Nosocomial respiratory infections with gram-negative bacilli. *Ann Intern Med* 77:701-706; 1972.
49. Johanson WG, Seidenfeld JJ, Gomez P, et al. Bacteriologic diagnosis of nosocomial pneumonia following prolonged mechanical ventilation. *Am Rev Resp Dis* 137:259-264; 1988.
50. Craven DE, Kunches LM, Kilinsky V, et al. Risk factors for pneumonia and fatality in patients receiving continued mechanical ventilation. *Am Rev Resp Dis* 133:792-796; 1986.
51. Meduri GU. Ventilator-associated pneumonia in patients with respiratory failure. *Chest* 97:1208-1219; 1990.
52. Joshi M, Ciesla N, Caplan E. Diagnosis of pneumonia in critically ill patients. *Chest* 94:4s; 1988.
53. Craven DE, Goularte TA, Make BJ. Contaminated condensate in mechanical ventilator circuits. *Am Rev Resp Dis* 129:625-628; 1984.
54. Stevens RM, Teres D, Skilman JJ, et al. Pneumonia in an intensive care unit. *Arch Intern Med* 134:106-111; 1984.
55. Chastre J, Fagon JY, Solar P, et al. Diagnosis of nosocomial bacterial pneumonia in intubated patients undergoing ventilation: comparison of the usefulncss of bronchoalveolar lavage and protected specimen brush. *Am J Med* 85:499-505; 1988.

56. Tuman KJ, Ivankovich AD. Bronchospasm during cardiopulmonary bypass. *Chest* 90:635-637; 1986.
57. Johnston WE, Moss J, Philbin DM, et al. Management of cold urticaria during hypothermic cardiopulmonary bypass. *N Engl J Med* 306:219-221; 1982.
58. Chenaueth DE, Cooper SW, Hugli TE, et al. Complement activation during cardiopulmonary bypass: evidence for generation of G3a and C5a anaphylatoxins. *N Engl J Med* 305:497-503; 1981.
59. Dinley AR. Dangers and difficulties from the rhinological aspect. *Br Med J* 1:693-696; 1943.
60. Zwillich C, Pierson DJ. Nasal necrosis: a complication of nasotracheal intubation. *Chest* 64:376-377; 1973.
61. Pinsky MR. The effects of mechanical ventilation on the cardiovascular system. *Crit Care Clin* 6:663-678; 1990.
62. Lodato RF. Oxygen Toxicity. *Crit Care Clin* 6:749-765; 1990.
63. Maroko PR, Radvany P, Braunwald E, et al. Reduction of infarct size by oxygen inhalation following acute coronary occlusion. *Circulation* 52:360-368; 1975.
64. Petty TL. Physical therapy. *Am Rev Resp Dis* 110:129-131; 1974.
65. Jones NL. Physical therapy. *Am Rev Resp Dis* 110:132-136; 1974.
66. Graham WB, Bradley DA. Efficacy of chest physiotherapy and intermittent positive-pressure breathing in the resolution of pneumonia. *N Engl J Med* 299:624-627; 1978.
67. Vraciu JK, Vraciu RA. Effectiveness of breathing exercises in preventing pulmonary complications following open heart surgery. *Phys Ther* 57:1367-1371; 1977.
68. Urban BJ. Avoidance of hypoxemia during endotracheal suctioning. *Anesthesiology* 31:473-475; 1969.
69. Shim C. Cardiac arrhythmias resulting from tracheal suctioning. *Ann Intern Med* 71:1149-1153; 1969.
70. Demers RR. Complications of endotracheal suctioning procedures. *Resp Care* 27:453-457; 1982.
71. Tobin MJ. Respiratory monitoring in the intensive care unit *Am Rev Resp Dis* 138:1625-1642; 1988.
72. Pologue JA. Pulse oximetry: technical aspects of machine design. *Int Anesth Clin* 25:137-153; 1987.
73. Niehoff J, DelGuericio C, LaMorte W, et al. Efficacy of pulse oximetry and capnometry in postoperative ventilatory weaning. *Crit Care Med* 16:701-705; 1988.
74. Saunders NA, Powles ACP, Rebuck AS. Ear oximetry: accuracy and practicability in the assessment of arterial oxygenation. *Am Rev Resp Dis* 113:745-749; 1976.
75. Chapman KR, Liu FLW, Watson RM, et al. Range of accuracy of two wave-length oximetry. *Chest* 89:540-542; 1986.
76. Palve H, Vuori A. Pulse oximetry during low cardiac output and hypothermia states immediately after open heart surgery. *Crit Care Med* 17:66-69; 1989.

77. Scheller J, Loeb R. Respiratory artifact during pulse oximetry in critically ill patients. *Anesthesiology* 69:602-603; 1988.
78. Wiedeman HP, McCarthy K. Noninvasive monitoring of oxygen and carbon dioxide. *Clin Chest Med* 10:239-253; 1989.
79. Jubran A, Tobin MJ. Reliability of pulse oximetry in titrating supplemental oxygen therapy in ventilator dependent patients. *Chest* 97:1420-1425; 1990.
80. Tobin MJ, Yang K. Weaning from mechanical ventilation. *Crit Care Clin* 6:725-747; 1990.
81. Tiep BL, Burns M, Kao D, et al. Pursed lip breathing training using ear oximetry. *Chest* 90:218-221; 1986.
82. Miyasaka K, Ohata J. Burn, erosion, and sun tan with the use of pulse oximetry in infants. *Anesthesiolosy* 67:1008-1009; 1987.
83. Carlon GC, Kay C, Miodowaik S, et al. Capnography in mechanically ventilated patients. *Crit Care Med* 16:550-556; 1988.
84. McLellan PA, Goldstein RS, Ramcharan V, et al. Transcutaneous carbon dioxide monitoring. *Am Rev Resp Dis* 124:199-203; 1981.
85. Shoemaker WC, Vidyasngar D. Physiological and clinical significance of $PtcO_2$ and $PtcCO_2$ measurements. *Crit Care Med* 9:689-690; 1981.
86. Tremper KK, Shoemaker WC. Transcutaneous O_2 monitoring of critically ill patients with and without low flow shock. *Crit Care Med* 9:706-709; 1981.
87. Tobin MJ. The pattern of breathing during successful and unsucccssful trials of weaning from mechanical ventilation. *Am Rev Resp Dis* 134:1111-1118; 1986.
88. Kimball WR, Leith DE, Robins AT. Dynamic hyperflation and ventilator dependence in chronic obstructive pulmonary disease. *Am Rev Resp Dis* 126:991-995; 1982.
89. Rochester DF, Briscoe AM. Metabolism of the working diaphragm. *Am Rev Resp Dis* 119:101-106; 1985.
90. Doekel RE, Zwillich CW, Scoggin CH, et al. Depression of hypoxic ventilatory response. *N Engl J Med* 295:358-361; 1976.
91. Agusti AG, Torres A, Estopa R, et al. Hypophosphatemia as a cause of failed weaning. *Crit Care Med* 12:142-143; 1984.
92. Aubier M, Viines N, Piquet J, et al. Effects of hypocalcemia on diaphragmatic strength generation. *J Appl Physiol* 58:2054-2061; 1985.
93. Molloy DW, Dhinga S, et al. Hypomagnesemia and respiratory muscle power. *Am Rev Resp Dis* 129:497-498; 1984.
94. Montgomery AB, Holle RH, Neagley SR, et al. Prediction of successful ventilatory weaning using airway occlusion pressure and hypercapnic challenge. *Chest* 91:496-499; 1987.
95. Estenne M, Yernault JC, DeSmet JM, et al. Phrenic and diaphram function after coronary artery bypass grafting. *Thorax* 40:293-299; 1985.
96. Wilcox P, Baile EM, Hands J, et al. Phrenic nerve function and its relationship to atelectasis after coronary artery bypass surgery. *Chest* 93:693-698; 1988.

97. Benotti PN, Bistrian B. Metabolic and nutritional aspects of weaning from mechanical ventilation. *Crit Care Med* 17:181-185; 1989.
98. Sahn SA, Lakshminarayan S, Petty T. Weaning from mechanical ventilation. *J Am Med Assoc* 235:2208-2212; 1976.
99. Tahvanainen J, Nikki P. The significance of hypoxemia with low inspired O_2 fraction before extubation. *Crit Care Med* 11:708-711; 1983.
100. Sahn SA, Lakshminarayan S. Bedside criteria for discontinuation of mechanical velitilation. *Chest* 63:1002-1005; 1973.
101. Radford EP, Ferris BG, Kriete BC. Clinical use of a normogram to estimate proper ventilation during artificial respiration. *N Engl J Med* 251:877-884; 1954.
102. Lecky JH, Ominsky AJ. Postoperative respiratory management. *Chest* 62:50-52; 1972.
103. Safar P, Kuekel HG. Prolonged artificial ventilation. *Resp Care* 1965:149-150.
104. Tahvanainen J, Salmenpera M, Nikki P. Extubation criteria after weaning from intermittent mandatory ventilation and continuous positive airway pressure. *Crit Care Med* 11:702-707; 1983.
105. Harris EA, Kenyon AM, Nisbet HD, et al. The normal alveolar-arterial oxygen tension gradient in man. *Clin Sci* 46:89-104; 1974.
106. MacIntyre NR. Respiratory function during pressure support ventilation. *Chest* 89:677-683; 1986.
107. Tomlinson JR, Miller KS, Lorch DG, et al. A prospective comparison of IMV and T-piece weaning from mechaniGal ventilation. *Chest* 96:348-352; 1989.
108. Groeger JS, Levinson MR, Graziano C, et al. Assist control versus synchronized intermittent mandatory ventilation during acute respiratory failure. *Crit Care Med* 17:607- 612; 1989.
109. Fleming WH, Bowen JC, Hatcher CA. Early complications of long term respiratory support. *J Thorac Cardiovasc Surg* 64:729-738; 1972.
110. Asmundsson T, Kilburn KH. Complications of acute reepiratory failure. *Ann Intern Med* 70:487-495; 1969.
111. Mertz JJ, Scharer L, McClement JH. A hospital outbreak of Klebsiella pneumonia from inhalation therapy with contaminated aerosol solutions. *Am Rev Resp Dis* 95:454-460, 1967.
112. Bonnet F, Richard C, Glaser P, et al. Changes in hepatic flow induced by continuous positive pressure ventilation in critically ill patients. *Crit Care Med* 10:703-705; 1982.
113. Robotham JL, Lixfeld W, Holland L, et al. The effects of positive end-expiratory pressure on right and left ventricular performance. *Am Rev Resp Dis* 121:677-683; 1980.
114. Guyton AC. *Circulatory Physiology: Cardiac Output and its Regulation.* Philadelphia, PA: WB Saunders; 1969:380-389.
115. Rasanen J, Downs JB, Stock MC. Cardiovascular effects of conventional positive pressure ventilation and airway pressure release ventilation. *Chest* 93:911-915; 1988.

116. Boldt J, Kling D, Bormann B, et al. Influence of PEEP ventilation immediately after cardiopulmonary bypass on right ventricular function. *Chest* 94:566-571; 1988.
117. Jardin F, Farcot JC, Gueret P, et al. Echocardiographic evaluation of ventricles during continuous positive pressure breathing. *J Appl Physiol* 56:619-627; 1984.
118. Lucas CE, Sugaiva G, Riddle J. Natural history and surgical dilemma of "stress" gastric bleeding. *Arch Surg* 102:266-273; 1971.
119. Peura DA, Johnson LF. Cimetidine for prevention and treatment of gastroduodenal mucosal lesions in patients in an intensive care unit. *Ann Intern Med* 103:173-177; 1985.
120. Shuman RB, Schuster DP, Zuckerman GR. Prophylactic therapy for stress ulcer bleeding: a reappraisal. *Ann Intern Med* 106:562-567; 1987.
121. Culpepper JA, Rinaldo JE, Rogers RM. Effect of mechanical ventilator mode on tendency towards respiratory alkalosis. *Am Rev Resp Dis* 132:1075-1077; 1985.
122. Strieter RM, Lynch JP. Complications in the ventilated patient. *Clin Chest Med* 9:127-135; 1988.
123. Marquez JM, Douglas ME, Downs JB. Renal function and cardiovascular response during positive airway pressure. *Anesthesiology* 50:393-398; 1979.
124. Martin RJ, Rogers RM, Gray BA. Mechanical aids to lung expansion: the physiologic basis for the use of mechanical aids to lung expansion. *Am Rev Resp Dis* 122:105-107; 1990.
125. Ali J, Serrette C, Wood LDH, et al. Effect of postoperative intermittent positive-pressure breathing on lung function. *Chest* 85:192-196; 1984.
126. Shapiro BA, Harrison RA, Kacmarck RM, et al. *Clinical Application of Respiratory Care*. Chicago Year Book Publ. 1985:123-132.
127. Burton GG, Gee GN, Hodgkin JE. *Respiratory Care*. 1977 Philadephia, PA: Lippincott; 1977:546-582.
128. Caro CG, Butler J, Dubois AB. Some effects of restriction of chest cage expansion on pulmonary function in man. *J Clin Invest* 39:573-583; 1960.
129. Dohi S, Gold MI. Comparison of two methods of postoperative reepiratory care. *Chest* 73:592-595; 1978.

Chapter 12

Cardiovascular Complications Following Open Heart Surgery

Pierre A. Casthely, MD, Haroutune Mekhjian, MD, and Thil Yoganathan, MD

The two most dangerous periods during any cardiovascular operation are the induction of anesthesia and the transfer of the patient from the operating room to the recovery room. One of the safest ways to transport the patient to the recovery room is to use ventilation with 100% oxygen and simultaneous arterial blood pressure and ECG monitoring. Initial postoperative care is very essential in decreasing the mortality and morbidity associated with open heart surgery.

Monitoring is one of the most important considerations involved in the management of the postoperative cardiac patients. It may be (a) continuous (ECG, arterial blood pressure, central venous pressure, pulmonary artery pressures); (b) hourly (temperature, cardiac output, urine, chest tube drainage); (c) intermittent (arterial blood gases, electrolytes, BUN, creatinine, glucose, hemo-

From Casthely PA, Bregman D, (eds): *Cardiopulmonary Bypass: Physiology, Related Complications, and Pharmacology.* Mount Kisco, NY, Futura Publishing Company, Inc., © 1991.

globin, hematocrit, prothrombin time and partial thromboplastin time, platelets, 12-lead ECG, chest X-ray).

This monitoring may vary depending on the patient's status. For example a patient with low cardiac output may require more vigilant cardiac output assessment.

The most common cardiovascular complications in the postoperative period are: (1) hypertension, (2) low output syndrome, (3) arrhythmias, (4) perioperative myocardial infarction (POMI), (5) postpericardiectomy syndrome (Table I).

Table I
Common Cardiovascular Complications in the Postoperative Period

— Hypertension
— Low output syndrome
— Arrhythmias
— Perioperative myocardial infarction (POMI)
— Post pericardiotomy syndrome

Hypertension

Increases in afterload are a common occurrence in the postoperative period. It is usually due to vasoconstriction, hypothermia, or low cardiac output and is treated with vasodilators, inotropic agents, and the insertion of an intra-aortic balloon pump. Hypertension following cardiac surgery occurs in 30% to 50% of patients undergoing coronary bypass, and in 5% of patients undergoing cardiac valve replacement.[1] The precise mechanisms remain unclear, but increased circulating catecholamines and increased renin-angiotensin activity are believed to play a role. Hypertension can increase myocardial oxygen demand, which in turn can lead to infarction of marginally ischemic areas and can also cause postoperative hemorrhage.

Hypoxia, hypercarbia, pain, bladder distension, and shivering may contribute to hypertension in the postoperative period and should be treated aggressively using vasodilators, analgesics, warming blankets, and adequate ventilation. These drugs may be used individually or in combination.

Intravenous Hypotensive Agents

The most commonly used hypotensive agents are sodium nitroprusside, nitroglycerin, trimetaphan, smooth-muscle relaxants, β-adrenergic blockers, labetalol and calcium channel blockers.

Sodium nitroprusside (SNP, nipride) continues to be the most widely used drug to treat hypertension in the open heart patient.[2] The solution of SNP is very sensitive to light and should be protected with aluminum foil. Fresh solutions should be made every 24 hours to prevent tachyphylaxis leading to cyanide intoxication. Sodium nitroprusside primarily dilates resistance vessels either by interfering with sulfhydryl groups or intracellular calcium activation. Its advantages are a very rapid onset and brief duration of action.

Cyanide (CN) is produced when SNP is metabolized. One milligram of SNP contains 0.44 mg of CN. The CN is eliminated by combining with methemoglobin or thiosulfate to form cyanomethemoglobin and thiocyanate respectively, which are excreted via the kidney. The remaining CN is metabolized through the rhodanase system in the liver, forming thiocyanate or it binds to the cytochrome oxidase in the tissue to cause CN toxicity. Recommended maximum dosage of 1.5 mg/kg for acute administration and 0.5 mg/kg/hour (8 μg/kg/min) for chronic administration appear to be safe guidelines.[3] Toxic blood levels (greater than 200 μg%) occur when greater than 1 mg/kg SNP is administered within 2½ hours. Death following SNP, secondary to CN, has been reported when the blood CN level was 400 μg%. Greater risk of CN toxicity exists in patients who are nutritionally deficient in the cobalamin (vitamin B^{12} compounds) or in dietary substances containing specific sulfur donors, or in patients who have an abnormal rhodanese system. Measurement of blood CN and pH will detect abnormalities in those patients at risk and determine in whom smaller amounts of SNP than previously recommended are used. Patients with end stage renal disease are usually more resistant to SNP toxicity because of the increased availability of sulfur donors. Signs of toxicity include: (1) severe metabolic acidosis because of increased anaerobic metabolism due to the binding of CN to the cytochrome oxidase of the tissues; and (2) an increase in mixed venous oxygen content because of decreased oxygen extraction. Treatment should consist of administration of intravenous thiosulfate, nitrates, methylene blue, and hydroxocobalamin.[4]

Thiocyanate levels increase when renal function is compromised and produces abnormal central nervous system (CNS) activity at levels greater than 5–10 mg/dL.

Rebound hypertension occurs following abrupt discontinuation of SNP. These complications result from increased plasma renin activity (PRA) from either ischemic or dilated renal vessels.[5] As we know, the plasma half-life of renin is greater than SNP (30 minutes vs 2 minutes). Gradual discontinuation of SNP, use of preoperative propranolol, and a converting enzyme inhibitor will attenuate this response until the increased PRA returns to normal.

Another adverse effect is the occurrence of abnormal blood coagulation following SNP-induced platelet disintegration and inhibition of platelet aggregation.[6] If hypotension occurs this may also result in increased pulmonary shunting in patients with normal pulmonary function. However, the pulmonary vessels of patients with chronic obstructive pulmonary disease (COPD) have little response to SNP, and shunting changes are not significant.[7]

Hypothyroidism may result from thiocyanate interference with thyroid iodide trapping mechanisms after chronic administration of SNP.[8]

Nitroglycerine is a predominant vasodilator with less marked effect on the arteries. It has many advantages over sodium nitroprusside. It does not produce toxic metabolites (although methemoglobin formation is a possible byproduct) and furthermore does not result in rebound hypertension. While nitroprusside may worsen myocardial blood flow in the ischemic region by reducing coronary perfusion pressure without augmenting collateral blood flow, nitroglycerin may improve ischemia by increasing flow through preexisting intracoronary collateral channels. The magnitude of ST segment elevation was increased with nitroprusside and improved with nitroglycerin.[9] Only nitroglycerin improved myocardial metabolism as measured by myocardial lactate utilization. Nitroglycerine is absorbed by various plastics especially polyvinylchloride plastic and should be given using a special administration set.

Trimetaphan is a ganglionic blocker that may be used if there is risk for developing toxicity to sodium nitroprusside. Trimetaphan also causes histamine release, tachyphylaxis, dilates the pupils, and has a slow onset of action. It is very seldom used to treat hypertension in the postoperative cardiac patient.

Hydralazine and diazoxide are smooth muscle relaxants. The therapeutic effect of 2.5 mg of hydralazine occurs within 10 minutes and its duration of action is approximately 4 hours. These agents cause reflex tachycardia, which may worsen myocardial ischemia.[10] Because of this side effect and its prolonged half-life its use has been completely abolished in the care of the postoperative open heart patient. Phentolamine, prazosin, and prostaglandin are not currently used vasodilators.

β-Adrenergic Blockers

A hyperdynamic cardiovascular function (increased cardiac output and systemic vascular resistance, sinus tachycardia) usually occurs during hypertension. β-Adrenergic blockade is particularly useful in these patients because they have increased catecholamine levels.[11] Intravenous propanolol is very effective in repeated doses of 1 mg. An ultrashort-acting β-adrenergic blocker, esmolol, appears to provide effective control of blood pressure and is gaining popularity. It is given in bolus of 25 mg followed by a continuous infusion of 50 to 250 μg/kg/min. It offers many advantages: (a) no increase in intrapulmonary shunting; (b) very short duration of therapeutic effect (2 minutes); (c) easily titratable; (d) only a small increase in pulse pressure, and (e) minimal decrease of cardiac output.[12–17] β-Adrenergic blockers should be used cautiously in patients with bronchospastic disorders.

Labetalol

Labetalol is an antihypertensive agent with both α- and β-blocking effects.[18] It is usually given in incremental doses of 10 to 30 mg followed by a continuous infusion of 2 mg/min. In one study, labetalol was successfully used in treating hypertension in 85% of the post-operative open heart patients.[19] It's mechanism of action appears to be negative inotropy and chronotropy. Like other β-blockers it should be used cautiously in patients with bronchospastic diseases.

Calcium Channel Blockers

The calcium channel blockers currently approved for use in the United States are diltiazem, nifedipine, nicardipine, and verapamil. All of these drugs have been used to treat postoperative hypertension. However, nicardipine holds the most promise for the future.[20] It is a short-acting, dihydropyridine, calcium entry blocker similar to nifedipine, but is stable in solution and can be administered intravenously.[21] It is unique among the calcium channel blockers in its consistent augmentation of coronary blood flow and ability to produce potent, subselective vasodilation in the coronary circulation. For postoperative hypertension, nicardipine can be administered as an intravenous loading infusion of 10 to 15 mg over 25 minutes, followed by a maintenance infusion of 3 to 5 mg/hr. Nicardipine offers many advantages: (a) a rapid onset of action (2.5 minutes); (b) short duration of therapeutic effect; (c) excellent titratability during the postoperative period. Nicardipine is as effective as nitroprusside in controlling blood pressure during coronary artery bypass surgery and it accomplishes this with fewer abnormal changes in the ST segments of the electrocardiogram.[22] Blood pressure is usually controlled within 6 to 7 minutes after intravenous administration of nicardipine to patients in the postoperative period without significant increases in heart rate.[23] It increased cardiac output more than nitroglycerin, but did not decrease filling pressures as much. It is very close to being the ideal antihypertensive drug for patients with coronary artery disease.

Low Output Syndrome

Low output syndrome is one of the major cardiovascular complications following cardiopulmonary bypass. It is usually due to myocardial damage (ischemia) or excessive workload (pressure or volume overload). The basic biochemical defect is usually due to impairment of calcium delivery and transport to the actin myosin contractile proteins.

The goal of therapy is to improve cardiac performance and reduce the heart's workload. This includes the augmentation of the preload by volume infusion, the use of inotropes, and the use of vasodilators. Mechanical interventions such as the insertion of an intra-aortic balloon pump can also be used and will be described in another chapter.

A balance must be maintained between the oxygen supply and demand of the heart. Factors affecting the oxygen supply include: hemoglobin, coronary artery patency, and the oxygen-hemoglobin dissociation curve. Factors affecting the oxygen demand of the heart include heart rate, preload, afterload, wall tension, and contractility.

Low preload is usually responsible for the low output syndrome seen in the postoperative period. This diagnosis can easily be made by interpreting the data obtained from a pulmonary artery catheter. The optimal value for preload is different before and after cardiopulmonary bypass. A high preload usually suggests over transfusion, impaired myocardial function, mitral valve dysfunction, or cardiac tamponade. The optimal preload is 10–16 mm Hg for normal ventricles and up to 22 mm Hg for ventricles with depressed function. These values can be increased by changing the intravascular volume via a colloid infusion, or decreased by vasodilators.

Cardiac output is the product of stroke volume and heart rate. An increasing heart rate should improve the output of the failing heart. Increasing the heart rate improves the cardiac performance most effectively in patients with wide pulse pressures. The inotropic effects of tachycardia decrease the heart size, thereby improving the subendocardial blood flow. The optimal heart rate in the postop open heart patient is usually between 80–100 beats/min. Bradycardia decreases cardiac output and should always be treated by pacing. Atrial pacing is preferable to ventricular pacing because the atrial kick accounts for 15% of the cardiac output. Patients with atrial fibrillation will not benefit from atrial pacing and therefore ventricular pacing is recommended. In the cases of heart block, atrioventricular sequential pacing should be used.

A variety of factors may be responsible for abnormal ventricular function following cardiac surgery. These include: abnormal myocardial protection, preexisting ventricular dysfunction, acute myocardial infarction, coronary air embolism, hypoxemia, and overdosing of antiarrhythmic medications. A low cardiac index is most often the earliest sign of ventricular dysfunction. Agents commonly used to treat abnormalities of cardiac contractility include: dopamine, dobutamine, epinephrine, norepinephrine, isoproterenol, amrinone, and calcium.

Dopamine

Dopamine is a naturally occurring precursor of norepinephrine and has both α and β receptor stimulating properties. It can specifically cause dilatation of the renal and mesenteric blood vessels in low doses (2–5 μg/kg/min) without any increases of heart rate or blood pressure. At higher doses (5–10 μg/kg/min) this drug has general β receptor stimulating properties on the heart that results in an increased cardiac output and tachycardia. At dosages greater than 10 μg/kg/min/min, dopamine stimulates α adrenergic receptors and results in peripheral vasoconstriction, which can be associated with significant dysrhythmia due to enhanced β stimulation.

Dobutamine

Dobutamine is a synthetic, inotropic catecholamine which produces myocardial β adrenergic stimulation and hence increases myocardial contractility.[24] Dobutamine exerts a favorable effect on coronary blood flow and myocardial oxygen consumption. It decreases wall stress while increasing mean systolic blood pressure.[25] Systemic and pulmonary vascular resistance decrease with dobutamine infusion. It does not stimulate renal dopaminergic receptors to cause vasodilatation. However, it usually increases renal blood flow by increasing cardiac output.[26] Administration of dobutamine for 24 hours may result in a tachyphylaxis effect. Unlike dopamine, dobutamine rarely causes tachycardia and produces little vasoconstriction at the usual therapeutic doses.

Epinephrine

Epinephrine continues to be a useful drug for treating low output failure following open heart surgery.[27,28] Epinephrine has prominent actions on the myocardium and the vascular smooth muscle stimulating both α and β adrenergic receptors. The result is increased heart rate and markedly increased cardiac work and oxygen consumption. In the heart and peripheral vascular beds, epinephrine at a dose of 1–2 μg/min primarily causes β_1- and β_2-adrenergic stimulation. At doses of 2–10 μg/min, the α-adrenergic stimulating effects become more prominent. Epinephrine is extremely valuable in the treatment of low output syndrome following cardiac surgery. Its usefulness can be limited by the development of tachycardia and dysarrhythmias. The addition of vasodilators to epinephrine can offset the splenic and renal vasoconstricting effects.

Norepinephrine

Norepinephrine, like epinephrine, stimulates both α- and β-adrenergic receptors. However, the α receptors stimulation of norepinephrine is apparent at a dosage lower than that needed for epinephrine. It is most useful to treat a high cardiac output associated with a low peripheral vascular resistance and low mean arterial blood pressure. Norepinephrine is also used to maintain adequate perfusion pressure in patients with low cardiac output following ventricular aneurysm resection. Low doses of dopamine can be added to the norepinephrine infusion to reduce renal vascular resistance and augment renal blood flow.[29]

Isoproterenol

Isoproterenol is the most potent synthetic catecholamine cardiac stimulant. It is a pure β drug. It causes marked dilatation of most vascular smooth muscle beds (kidneys, brain, coronary arteries, lungs).[30] Isoproterenol has a marked potential for inducing tachycardia and ventricular ectopic beats both by its direct action and its peripheral vasodilatation. It is useful in stimulating cardiac pacemaker cells in patients with bradycardia and atrioventricular block and after cardiac transplantation.[31] It is also useful in decreasing pulmonary vascular resistance in patients with primary or secondary pulmonary hypertension.

Amrinone

Amrinone is a newly synthesized dypyridine ring that possesses a potent inotropic effect. It is neither a catecholamine nor a digitalis glycoside. It acts by inhibiting phosphodiesterase, thereby increasing cellular levels of cyclic AMP. However, the hemodynamic and clinical benefits of amrinone have been complicated by a variety of side effects including: dose-related thrombocytopenia, hepatotoxicity, and fever. Amrinone therapy usually begins with a bolus of 1 mg/kg administrated over 3–5 minutes period following by a maintenance infusion of 5 μg/kg/min. It is very useful in patients with right ventricular failure and pulmonary hypertension.[32]

Calcium

Calcium is critical for excitation-contraction coupling in cardiac muscle.[32] The ionized or free calcium is the only form that is available for physiological activity. Low calcium ion concentration is usually associated with a decrease in peripheral vascular resistance and significant depression of ventricular function. Calcium appears to be essential for the action of most of the vasoactive drugs including sympathomimetic amines.

Cardiopulmonary bypass may lead to hypocalcemia. Among the events associated with cardiopulmonary bypass that may cause changes in calcium ion concentration are: use of citrated blood products,[33] heparin administration,[34] and albumin administration.[35] Prostacyclin may also modulate the vascular actions of calcium in humans.[36] The importance of the interactions between the prostanoids and serum calcium is presently unknown. It is not known at the present time if calcium can overcome the negative inotropism associated with the administration of calcium channel blockers to cardiac surgical patients.[37,38]

Calcium can also be detrimental in the presence of global and regional myocardial ischemia. However, calcium is potentially useful to restore normal intravascular calcium levels after open heart surgery. It has short-lived beneficial effects on cardiac performance[39] and transiently raises systemic vascular resistance[40,41] and blood pressure.[42] It increases left ventricular dp/dt, cardiac index, and stroke volume, which appears to be related to the initial calcium level. It reverses the hypotension induced by protamine, and may precipitate arrhythmias in patients taking digitalis. Long-term infusions do not sustain the beneficial effects of calcium administration.[39] Administration of calcium chloride can temporarily improve ventricular function and blood pressure and afford time to administer definitive therapy.

Rational Selection of Inotropic Drugs

The desired response in heart rate, filling pressures, pulmonary and systemic pressures must be evaluated before selecting an inotropic drug. Dopamine and dobutamine are the agents of first choice in the postoperative cardiac patients who require inotropic support. Both of these agents are equally effective in increasing cardiac output. However, they have different effects on the peripheral vasculature and myocardial oxygen consumption. Dobutamine appears to be most useful in patients in whom reductions in afterload and preload are indicated. A fall in mean arterial pressure must be expected, or at least anticipated after dobutamine infusion, but the oxygen consumption is reduced.

Dopamine is particularly advantageous in contracting the reperfused, salvaged, stunned myocardium following acute ischemia.[11,43] It increases myocardial oxygen consumption and mean arterial pressure. Dopamine enhances urine output by increasing renal blood flow at doses of 2–5 μg/kg especially in patients with underlying renal abnormalities and abnormal ventricular function.[44]

A combination of low dose dopamine for its specific renal effects, and dobutamine for its inotropic effects, may be useful to maximize the benefit of these agents, while decreasing their undesirable side effects.[45]

The combination of inotropic drugs and vasodilators is more often effective.[46–49] Epinephrine is very effective in patients with severe impairment of left ventricular function. It can be used in combinations with dopamine and dobutamine. If often produces metabolic acidosis by increasing blood glucose levels when used in high doses.

Isoproterenol is almost totally reserved for patients with extreme pulmonary hypertension and right ventricular failure due to mitral valve disease. It can also be used after cardiac transplantation and before stable endogenous pacemakers are established in the transplanted heart.

Amrinone's role in the treatment of low cardiac output is not completely established. It may be useful in situations where dobutamine is indicated and tachycardia is unwanted. Hypotension may follow its use.

Calcium has no role in maintenance of inotropism in the postoperative cardiac patients. It may be used as a temporary measure to raise the blood pressure until the diagnosis is made and definitive treatment established.

Combination therapy with an inotrope and a vasodilator offers many advantages over the inotrope alone: (1) a greater augmentation of cardiac output and blood pressure, (2) vital organ functions are better maintained, (3) fewer side effects are evident. In acute ventricular failure, therapy with inotropes and vasodilators can achieve dramatic short-term benefits while allowing "stunned" myocardium to recover. Combined inotrope and vasodilator therapy, has markedly contributed to decreased morbidity and mortality from the low output syndrome in conjunction with CHF after cardiac surgery.[50]

Cardiac Tamponade

Cardiac tamponade is also a cause of low output syndrome following open heart surgery. It occurs in 3%–15% of patients following cardiac surgery.[51,52] Closure of the pericardium is not associated with a higher incidence of postoperative tamponade. It can occur even if the pericardium is not closed and the chest tubes are draining adequately. Most of the time it occurs in the first postoperative hours or day, and is usually recognized and adequately treated.

A very high index of suspicion must exist for the early diagnosis of cardiac tamponade. It should be the first diagnosis to be considered in a postoperative cardiac patient with evidence of bleeding and low output syndrome. It should also be considered in any patient with rapid deterioration of this cardiovascular status and cessation or abrupt slowing of chest tube drainage or increase of bleeding.

Tamponade delayed by several days is less common.[53–56] The classical signs of cardiac tamponade: pulsus paradoxicus, equalization of pulmonary capillary wedge pressure and central venous pressure, and echocardiographic criteria may be absent. The diagnosis is particularly difficult when compression of the heart is not generalized but localized because a clot is compressing one or two chambers of the heart.[57] When the left-sided chambers are compressed, right atrial pressure, although elevated, does not rise sufficiently to equal the left ventricular filling pressure.

Cardiac tamponade is readily reversible. Satisfactory echocardiograms are technically difficult and do not offer much help in the diagnosis of delayed cardiac tamponade. However, contrast enhanced computerized tomography will demonstrate the pericardial effusion when the echocardiography fails to do so.

Treatment consists of immediate evacuation of the tamponade. This can be done through the subxiphoid approach under local anesthesia or through median sternotomy. Pericardiocentesis under fluoroscopy has also proven to be effective in rare cases.

Arrhythmias

Arrhythmias can occur in up to 50% of patients after cardiac surgery (Table II). The etiology is multifactorial and includes: the trauma of surgery, endogenous and exogenous catecholamines, drugs, hypoxia, electrolyte and acid-base abnormalities, and the

Table II
Factors Predisposing Arrhythmias

— Recent myocardial infarction
— Severe myocardial ischemia
— Poor ventricular function
— Incomplete revascularization
— Duration of aortic cross clamping time
Inadequate myocardial protection

underlying cardiac disease (Table II). The most common arrhythmias are enumerated in Table III.

Premature Ventricular Contractions

Premature ventricular contractions are common, but in the postoperative cardiac patient they are important because they may serve as a warning of impending ventricular tachycardia and fibrillation. They must be treated aggressively. Their incidence is greatest following aortic valve replacement and coronary artery bypass surgery. Indications for treatment include premature ventricular contractions that occur six or more times per minute, those that are multifocal, and those that occur close to the preceding T wave.

Should the underlying cardiac rate be slow, then overdrive pacing using atrial or ventricular wires may suppress the premature ventricular contractions. Temporary pacing wires left on the atrium and ventricle at the completion of cardiac surgery allow convenient access.

Table III
Common Arrhythmias Following Open Heart Surgery

— Premature ventricular contractions
— Ventricular tachycardia and fibrillation
— Sinus tachycardia
— Sinus bradycardia
— Supraventricular dysarrhythmias
— Heart block and nodal rhythm

Lidocaine is the drug most commonly used to treat premature ventricular contractions. A loading dose of 1 mg/kg intravenously is given initially, followed by maintenance doses of 1 to 4 mg per minute. Procainamide is often the second drug of choice when premature ventricular contractions are refractory to lidocaine. An initial loading dose of 5 mg/kg followed by an continuous infusion of 1 to 4 mg/min is often sufficient. Side effects include peripheral vasodilation and depression of cardiac contractility. Quinidine may raise serum digoxin levels, and appropriate dosage adjustments in digoxin may be required.

Potassium may be very effective in suppressing premature ventricular contractions, particularly in patients on digitalis therapy. Ideally, the serum potassium concentration should be maintained between 4–5 mEq/L throughout the postoperative period. Potassium will counteract the dysrhythmic effects of digitalis without suppressing its inotropic effects. However, potassium should not be used when prolonged atrioventricular conduction is observed, because it may cause conversion to complete heart block.

Bretylium tosylate is highly effective in reducing ventricular irritability, and it may be particularly useful in cases in which such irritability has been refractory to treatment with other drugs. Peripheral vasodilation and hypotension may be seen unless it is given slowly. The usual dosage is 7 mg/kg IV followed by a continuous infusion of 1 to 4 mg/min.

Phenytoin sodium is particularly effective in suppressing the premature ventricular contractions that are caused by digitalis toxicity.

Patients requiring drug treatment for premature ventricular contractions within the first week of cardiac surgery are generally discharged home on a long-term regimen of antidysarrhythmic therapy.

Ventricular Tachycardia and Fibrillation

Ventricular tachycardia accompanied by hypotension is treated with electrocardioversion. Ventricular tachycardia without hypotension may be treated with lidocaine and, if that is unsuccessful, by electrocardioversion. Should lidocaine fail to control recurring ventricular tachycardia, then procainamide and bretylium will generally be the drugs of choice. It should be noted, however, that procainamide and related drugs can cause prolongation of the QT interval and may precipitate ventricular tachycardia. Ventricular fibrillation is treated by electrocardioversion followed by lidocaine, procainamide, or bretylium infusion.

Sinus Tachycardia

Sinus tachycardia is usually due to fever, hypoxia, hypovolemia, and tamponade. It increases the oxygen demand of the heart and may precipitate myocardial ischemia. After treating the underlying cause, small doses of propranolol or esmolol may help by decreasing the heart rate.

Sinus bradycardia may be severe enough to produce hypotension. Atrial pacing or infusion of dopamine and isuprel may be required.

Supraventricular Dysrhythmia

Supraventricular dysrhythmia are commonly seen following cardiac surgery. Supraventricular dysrhythmia with aberrant conduction may closely resemble ventricular tachycardia, and the nature of any tachycardia following cardiac surgery must be determined as soon as possible. Maneuvers to slow the ventricular rate include: massage of the carotid sinus, applying pressure to the eyeball, and the Valsalva maneuver. Most of those patients require prompt administration of digitalis, calcium channel blockers, or both. Edrophonium chloride (10 mg intravenously in adults) may also slow any ventricular response to supraventricular tachycardia. These maneuvers may facilitate analysis of the dysrhythmia. When epicardial atrial wires have been left in place after cardiac surgery, the recording of electrocardiographic activity from these leads may help to differentiate underlying dysrhythmia.

The occurrence of atrial fibrillation frequently results in decreases in cardiac output that are detrimental to the cardiac surgical patient. Atrial fibrillation or flutter may be converted quickly to sinus rhythm by electrical stimulation of the atrium utilizing atrial electrodes. Capture of the atrium and breaking up the reentry circuits may result from atrial pacing as rapidly as 300 beats/min. When rapid supraventricular tachycardia is accompanied by hypotension, electric cardioversion should be done immediately.

β-Adrenergic blocking drugs are effective in the treatment of supraventricular tachyarrhythmias (SVT). They prolong the condition time through the AV node, thereby reducing the ventricular rate and improving ventricular function. The occurrence of SVT in patients with underlying coronary artery disease may have serious consequences due to the rapid rate increasing the myocardial oxygen demand. Although β-blockers are beneficial in this setting, the relatively long duration of the older drugs limits their use during acute situations. However, esmolol may prove useful because of its unique pharmacokinetic profile. The efficacy and safety of esmolol in patients with SVT (atrial fibrillation, atrial flutter, and sinus tachycardia) have been demonstrated in clinical studies. The efficacy of esmolol was compared with that of IV verapamil in patients with either recent onset or previous onset atrial fibrillation or flutter.[58] The mean reduction of heart rate with esmolol and verapamil was 24% and 31%, respectively. Hypotension occurred with equal frequency between those treated with esmolol or verapamil, but was more readily controllable in the patients treated with esmolol than in those treated with intermittent doses of verapamil (5 to 10 mg). Discontinuing or lowering the esmolol infusion dosage caused the hypotension to resolve within 5 to 20 minutes. Because esmolol and verapamil have been shown to be equally effective in patients with atrial fibrillation or flutter, and because of the obvious advantage of the short duration of action of esmolol, it appears to be safer as the first-line drug. The other major advantage appears to be a higher conversion rate to normal sinus rhythm during titration. In one study, 36% of the esmolol-treated patients were found to convert to normal sinus rhythm versus only 12% with verapamil.[58]

Verapamil can slow the ventricular response to atrial fibrillation and frequently convert paroxysmal supraventricular tachycardia or atrial flutter to a sinus rhythm, but side effects like peripheral vasodilation and cardiac depression can be detrimental in the postoperative cardiac surgical patient.

Verapamil, 75 μg/kg, is usually very effective in reducing the ventricular rate within several minutes, but conversion is rare. Intravenous bolus therapy of verapamil may result in hypotension that may be prevented by the slow administration of verapamil (mg/min) or by pretreatment with an intravenous dose of calcium. Calcium therapy reverses the hemodynamic effects of verapamil but does not reverse the electrophysiologic effects. Frequently, a 30% reduction in the ventricular rate can be achieved with the initial dose of verapamil, but maximal clinical effects last only 30–45 minutes. To maintain this reduction of the heart rate, intravenous digoxin is necessary after successful rate reduction with verapamil. However, digoxin is not as effective as verapamil and may lack effectiveness in rate control during the stress of the perioperative period.

Digoxin has a slower onset of action than verapamil but is more useful for chronic treatment. One half of a digitalizing dose may be safely given over 5 minutes, with two additional doses of one quarter the digitalizing dose given over the next two to three hours. Additional doses can be based on the ventricular response.

Recently, procainamide and esmolol have demonstrated effectiveness in the conversion of atrial fibrillation to sinus rhythm. Esmolol in several studies has shown a 50% success rate in converting this arrhythmia to sinus rhythm. Patients who are successfully cardioverted electrically usually have atrial fibrillation of less than 1 year's duration, a left atrial dimension of less than 45 mm by echocardiography, no ventricular enlargement, and have had prior successful treatment of the precipitating factor. Anticoagulation should be considered prior to cardioversion in patients in atrial fibrillation longer than 4 to 5 days and maintained for several weeks after establishment of sinus rhythm.

Atrial Flutter

Atrial flutter is much less common than atrial fibrillation but shares the same predisposing factors. Atrial flutter is categorized into two types: type I and type II. Type I atrial flutter usually occurs at a rate of 300 beats/min with a ventricular rate of 150 beats/min. The flutter waves are of a typical sawtooth or biphasic appearance in the inferior leads and are usually converted by rapid atrial pacing. Type II atrial flutter exhibits a flat baseline with a positive flutter waves in the inferior leads with a rate usually greater than 350 beats/min. Type II atrial flutter frequently cannot be converted by rapid atrial pacing.

Rapid Atrial Pacing (Overdrive Suppression)

Atrial flutter compared to fibrillation is usually more difficult to treat. However, rapid atrial pacing in type I atrial flutter is effective. Rapid atrial pacing should proceed at a rate approximately 20% faster than the flutter rate. During rapid atrial pacing, a change in the morphology of the flutter pattern or a change in the ventricular response is a sign of overdrive suppression. In addition, there is a critical duration of rapid atrial pacing required to convert atrial flutter. After interruption of atrial flutter, pacing should continue for approximately 30 seconds; pacing for shorter amounts of time may not be successful. Because atrial pacing thresholds are usually higher in atrial flutter and determination of capture is difficult, maximal current (usually 20 milliamps on temporary pacemakers) is necessary for overdrive suppression. If suppression does not occur, it is usually because of inadequate rate, pacing duration, or current threshold.

Adenosine

Adenosine is an endogenous nucleoside occurring in all cells of the body. It slows conduction time through the AV node and can interrupt the reentry pathways through the AV node and restore normal sinus rhythm in patients with paroxysmal supraventricular tachycardia. It has a very short half-life (10 seconds), has similar activity to verapamil and is ten times more expensive. The initial dose is 6 mg IV bolus over 2 seconds that can be repeated 2 minutes later. Doses greater than 12 mg are not recommended. At the time of conversion to normal sinus rhythm a variety of new rhythms may appear on the electrocardiogram. They generally last only a few seconds. The most common ones are premature ventricular contractions, atrial premature contractions, sinus bradycardia, sinus tachycardia and varying degrees of AV nodal block.

Intravenous adenocard is absolutely contraindicated in second or third-degree AV block, sick sinus syndrome, atrial flutter, atrial fibrillation, ventricular tachycardia.

The effective use of digoxin and propranolol to prevent the dysrhythmia that commonly follow coronary artery bypass grafting has been reported.[59] Patients are usually given digoxin 1 mg intravenously over 24 hours, followed by a maintenance dose of 0.25 mg per day orally, and propranolol 10 mg every 6 hours starting 6 hours after surgery that results in decrease ventricular and supraventricular arrhythmias. No adverse reactions were noted. The postoperative use of propranolol as a single agent in prophylaxis of these dysrhythmia has also been effective.

Heart Block and Nodal Rhythms

First-degree heart block occurs in virtually every patient following a cardiac procedure in which cardioplegia solution is used to protect the myocardium. Second-degree heart block and nodal rhythms are also common. While each of these problems is usually well tolerated, the contribution of atrial systole to overall cardiac output may be particularly important in some patients. In these patients, if the atrium is responsive to stimulation, atrial pacing may be beneficial. Atropine or isoproterenol may also prove effective. Third-degree heart block is uncommon. The use of temporary atrial and ventricular pacing electrodes with sequential atrial and ventricular pacing is appropriate treatment. Occasionally, third-degree heart block is transient and may be the result of edema or hemorrhage in the region of the conduction system. Persistence of the conduction defect for five to seven days generally indicates the need for a permanent pacemaker.

Perioperative Myocardial Infarction

Perioperative myocardial infarction (POMI) remains a major cause of death following coronary artery bypass surgery. The mechanism responsible for myocardial necrosis include for: graft occlusion, reperfusion injury, coronary artery spasm, and imbalance in the oxygen supply and demand of the heart.[60,61] There are several factors that predispose patients to perioperative myocardial infarction: severe myocardial ischemia,[62] severe diffuse, multiple vessel coronary artery disease, aortic cross clamp time, left main coronary artery disease, inadequate myocardial protection, and incomplete revascularization. The adequacy of myocardial cooling may be the most important factor in successful myocardial protection.[63] The pathophysiology of perioperative myocardial damage is often unclear and prompt assessment of the situation should be performed (Table IV). The clinical syndrome carries a high mortality rate despite the use of new inotropic agents, intra-aortic balloon pumping, secondary cardioplegia, and additional coronary artery bypass grafting. In a few cases left atrial-femoral artery or right atrial-pulmonary artery bypasses have also been used.

Malignant ventricular arrhythmias including ventricular tachycardia or fibrillation in the early postoperative period usually suggest perioperative myocardial infarction.

The electrocardiogram is the monitor routinely used to diagnose perioperative myocardial infarction. Persistent Q waves of 0.04 seconds or longer duration or new QS deflections associated with ST segment depressions greater than 2 mm in the left ventricular leads and T wave inversion, ventricular tachycardia or fibrillation, and new left bundle branch blocks are very likely to be diagnostic of POMI.[64]

Electrocardiogram changes have their limitation. New Q waves are not always associated with new areas of ventricular asynergy by ventriculogram, implying a POMI.[65] Sometimes new Q waves develop in association with improved ventriculogram and patent grafts.[66] ST segments and T waves changes are not specific and

Table IV
Assessments of Postoperative Myocardial Infarction

— Electrocardiogram
— CPK MB levels
— Infarct avid myocardial imaging
— Myocardial perfusion imaging

may be due to pericarditis, electrolytes imbalance, hypothermia, hypoglycemia, pancreatitis, or delayed ventricular conduction.[67]

Traditionally levels of the standard serum enzymes, serum glutamic oxaloacetic transaminase, creatine phosphokinase and lactic dehydrogenase have been used to indicate the presence and extent of POMI. These serum enzyme levels have lacked sensitivity and specificity because of a multiplicity of factors contributing to increased enzyme values after cardiac surgery.[68–70] The myocardial specific isoenzyme CK (CKMB) has proved useful in the diagnosis of acute myocardial infarction.[71] When CKMB levels were used together with electrocardiographic and scintigraphic methods, a greater diagnostic accuracy in detecting perioperative myocardial infarction was achieved.[72,73]

However, global myocardial ischemia and multiple defibrillations can also increase CKMB titers. A profile of serum CKMB activity based on frequent perioperative blood samples may prove to be a most discriminating technique in separating abnormal liberation of isoenzyme secondary to myocardial infarction from the ordinary elevation observed secondary to general surgical trauma. A serum CKMB curve with a prolonged plateau or perhaps a second peak may suggest myocardial damage. The values of serum CKMB still remains inconclusive. There is no correlation between the peak amount of serum CKMB and the size of myocardial infarction.

Abnormal postoperative serum CKMB levels may not be associated with a depression in the global left ventricular ejection fraction early after coronary artery bypass surgery unless the patient has low cardiac output.[74]

Infarct Avid Myocardial Imaging

Visualization of areas of myocardial necrosis by radiopharmaceutical uptake has gained popularity.[73,75] The most commonly used hot-spot imaging agent has been technetium-^{99m} pyrophosphate. Those scintigrams become positive approximately 12 hours after acute myocardial infarcts reaching a peak 72 hours after the event.[76] Most positive scintigrams fade 6–10 days after myocardial infarction, although a large perioperative myocardial infarction may remain positive longer. False-positive scan can be due to ventricular aneurysm,[77] cardioversion,[78] old myocardial infarction,[79] and bacterial endocarditis.

Myocardial scintigraphy following coronary artery bypass grafting reveals a higher incidence of POMI changes than ECG alone.[80] If only the scintigram is positive as diagnosis of POMI there is no related depression of the left ventricular ejection fraction either early or late in the postoperative period.[81] CKMB levels used concomitantly with myocardial scintigraphy may improve diagnosis accuracy.[82]

Myocardial Perfusion Imaging

Myocardial perfusion imaging (cold spot) has found wide application in the clinical evaluation of patients with ischemic heart disease[83] and the detection of acute myocardial infarction. Improvement in myocardial perfusion occurs in most cases following CABG surgery.[84]

The incidence of POMI has decreased in recent years. This may be due to the improvement in myocardial preservation techniques (cold cardioplegia), better intraoperative monitoring (pulmonary artery catheter, two-dimensional echocardiography, two-channel EKG monitoring) better anesthetic technique (sulfentanyl or fentanyl versus halothane, ethrane, or isoflurane). The treatment is aimed in optimizing the oxygen supply demand ratio of the myocardium. Hypertension, hypotension and tachycardia should be avoided at any cost. Judicious use of inotropic, vasodilator, β blockers, calcium channel blocker, and antiarrhythmic medications and the intra-aortic balloon will help decrease the mortality rate associated with POMI.

Nicardipine

Nicardipine, as well as other calcium channel blockers, has been shown to have beneficial effects on the ischemic myocardium when therapy is initiated before or immediately after the onset of ischemia.[85,86] Treatment late in the ischemic period or during reperfusion does not reverse ischemic injury.[85] During acute coronary artery occlusion in dogs, nicardipine increased regional myocardial oxygen tension, and preservation of function.[87] A direct cytoprotective effect of nicardipine against anoxic damage in myocardial cells has also been demonstrated.[88]

Intravenous nicardipine has been shown to consistently increase cardiac index in healthy volunteers and in patients. This action is primarily attributed to its effect on systemic vascular resistance (SVR). Following nicardipine administration, SVR is reduced to approximately half the control value. The correlation between increases in cardiac index and decreases in SVR suggests that afterload reduction might be responsible for improved cardiac pumping activity.

Nicardipine has also been shown to produce beneficial cardiac hemodynamic effects in patients with mild to moderate heart failure.[89] In patients with resting ejection fractions ranging from 20% to 40%, acute administration of nicardipine, 10 to 20 mg, significantly reduced SVR with a concomitant increase in cardiac index. The net effect of nicardipine in these patients is to improve left ventricular function, presumably due to reduction of left ventricular afterload.

In a study comparing the cardiac hemodynamic effects (rest and exercise) of verapamil and nicardipine at doses selected to produce equal reductions in SBP, it was shown that cardiac function was significantly depressed following verapamil, but not nicardipine.[90]

Favorable hemodynamic effects were reported in CAD patients receiving nicardipine and β-blockers. In a study evaluating the combination therapy of nicardipine and metoprolol, it was found that addition of nicardipine countered the increase in SVR and cardiac depressant effects of metoprolol.[91]

Nicardipine is a potent coronary vasodilator as demonstrated by increased coronary blood flow and decreased coronary vascular resistance in patients with CAD.[92] The effect on coronary vascular resistance is greater than on SVR. Intravenous nicardipine has been shown to reduce ventricular lactate production in patients with angina pectoris, suggesting that nicardipine improves perfusion and aerobic metabolism in chronically ischemic areas. Similarly, intracoronary injection of nicardipine in patients undergoing percutaneous transluminal coronary angioplasty resulted in reduced lactate production and accelerated lactate extraction, indicating a protective effect on the ischemic myocardium.[93,94]

Postpericardiotomy Syndrome

The postpericardiotomy syndrome is characterized by the appearance of pericarditis 1 week or longer after open heart surgery. The findings include: fever, chest pain, malaise, pericardial and pleural effusions, dyspnea, leukocytosis, pericardial rub, and atypical lymphocytes. Electrocardiograms may show the reappearance of ST segment and T wave changes consistent with pericarditis. Rarely the syndrome leads to cardiac tamponade.

The cause of postpericardiotomy syndrome is not known. But there is evidence that strongly suggests that it is triggered by a combination of an autoimmune reaction to injury coupled with viral infection.[95–99] The post pericardiotomy syndrome, being an autoimmune reaction, responds well to treatment with antiinflammatory agents. Steroids should be avoided whenever possible by giving antiinflammatory drugs such as indomethacin, motrin, and ASA. Because of the recurrent nature of the disease the medications should be continued for several weeks (4–6 weeks). When symptoms recur prednisone 80 mg daily should be given.

REFERENCES

1. Estafanous FG, Tarazi RF. Systemic arterial hypertension associated with cardiac surgery. *Am J Cardiol* 46:685-692, 1980.
2. Roberts AJ, Niarchos AP, Subramanian VA. Systemic hypertension associated with coronary artery surgery: predisposing factors, hemodynamic characteristics, humoral profile and treatment. *J Thorac Cardiovasc Surg* 86:47-56, 1983.
3. Michenfelder TD, Tinker JH. Cyanide toxicity and thiosulfate protection during chronic administration of sodium nitroprusside in the dog: correlation with a human case. *Anesthesiology* 47:441-447, 1977.
4. Cottrell JE, Casthely PA, Brodie JD, et al. Prevention of nitroprusside-induced cyanide toxicity with hydroxocobalamin. *N Engl J Med* 298:809-811, 1978.
5. Cottrell JE, Ullner P, Kittay MJ, et al. Rebound hypertension after sodium nitroprusside-induced hypotension. *Clin Pharmacol Ther* 27:32-36, 1980.

6. Allen FB, Gerson JI, Davis FG. Platelet inhibition by nitroprusside and nitroglycerin. *Anesthesiology* 51:575, 1979.
7. Casthely PA, Lear S, Cottrell JE, et al. Intrapulmonary shunting during induced hypotension. *Anesth Analg* 61:231-235, 1982.
8. Tinker JH, Michenfelder JD. Sodium nitroprusside. *Anesthesiology* 45:340-354, 1982.
9. Chiarello M, Gold HK, Leinback RC, et al. Comparison between the effects of nitroprusside and nitroglycerin on ischemic injury during acute myocardial infarction. *Circulation* 54:766-773, 1976.
10. Gabrielson G, Dimich L, Lingham R, et al. Comparative effects of labetalol and hydralazine in the treatment of postoperative hypertension. *J Clin Anesth* 1:201-204, 1989.
12. Turlapaty P, Laddu A, Murthy VS, et al. Esmolol: A titratable short-acting intravenous β-blocker for acute critical care settings. *Am Heart J* 114:866, 1987.
13. Erhardt PW, Woo CM, Gorczynski RJ, et al. Ultrashort-acting β-adrenergic blocking agents. *J Medkem* 25:1402, 1982.
14. Lowenthal DT, Porter RS, Saris SD, et al. The clinical pharmacology of an ultrashort-acting β-blocker, esmolol. In Kaplan JA ed. *Esmolol and the Adrenergic Response to Perioperative Stimuli.* New York, BMI, 1985:31-35.
15. Lowenthal DT, Porter RS, Saris SD, et al. Clinical pharmacology, pharmacodynamics, and interactions with esmolol. *Am J Cardiol* 56:14F-18F, 1985.
16. Sum CY, Yacobi A, Kartzinel R, et al. Kinetics of esmolol, an ultra-short-acting β-blocker, and its major metabolite. *Clin Pharmacol Ther* 34:427-434, 1983.
17. Kaplan JA. Role of ultra-short acting β-blockers in the perioperative period. *J Cardiothorac Anesth* 2:683-691, 1988.
18. Morel DR, Foster A, Suter PM. Intravenous labetalol in treatment of hypertension following coronary artery surgery. *Br J Anaesth* 54:1191-1196, 1981.
19. Sladen RN, Klamerus KJ, Swafford MWG, et al. Labetalol for the control of elevated blood pressure following coronary artery bypass grafting. *J Cardiothorac Anesth* 4:210-221, 1990.
20. Kaplan JA. Clinical considerations for the use of intravenous nicardipine in the treatment of postoperative hypertension. *Am Heart J* 119:443-446, 1990.
21. Turlapaty P, Vary R, Kaplan JA. Nicardipine, a new intravenous calcium antagonist: review of its pharmacology, pharmacokinetics, and perioperative applications. *J Cardiothorac Anesth* 3:334-355, 1989.
22. Van Wezel HB, Koolen JJ, Viser CA, et al. The efficacy of nicardipine and nitroprusside in preventing post-sternotomy hypertension. *J Cardiothorac Anesth* 3:700-706, 1989.
23. Chelly JE, Pool JL, Casar G, et al. Treatment of postoperative hypertension with intravenous nicardipine. *Clin Pharmacol Ther* 41:209-213, 1987.
24. Leier CV, Unverferth DV. Dobutamine. *Ann Intern Med* 99:490, 1983.

25. Amin DK, Shah PK, Shellock FG, et al. Comparative hemodynamic effects of intravenous dobutamine and MDL-17,043, a new cardioactive drug in severe congestive heart failure. *Am Heart J* 109:91-98, 1985.
26. Leier CV, ed. *Cardiotonic Drugs. A Clinical Survey.* New York, NY: Marcel Dekker, 1986:90-97.
27. Steen PA, Tinker JH, Pluth JR, et al. Efficacy of dopamine, dobutamine, and epinephrine during emergency from cardiopulmonary bypass in man. *Circulation* 57:378-384, 1978.
28. Tinker JH. Strong inotropes (e.g., epinephrine) should be drugs of first choice during emergence from cardiopulmonary bypass. *J Cardiothorac Anesth* 1:24-28, 1987.
29. Schaer GL, Fink MP, Parrillo JE. Norepinephrine alone versus norepinephrine plus low-dose dopamine: enhanced renal blood flow with combination pressor therapy. *Crit Care Med* 13:492-496, 1985.
30. Succhesi BR. Inotropic agents and drugs to support the failing heart. In: Antonaccio M, ed. *Cardiovascular Pharmacology.* New York, NY: Raven Press, 1977: 337-375.
31. Cannon DS, Rider AK, Stinson EB, et al. Electrophysiologic studies in the denervated transplanted human heart. Response to norepinephrine, isoproterenol and propanolol. *Am J Cardiol* 36:859-866, 1975.
32. Ducharne A. Amrinone efficacy in experimental cardiac transplantation: preliminary report. Transplant Proc 21(2):3344-3346, 1989.
33. Drop LJ, Scheidegger D. Plasma ionized calcium concentration. *J Thorac Cardiovasc Surg* 79:425, 1980.
34. Urban P, Scheidegger D, Buchmann B, et al. The hemodynamic effects of heparin and their relation to ionized calcium levels. *J Thorac Cardiovasc Surg* 91:303, 1986.
35. Kovalik SG, Ledgerwood AM, Lucas CE, et al. The cardiac effect of altered calcium hemostasis after albumin resuscitation. *J Trauma* 21:275, 1981.
36. DeSasa VJ, Huval W, Lelcuk S, et al. Disadvantages of prostacyclin infusion during cardiopulmonary bypass: a double-blind study of 50 patients having coronary revascularization. *Ann Thorac Surg* 38:514, 1984.
37. Walsh RA, Clearly FX, O'Rourke RA. Effects of calcium entry blockade on left ventricular dynamics in exercising dogs. *Am Physiol Soc* 656, 1986.
38. Godfraind T, Morel N, Wibo M. The heterogeneity of calcium movements in cardiac and vascular smooth muscle cells. *Scand J Clin Lab Invest* 180:29, 1986.
39. Shapira N, Schaff HV, White RD, et al. Hemodynamic effects of calcium chloride injection following cardiopulmonary bypass: response to bolus injection and continuous infusion. *Ann Thorac Surg* 37:133, 1984.
40. Auffant RA, Downs JB, Amick R. Ionized calcium concentration and cardiovascular function after cardiopulmonary bypass. *Arch Surg* 116:1072, 1981.

41. Gallagher JD, Geller EA, Moore RA, et al. Hemodynamic effects of calcium chloride in adults with regurgitant valve lesions. *Anesth Analg* 63:723, 1984.
42. Scheidegger D, Drop LJ, Schellenberg JC. Role of the systemic vasculature in the hemodynamic response to changes in plasma ionized calcium. *Arch Surg* 115:206, 1980.
43. Ellis SG, Wynne J, Braunwald E, et al. Response to reperfusion-salvaged, stunned myocardium to inotropic stimulation. *Am Heart J* 107:13, 1984.
44. Davis RF, Lappas DG, Kirklin JK, et al. Acute oliguria after cardiopulmonary bypass: renal functional improvement with low-dose dopamine infusion. *Crit Care Med* 10:852, 1982.
45. Richard C, Ricome JL, Rimailho A, et al. Combined hemodynamic effects of dopamine and dobutamine in cardiogenic shock. *Circulation* 67:620, 1983.
46. Miller DC, Stinson EB, Oyer PE, et al. Postoperative enhancement of left ventricular performance by combined inotropic-vasodilator therapy with preload control. *Surgery* 88:108, 1980.
47. Verma SP, Silke B, Nelson GIC, et al. Haemodynamic advantages of a combined inotropic/venodilator regimen over inotropic monotherapy in acute heart failure. *J Cardiovasc Pharmacol* 7:943, 1985.
48. Dell'Italia LJ, Starling MR, Blumhardt R, et al. Comparative effects of volume loading, dobutamine, and nitroprusside in patients with predominant right ventricular infarction. *Circulation* 72:1237, 1985.
49. O'Brodovitch H, Coates G. Effect of isoproterenol or exercise on pulmonary lymph flow and hemodynamics. *J Appl Physiol* 60:38, 1986.
50. Abrams J. Vasodilator therapy for congestive heart failure. *J Am Med Assoc* 254:3070-3074, 1985.
51. Weeks KR, Chatterjee K, Block S, et al. Bedside hemodynamic monitoring: its value in the diagnosis of tamponade complicating cardiac surgery. *J Thorac Cardiovasc Surg* 71:250-252, 1976.
52. Nelson RM, Jenson CB, Smoot WM II. Pericardial tamponade following open-heart surgery. *J Thorac Cardiovasc Surg* 58:510-516, 1969.
53. Fernando HA, Friedman HS, Lejam F, et al. Late cardiac tamponade following open-heart surgery: detection by echocardiography. *Ann Thorac Surg* 24:174, 1977.
54. Merrill W, Donahoo JS, Brawley RK, et al. Late cardiac tamponade. A potentially lethal complication of open-heart surgery. *J Thorac Cardiovasc Surg* 72:929-932, 1976.
55. Hill JD, Johnson DC, Miller GE, et al. Latent mediastinal tamponade after open-heart surgery. *Arch Surg* 99:808, 1969.
56. Prewitt TA, Rackley CE, Wilcox BR, et al. Cardiac tamponade as a late complication of open-heart surgery. *Am Heart J* 76:139, 1968.
57. Bateman T, Gray R, Chaux A, et al. Right atrial tamponade complicating cardiac operation: clinical, hemodynamic, and scintigraphic correlates. *J Thorac Cardiovasc Surg* 84:413-419, 1982.

58. Michelson EL, Porterfield JK, Das G, et al. A comparison of esmolol and verapamil in the treatment of atrial fibrillation/flutter. *J Am Coll Cardiol* 7:157A, 1986.
59. Mills SA, Poole GV, Breyer RH. Digoxin and propranolol in the prophylaxis of dysarrhythmias after coronary artery bypass grafting. *Circulation* 68:222-225, 1983.
60. Roberts AJ, Lichtenthal PR, Spies SM, et al. Perioperative myocardial damage in coronary artery bypass graft surgery: analysis of multifactorial etiology and evaluation of diagnostic techniques. In: Moran JM, Michaelis LL, eds. *Surgery for the Complications of Myocardial Infarction.* New York, NY: Grune & Stratton; 1980:67-92.
61. Baur HR, Peterson TA, Arnar O, et al. Predictors of perioperative myocardial infarction in coronary artery operation. *Ann Thorac Surg* 31:36, 1981.
62. Flemma RJ, Singh HM, Tector AJ, et al. Factors predictive of perioperative myocardial infarction during coronary operations. *Ann Thorac Surg* 21:215-220, 1976.
63. Jacocks MA, Fowler BN, Chaffin JS, et al. Hypothermic ischemic arrest versus hypothermic potassium cardioplegia in human being. *Ann Thorac Surg* 34:157, 1981.
64. Roberts AJ. Perioperative myocardial infarction and changes in left ventricular performance related to coronary artery bypass graft surgery. *Ann Thorac Surg* 35:208-225, 1983.
65. Warren SG, Wagner GS, Bethea CF, et al. Diagnostic and prognostic significance of electrocardiographic and CPK isoenzyme changes following coronary bypass surgery: correlation with findings at one year. *Am Heart J* 93:189, 1977.
66. Berger BC, Watson DD, Burwell LR, et al. Redistribution of thallium at rest in patients with stable and unstable angina and the effect of coronary artery bypass surgery. *Circulation* 60:1114, 1979.
67. Roberts AJ. Perioperative myocardial infarction associated with coronary artery bypass graft surgery. *Cardiovasc Rev Rep* 3:1760, 1982.
68. Galen RS. Myocardial injury during open heart surgery. *Lancet* 1:1085, 1976.
69. Hultgren MN, Miyagawa M, Buck W, et al. Ischemic myocardial injury during coronary artery surgery. *Am Heart J* 62:624, 1971.
70. Klein MS, Shell WE, Sobel BE. Serum creatine phosphokinase CPK isoenzymes following intramuscular injection, surgery and myocardial infarction: experimental and clinical studies. *Cardiovasc Res* 7:412, 1972.
71. Roberts R, Sobel BE. Creatine kinase isoenzymes in the assessment of heart disease. *Am Heart J* 95:521, 1978.
72. Kausner SC, Botvinick EH, Shames D, et al. The application of radionuclide infarct scintigraphy to diagnose perioperative myocardial infarction following revascularization. *Circulation* 56:173-181, 1977.
73. Crowley MJ, Mantle JA, Rogers WJ, et al. Technetium-^{99m} stannous pyrophosphate myocardial scintigraphy: reliability and limitations in assessment of acute myocardial infarction. *Circulation* 56:192, 1977.

74. Roberts AJ. Perioperative myocardial infarction and changes in left ventricular performance related to coronary artery bypass graft surgery. *Ann Thorac Surg* 35:208-255, 1983.
75. Lowenthal IS, Parisi AF, Tow DE, et al. Diagnosis of acute myocardial infarction in patients undergoing open heart surgery: a comparison of serial myocardial imaging with cardiac enzymes, electrocardiography, and vectorcardiography. *J Nucl Med* 18:770, 1977.
76. Buja LM, Parkey RW, Dees JH, et al. Morphologic correlates of technetium-99m stannous pyrophosphate imaging of acute myocardial infarcts in dogs. *Circulation* 52:596, 1975.
77. Ahmad M, Dubiel J, Verdon TA, et al. Technetium-99m stannous pyrophosphate myocardial imaging in patients with and without left ventricular aneurysm. *Circulation* 53:833, 1976.
78. Pugh BR, Buja LM, Parker RW, et al. Cardioversion and "false positive" technetium-99m stannous pyrophosphate myocardial scintigram. *Circulation* 54:399, 1976.
79. Olson HG, Lyons KP, Aronow WS, et al. Prognostic value of a persistently positive technetium-99m stannous pyrophosphate myocardial scintigram after myocardial infarction. *Am J Cardiol* 43:889, 1979.
80. Hung J, Kelly DT, McLaughlin AF, et al. Perioperative and postoperative technetium-99m pyrophosphate myocardial scintigraphy in the assessment of operative infarction in coronary artery surgery. *J Thorac Cardiovasc Surg* 78:68, 1979.
81. DiLuzio V, Roy PR, Sowton E. Angina in patients with occluded aortocoronary vein grafts. *Br Heart J* 36:139, 1974.
82. Roberts AJ, Jacobstein JG, Combes JR, et al. ^{99m}Tc-labeled glucoheptonate myocardial infarct imaging in patients undergoing coronary artery revascularization. *J Surg Res* 25:83, 1978.
83. Hamilton GW. Myocardial imaging with thallium-201: the controversy over its clinical usefulness in ischemic heart disease. *J Nucl Med* 20:1201, 1979.
84. Ritchie JL, Narahara KA, Trobaugh GB, et al. Thallium-201 myocardial imaging before and after coronary revascularization: assessment of regional myocardial blood flow and graft patency. *Circulation* 56:830, 1977.
85. Nayler WG, Ferrari R, Williams A. Protective effect of pretreatment with verapamil, nifedipine, and propranolol on mitochondrial function in the ischemic and reperfused myocardium. *Am J Cardiol* 46:242-248, 1980.
86. Endo T, Nejima J, Fujita S, et al. Comparative effects of nicardipine, a new calcium antagonist, on size of myocardial infarction after coronary artery occlusion in dogs. *Circulation* 74:420-430, 1986.
87. Hashimoto H, Asano M, Takiguchi Y, et al. Effects of nicardipine, a dihydropyridine calcium antagonist, on regional myocardial blood flow, myocardial oxygen tension, and electrical abnormalities during acute coronary artery occlusion in dogs. *J Cardiovasc Pharmacol* 7:613-621, 1985.

88. Hashimoto H, Asano M, Takiguchi Y, et al. Effects of nicardipine, a dihydropyridine calcium antagonist, on regional myocardial blood flow, myocardial oxygen tension, and electrical abnormalities during acute coronary artery occlusion in dogs. *J Cardiovasc Pharmacol* 7:613-621, 1985.
89. Lahiri A, Robinson CW, Caruana MP, et al. Acute and chronic, effects of nicardipine on systolic and diastolic left ventricular performance in patients with heart failure: a pilot study. *Clin Cardiol* 9:257-261, 1986.
90. Silke B, Verma SP, Hussain M, et al. Comparative hemodynamic effects of nicardipine and verapamil in coronary artery disease. *Herz* 10:112-119, 1985.
91. Silke B, Verma SP, Frais MA, et al. Hemodynamic analysis of the effects of nicardipine and metoprolol alone and in combination in coronary artery disease. *Eur Heart J* 6:930-938, 1985.
92. Pepine CJ, Lambert CR. Effects of nicardipine on coronary blood flow. *Am Heart J* 116:248-254, 1988.
93. Hanet C, Rousseau MF, Vincent MF, et al. Myocardial protection by intracoronary nicardipine administration during percutaneous transluminal coronary angioplasty. *Am J Cardiol* 59:1035-1040, 1987.
94. Feldman RL, MacDonald RG, Hill J, et al. Effect of nicardipine on determinants of myocardial ischemia occurring during acute coronary occlusion produced by percutaneous transluminal coronary angioplasty. *Am J Cardiol* 60:267-279, 1987.
95. Engle MA, Zabriskie JB, Senterfit LB, et al. Vital illness and the post-pericardiotomy syndrome. A prospective study in children. *Circulation* 62:1151, 1980.
96. Ito T, Engle MA, Goldbert HP. Post-pericardiotomy syndrome following surgery for non-rheumatic heart disease. *Circulation* 17:549, 1958.
97. Engle MA, Ito T. The post-pericardiotomy syndrome. *Am J Cardiol* 7:73, 1961.
98. Engle MA, Gay WA Jr, Kaminsky ME, et al. The post-pericardiotomy syndrome then and now. In: *Current Problems in Cardiology.* Vol. 3, no. 2. Chicago, IL: Chicago Year Book Medical Publishers; 1978:35.
99. Engle MA, Zabriskie JB, Senterfit LB, et al. Immunologic and virologic studies in the post-pericardiotomy syndrome. *J Pediatr* 87:1103, 1975.

Chapter 13

Antiarrhythmic Therapy

Robert C. Mayer, MD
and Bruce Kleinman, MD

This chapter will provide an overview of the current state of antiarrhythmic agents and therapy. An understanding of normal cardiac cellular electrophysiology and arrhythmogenic mechanisms becomes necessary to comprehend the rational selection of antiarrhythmic agents. These topics will be briefly reviewed.

Cardiac Electrophysiology

The electrical events occurring in cardiac tissues can be recorded for single cells by means of microelectrodes that penetrate cell membranes. The action potential (AP) waveform is the electrical pulse recorded from intracellular microelectrodes. Most of the cells of the cardiac specialized conduction system and myocardium have an isoelectric resting membrane potential with negativity below −80 mV. The cells of the sinoatrial (SA) and atrioventricular (AV) nodes are exceptions as they have membrane potentials of −70 mV or less. In contrast to the cells of the myocardium, the

From Casthely PA, Bregman D, (eds): *Cardiopulmonary Bypass: Physiology, Related Complications, and Pharmacology.* Mount Kisco, NY, Futura Publishing Company, Inc., © 1991.

nodal cell membranes are more permeable to ions and do not maintain an isoelectric potential (Fig. 1).

The resting membrane potential (RMP) is maintained by energy provided by the hydrolysis of ATP via the Na-K-ATPase component of a membrane bound electrogenic pump.[1] As the RMP approaches a threshold potential, a few channels open allowing cations to enter the cell. This causes the intracellular environment to become less negatively charged. When the RMP is reduced to the threshold potential, many cation channels open. There is a massive flow of cations into the cell and the intracellular environment becomes positively charged. This sequence results in an action potential upstroke (phase 0) and the cell is now in a state of depolarization. The AP is propagated by the flow of current into adjacent nondepolarized areas of the membrane. This lowers the local adjacent potential to threshold initiating depolarization.[2]

The initial membrane potential is a major determinant of the type of ionic channels that open and type of AP generated. For example, stimulation of the Purkinje fibers or myocardium, which have high (> -80 mV) membrane potentials, induces the rapid entry of sodium ions through specific "fast" sodium channels. Hence, depolarizations in these "fast response" cells is sodium dependent. In nodal cells, which have lower (-65 mV) membrane potentials, depolarization results from calcium entry. The entry of calcium that characterizes nodal cell depolarization is relatively

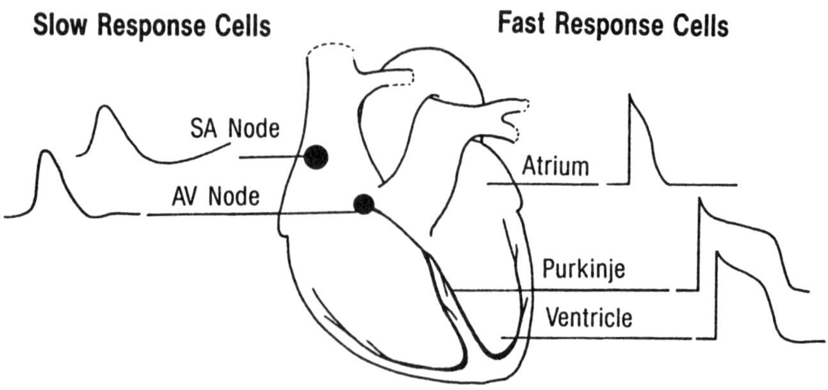

Figure 1. Slow upstroke action potentials of nodal cells contrasted with those of Purkinje fibers and myocardial cells.

much slower compared to sodium dependent depolarization. Hence, the SA and AV nodes are referred to as "slow response" cells. "Fast response" sodium channels are inactivated at the relatively low membrane potentials maintained in the SA and AV nodes.[3] Figure 1 contrasts the action potential recorded from nodal cells with those of Purkinje and myocardium cells.

Five phases (0–4) comprise the cardiac action potential in fast myocardial cells[4] (Fig. 2). A rapid influx of sodium ions through the cell membrane creates phase 0. Maximum amplitude and rate of rise (maximum velocity = $\dot{V}_{max}$) quantitatively describe phase 0 of the AP. Closing of the sodium channels ends phase 0 and makes these cells refractory to further stimulation. Repolarization begins with closure of the fast sodium channel which produces a brief period when the membrane potential returns toward 0 (phase 1).

During phase 2, there is a balance between calcium entrance and potassium extrusion such that the transmembrane potential does not change (plateau phase). During this plateau phase cells

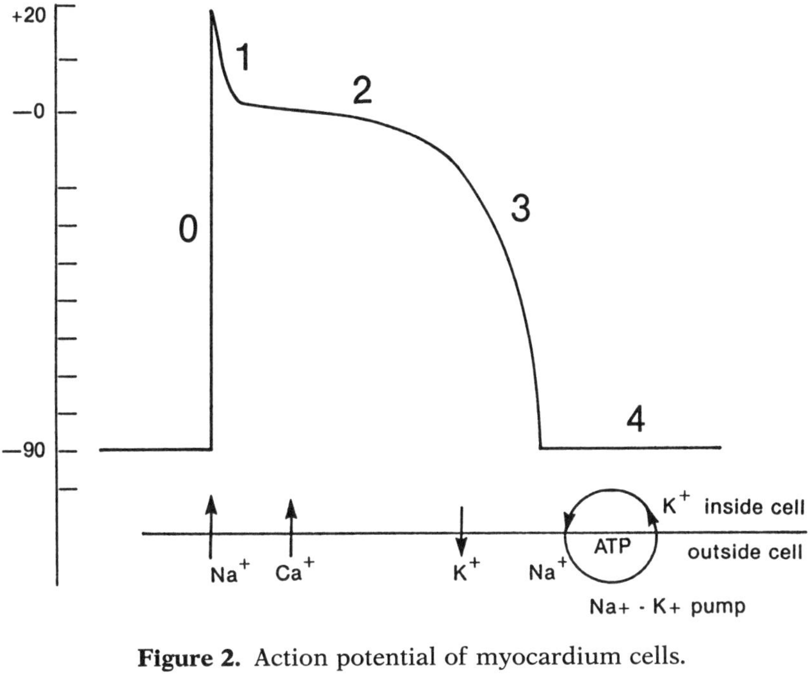

Figure 2. Action potential of myocardium cells.

are absolutely refractory, that is they cannot be reexcited regardless of stimulus strength. There is a progressive lengthening of phase 2 from the atrium to the Purkinje fiber and then shortening in ventricular muscle (Fig. 1). The lengthening of the plateau phase in ventricular Purkinje fibers compared with ventricular muscle protects the ventricular muscle from reexcitation. Phase 3 repolarization occurs when the slow inward flow of calcium ions diminishes and the outward potassium (K^+) efflux continues. This potassium efflux constitutes the major repolarization current. It probably involves several types of potassium currents. This results in a progressively more negative intracellular potential. During phase 3, the cell transforms from being absolutely refractory to being relatively refractory. This relative refractory period implies a larger than usual stimulus may produce reexcitation. Phase 3 repolarization is complete when the RMP is reestablished.

During phase 4, electrical diastole, myocardial cells maintain the RMP. However, during this isoelectric phase normal ionic gradients are reestablished. This involves ionic transport of sodium and potassium. The membrane bound energy dependent Na^+-K^+-ATP pump extrudes sodium and returns potassium into the cell.

In contrast to the contracting myocardial cells, other specialized cells undergo spontaneous phase 4 depolarization. This property is termed automaticity. Because the rate of rise of phase 4 is faster in the SA node than any other automatic cells, this area reaches its depolarization threshold potential the quickest. Thus the SA node becomes the hearts' dominant pacemaker; this is termed normal automaticity. Automatic cells with slower diastolic depolarization than the SA node may assume a primary pacemaker function if the SA node slows sufficiently or has no conducted impulse. Normal atrial and ventricular myocardial cells are not automatic, i.e., they are not capable of spontaneous phase 4 depolarization. However, certain pathologic conditions may result in abnormal automaticity in these cells. Abnormal automaticity is one possible mechanism of arrhythmias and will be discussed in the subsequent section.

Mechanisms of Arrhythmias

Cardiac arrhythmias may be broadly classified as either abnormalities of automaticity or conduction.[5] They may also be classified as abnormalities of both automaticity and conduction. Although one can distinguish these mechanisms in isolated heart tissue, distinction becomes far more difficult in the intact heart or clinical situation. Normal impulse initiation occurs during spontaneous phase 4 depolarization in the SA node and is called normal automaticity. Automaticity is a property of the specialized conduction cells of the heart.

Abnormalities of Automaticity

Specialized automatic cells include the SA and AV nodes, bundle of His, bundle branches, and Purkinje fibers. The intrinsic rate of impulse initiation in the sinus (SA) node is faster than in other specialized automatic cells. This explains the function of the SA node as the primary cardiac pacemaker.[6,7] Other automatic cells are masked by the impulse from the SA node that has an automatic rate of 60–100 depolarizations per minute. However, when the SA node fails to initiate an impulse or its propagation is blocked, other automatic sites assume the pacemaker function. "Secondary" pacemaker intrinsic rates are 40–60 and 20–40 depolarizations per minute in the AV node and Purkinje fibers, respectively. Normal automaticity in any tissue of the heart occurs at a membrane potential and rate normal for that tissue. If the functional primary pacemaker is depolarizing at an abnormal rate this condition is termed "altered normal automaticity". Examples of altered normal automaticity are sinus bradycardia, junctional tachycardia, or junctional escape beats.[8]

Normal atrial and ventricular myocardial cells do not display automaticity. However, changing the RMP to a less negative potential, (−60 mV) as can occur in ischemia, creates a condition of abnormal automaticity. This will initiate spontaneous depolarizations from ectopic foci and may be one mechanism of premature beats during ischemia.[8] Regardless of the mechanism for automaticity (normal or abnormal), the rate of automaticity is affected by changes in membrane resting potential (MRP), threshold potential, and the rate of rise of phase 4 depolarization.[6]

Another mechanism responsible for abnormal automaticity is the afterdepolarization (AD) that may be categorized as early (EAD) or delayed (DAD). Afterdepolarizations are oscillatory currents in transmembrane potential that can trigger another action potential[9] (Fig. 3). This arrhythmogenic mechanism is termed triggered automaticity. The major difference between triggered automaticity from other types of automaticity is that triggered automaticity is dependent on a preceding AP in contrast to other spontaneous forms. Early afterdepolarizations occur during phase 2 or 3, and DAD occur in phase 4 of the preceeding AP. The molecular mechanism for DAD remains unknown; however, DAD occur in a variety of conditions in which there appears to be excessive accumulation of intracellular calcium stores.[5] These conditions include toxic levels of digitalis and exposure to excessive levels of catecholamines.[6]

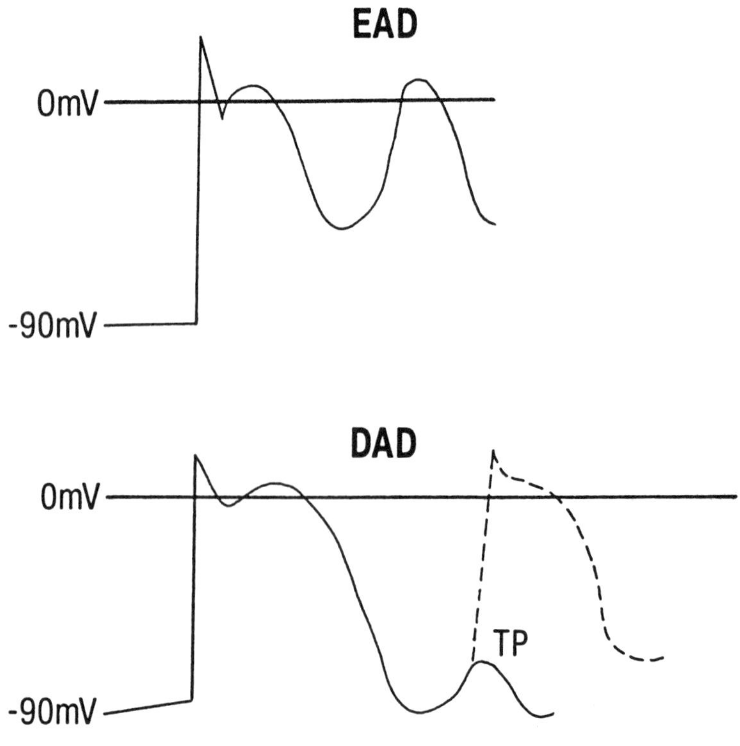

Figure 3. Schematic drawing of early afterdepolarizations (EAD) and delayed afterdepolarizations (DAD). Exceeding the threshold potential (TP) results in the triggering of another action potential.

It is possible that this mechanism is responsible for digitalis-induced arrhythmias, reperfusion arrhythmias, or exercise-induced VT in patients without coronary artery disease.[8,10]

Abnormalities of Conduction

Among abnormalities of impulse conduction, the mechanisms most widely referred to are reentry and reflection.[11] Reentrant conduction results in an abnormal self-propagating circuit. Formation of this abnormal circuit requires: (1) a unidirection block, (2) slow conduction in an alternate pathway, and (3) a short refractory period at the site of origin. This slowed conduction allows tissue proximal to the unidirectional block to recover from refractoriness. The slowed current can travel retrograde through the unidirection block and reenter tissue proximal to the block (Fig. 4). It is important to understand that for an impulse to travel continuously around a reentrant loop, the conduction time around the loop must exceed the refractory period. If the conduction time is too fast,

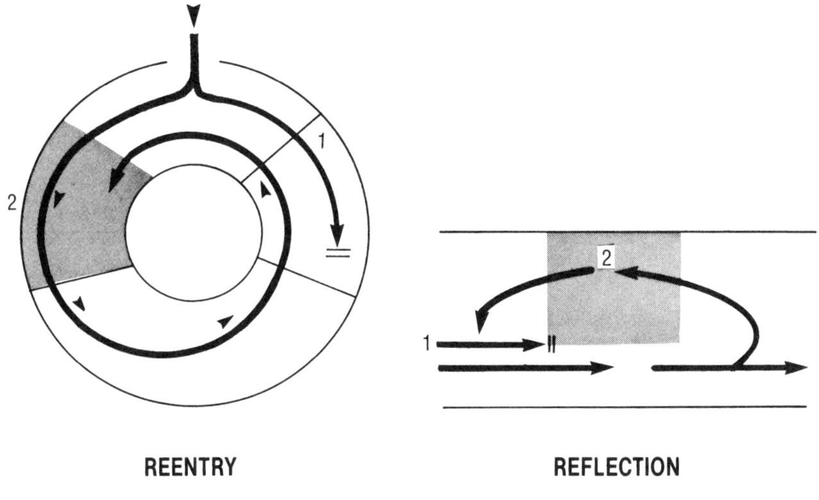

Figure 4. Reentry and reflection. These mechanisms can occur when an area of unidirectional conduction block (1) is coupled with depressed conduction (2).

when the impulse returns to its starting point, it will encounter refractory tissue. A bidirectional block would not allow the slowed current retrograde access to reexcitate proximal tissue. Antiarrhythmic drugs act by these mechanisms; they increase or decrease conduction to terminate reentry loops. Reentry is believed to be the most common etiology of many clinical arrhythmias, especially those associated with myocardial ischemia. Examples of reentrant arrhythmias include some forms of paroxysmal supraventricular tachycardia (PSVT), atrial fibrillation, atrial flutter, and ventricular tachycardia.[8,12]

Reflection is a type of reentry occurring in longitudinally conducting fibers when a zone of depressed conduction separates two segments of normally conducting tissue. Once an impulse transverses this depressed area, it would not normally retrogradely conduct to the proximal segment. However, it has been demonstrated, in vitro, that retrograde transmission along the same pathway initially travelled can occur and reexcite the proximal segment[13,14] (Fig. 4).

Pharmacologic Treatment of Chronic Arrhythmias

Ventricular arrhythmias are classified according to mortality risk as benign, potentially malignant, and malignant. Data to be considered when attempting to classify a patient's risk include consideration of coexisting heart disease, frequency and complexity of ventricular ectopy, and the patient's symptoms. This classification appears in Table I and is used to aide in treatment decisions.[15,16]

However, a consensus as to what should be treated exists only at the extremes of the ventricular arrhythmia spectrum. Obviously, physicians immediately treat acute life-threatening arrhythmias; however, there is no uniformity of opinion about the treatment of non-life-threatening ventricular arrhythmias. Reasons for concern about pharmacologic treatment include the significant adverse cardiac and noncardiac side effects associated with antiarrhythmic therapy. The recent data from the Cardiac Arrhythmia Suppression Trial (CAST) demonstrate this point and have fueled much controversy.

It is important to realize that the three clinical classes in Table I are not distinct, and numerous exceptions exist. To illustrate

Table I
Clinical Classification of Ventricular Arrhythmia

	Benign	*Potentially Malignant*	*Malignant*
Mortality Risk	very low	moderate	high
Heart Disease	no	no or yes	yes
PVC Frequency	low	moderate	high
Unsustained VT (< 30 seconds)	no	yes	yes
Sustained VT	no	no	yes
Symptoms	none or palpitations	none or palpitations	palpitation syncope, cardiac arrest

VT = ventricular tachycardia. PVC = premature contraction.

this point, one need only consider the prevalence of ventricular arrhythmias in the normal population. Studies utilizing Holter monitoring have provided much information concerning the prevalence, complexity, and prognosis of ventricular ectopic activity (VEA) in normal adults[17-20] (Table II). The prevalence of VEA as detected by exercise stress testing, is greater than that reported by Holter monitoring.[21,22] Normal people in these studies were defined as active men and women with no evidence of overt heart disease by history and physical examination. Based on this information (Table II), one can see a significant percentage of healthy patients will have VEA that would be classified as potentially malignant.

The overall mortality of normal adults with frequent and complex VEA is similar to an age-matched control group without VEA.[23] Therefore, distinguishing patients with a significant mortality risk

Table II
Prevelence of Ventricular Ectopy Activity (VEA) in Normal Adults Detected by Holter Monitoring

Age (yrs)	*VEA*	*Frequent VEA (> 10 PVCs/hr)*	*Unsustained VT*
< 30	50%–55%	2%–6%	2%
40–60	64%–73%	7%–24%	2%

from those with "benign" but frequent VEA is particularly important but exceedingly difficult. Difficulty in clearly defining a patient's risk and consequently lack of a quantifiable risk-benefit ratio further contribute to the present controversy over which patients to treat.

The primary indications for drug therapy are to reduce the risk of sudden death or to control symptoms. Symptomatic patients with benign arrhythmias frequently respond to lifestyle changes without the need for drug therapy. Reduction in caffeine, tobacco, or body weight may be all that is necessary. Patients with potentially malignant arrhythmias usually complain of palpitations or are asymptomatic. A majority of patients in this group have structural heart disease. Treatment of this group of patients is especially controversial.

Two well-studied subgroups are postinfarction patients and patients with congestive heart failure. These patients are frequently diagnosed during exercise stress testing or during 24-hour Holter monitoring. Several large studies have demonstrated that postinfarction patients with potentially malignant arrhythmias are at increased risk of sudden death.[24–27] Based on this information, many clinicians treat patients with asymptomatic arrhythmias and coexisting heart disease. However, because treatment has not yet been demonstrated to reduce mortality, many clinicians avoid treating asymptomatic patients. It is not yet clear how unsustained potentially malignant arrhythmias seen after infarctions are linked to sustained malignant arrhythmias that cause sudden death.

Ventricular ectopy has been identified as an independent risk factor that causes cardiac mortality following acute myocardial infarction (MI).[24,25] Among cardiologists, it had long been assumed, but not proven, that suppression of post-MI ventricular ectopy would improve postinfarction mortality. The Cardiac Arrhythmia Pilot Study (CAPS) investigated the treatment of these potentially malignant postinfarction ventricular arrhythmias with newer class IA and IIC antiarrhythmic drugs.[28] CAPS demonstrated the new IC agents, flecanide and encainide, had an efficacy of suppressing postinfarction premature ventricular contractions (PVC) of greater than 79% and 83%, respectively. This compared to the placebo rate of 37% during the first year after infarction. These agents also had a very low (6%) incidence of adverse side effects. However, CAPS did not use mortality as an end point. Among cardiologists, it had long been hypothesized that suppression of post-MI ectopy would improve postinfarction mortality. Therefore, based on this reported efficacy and safety, the CAPS investigators determined it was feasible to carry out a human study. This study would test the hypothesis that suppression of postinfarction ectopy would improve mortality; hence Cardiac Arrhythmia Suppression Trial (CAST).

With mortality as an end point, CAST enrolled only postinfarction patients who responded to treatment with the newer agents (defined as a 80% reduction of ventricular ectopy). Patients were randomly placed into drug or placebo groups. Four thousand patients were to be enrolled, but by the time CAST evaluated 1,455 patients, sufficient statistical significance existed to refute their hypothesis. Figure 5 summarizes this data.[29] Despite suppression of postinfarction arrhythmias, flecanide and encainide increased the incidence of cardiac death due to arrhythmia. This increase in mortality is presumably from the proarrhythmic side effects of

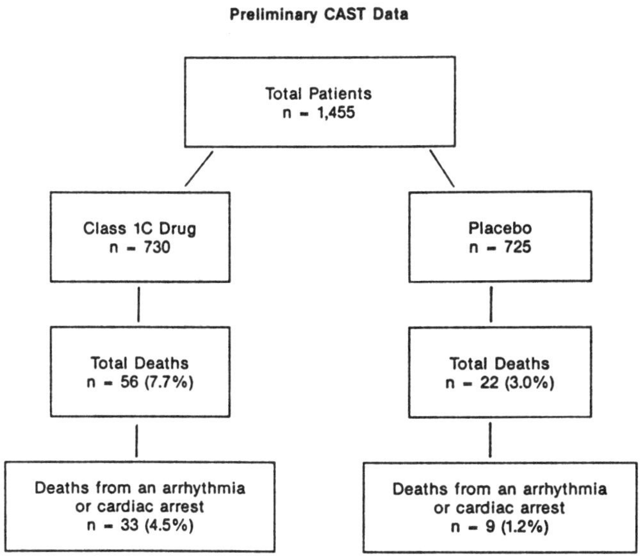

Figure 5. Preliminary CAST data demonstrating a significantly higher cardiac death rate in those taking class IC antiarrhythmic agents.

these drugs. Conclusions from the preliminary report from the CAST investigators are that neither flecainide or encainide should be used in post-MI patients who have ventricular arrhythmias and are asymptomatic or minimally symptomatic.[29] This data caused the FDA to cancel encainide and flecanide components of the CAST and promptly narrow the indications for these agents to refractory life-threatening arrhythmias.

A random survey of the practice habits of United States cardiologists was completed prior to the CAST results.[30] In this survey of 252 respondents, only 1% treated patients with asymptomatic VPCs and no heart disease, but 17% treated these patients if unsustained VT (defined as less than 30 seconds) was present. The treatment rate among cardiologists increased to 38% when coronary artery disease with LV dysfunction was present in patients with asymptomatic VPCs. The presence of any heart disease and symptomatic ventricular arrhythmias increased the treatment rate to 80% to 100%.

With the results of the CAST study, physicians may change their habits somewhat as the study has created considerable controversy. Indeed, the CAST study refutes the beneficial presumption accorded post-MI suppression of ventricular arrhythmias. However, the risks from the proarrhythmic effects of drug treatment weighed against the efficacy of treating potentially malignant ventricular arrhythmias has not been quantified. Further controlled studies are needed to determine this risk-benefit ratio.

Malignant ventricular arrhythmias require immediate treatment. Subsequently, these patients are evaluated, invasively or noninvasively, for arrhythmia control with pharmacologic agents. Both invasive electrophysiologic stimulation (EPS) testing methods and noninvasive methods (electrocardiographic Holter monitoring or exercise testing) are useful. A study called ESVEM (Electrophysiologic Studies Versus Electrocardiographic Monitoring) is underway.[31] The purpose of the ESVEM trial is to determine whether EPS or electrocardiographic Holter monitoring more accurately predicts drug efficacy in patients with aborted sudden death or sustained ventricular arrhythmias. The end point of EPS studies is inducible VT. The patient who is uninducible with drug therapy has a low probability of dying or developing symptomatic sustained ventricular arrhythmias.[32] However, some patients have inducible ventricular tachycardia (VT) despite multiple drug trials. These patients are considered refractory to drug therapy and are candidates for automatic implantable cardioverter defibrillator (AICD) implantation.

Basic Measures for Treatment of Acute Arrhythmias

Implicit in the treatment of all acute arrhythmias is that the underlying cause of the arrhythmias should be treated. It is important to remember that an arrhythmia in an operating room or in intensive care unit is frequently a warning of an underlying problem. With a life-threatening arrhythmia, simultaneous IV drug therapy and metabolic normalization must be undertaken. In a patient being mechanically ventilated, evaluation of airway, breathing, and circulation as a first priority must never be overlooked. Hypoxia or hypercarbia resulting in myocardial ischemia are common underlying causes of arrhythmias. Correction of the pH, $PaCO_2$ and PaO_2 should be accomplished by normalization of ventilation and appropriate oxygen therapy. Hyper- or hypoventilation will cause alterations in pH and result in intracellular or extracellular shifts in serum electrolytes. These shifts can result in abnormal myocardial membrane potentials thus predisposing to arrhythmias. Metabolic abnormalities may cause arrhythmias to be refractory to treatment. These abnormalities need to be evaluated and corrected in all patients with acute arrhythmias. Serum potassium and magnesium have received much attention for their roles in arrhythmogenesis and will be briefly discussed.

The resting potential is determined primarily by the potassium gradient across the membrane. Hypokalemia decreases the resting membrane potentials of cells and predisposes to abnormal automaticity and ectopic foci. Hypokalemia also augments automaticity by increasing the slope of phase 4.[33] In patients who sustain a perioperative MI, there is considerable evidence that hypokalemia might contribute to an early mortality.[34,35] Therefore, for surgical patients with serious cardiac disease, the risk of hypokalemia may be significant. Potassium levels also influence the magnitude of digitalis-induced delayed afterdepolarizations and permit the threshold potential to be reached, thereby triggering digitalis toxic arrhythmias.[36] Correction of serum potassium levels can eliminate ectopic ventricular foci. In addition, correction of hyper- or hypokalemia can suppress digitalis toxic arrhythmias.

Remember, however, that many patients on chronic diuretic therapy may have a substantial reduction in both total body and extracellular potassium. Correction of serum levels may not restore normal cellular ionic gradients. While normal serum levels are 3.5–5.5 mmol/L, the serum levels in patients with rhythm disturbances are commonly maintained above 4.0 mmol/L. A high normal level of potassium may help replete the total body potassium and result in resolution of the arrhythmia.

The significance of potassium for the control of arrhythmias has long been appreciated. However, many clinicians are less aware of the role of magnesium.[37,38] Magnesium has direct electrophysiologic effects on myocardial cells and is also closely linked to potassium homeostasis. Electrophysiologic studies in humans have shown the predominant effect of magnesium to be an increase in the AV node refractory period.[39–41] On a cellular level, magnesium is required as a cofactor for the Na^+-K^+ membrane bound pump. Low serum magnesium levels reduce Na^+-K^+ pump activity. This results in reduced intracellular potassium concentration. Experimental and clinical observations demonstrate the inability to replete intracellular potassium in the presence of ongoing magnesium deficiency.[42,43] Importantly, potassium repletion cannot be accomplished without simultaneous magnesium therapy.

Hypomagnesemia as an etiology of refractory hypokalemia is difficult to recognize clinically. This is because it is not observed in serum magnesium levels. Because less than 1% of magnesium is extracellular, the serum level does not always accurately reflect intracellular magnesium stores. Intracellular stores are estimated clinically by lymphocyte or mononuclear cell magnesium (Mg) content (mMg). A recent investigation has shown 53% of 104 patients admitted to the CCU had low mMg.[44] Only 7% of these patients had low serum magnesium levels. Investigators speculate that low mMg levels may contribute to cardiac morbidity. Mononuclear Mg levels are not readily available to the clinician. A study to identify markers of serum hypomagnesemia concluded hypokalemia, hypophosphatemia, hyponatremia, and hypocalcemia were frequently associated.[45] The clinical implication of this study is that low levels of one electrolyte necessitates investigation of all electrolytes. Chronic magnesium depletion occurs in diuretic usage, aminoglycoside therapy, alcohol abuse, secondary aldosteronism, and malabsorption syndromes. With chronic depletion, serum magnesium levels will not reflect intracellular magnesium levels. Bolus administration of magnesium to patients on diuretic treatment, for chronic heart failure, has terminated digitalis toxic arrhythmias despite normal serum magnesium.[46] This effect of magnesium may be related to the activation of the Na^+-K^+-ATP pump that is inhibited by digitalis.[47] Drug-induced torsade de pointes (discussed later) has been successfully terminated by magnesium administration. Experimental studies support that magnesium suppresses the early afterdepolarizations responsible for this arrhythmia.[48]

Magnesium has been reported to treat digitalis successfully induced arrhythmias, torsade de pointes, and supraventricular tachyarrhythmias. Despite demonstrated AV nodal effects, the efficacy of magnesium treatment for AV nodal reentrant paroxysmal supraventricular tachycardia (PSVT) is not proven. Some investigators have demonstrated conversion to sinus rhythm after Mg treatment while others note only a slowing heart rate.[49,50] A cardioprotective effect of magnesium in patients with acute MI has also been recently suggested. Rasmussen et al.[51] gave Mg infusions to patients admitted with an MI and demonstrated fewer arrhythmias and decreased early mortality. Although the mechanism of magnesium's cardioprotective effect is unclear and may be mediated by potassium, laboratory studies of ischemic myocardium have supported the hypothesis that hypomagnesium predisposes patients to ischemic ventricular arrhythmias.[52]

The role of magnesium for the treatment of arrhythmias has not been clearly defined. There are many successful case reports but standard dosages are lacking as are large scale studies. Magnesium is also a viable treatment for therapy of refractory ventricular and supraventricular tachyarrhythmias. In the unstable ICU patient or postcardiopulmonary bypass patient with refractory ventricular arrhythmias, we administer 2 g of magnesium sulfate ($MgSO_4$) intravenously over 2 minutes prior to repeated treatment with lidocaine if necessary. A continuous infusion is begun with 10 g of $MgSO_4$ over 5 hours. If the arrhythmias subside, a second 10 g over 10 hours restores intracellular magnesium levels. Serum K^+ and Mg^{++} levels are monitored during $MgSO_4$ infusions. Flushing and nausea occur in about 10% of patients during bolus administration. Transient hypotension uncommonly occurs and is easily reversed by fluid administration or small doses of calcium chloride. This is similar to other reported treatment protocols.[53]

Digitalis Glycosides

Digitalis glycosides have been used in clinical medicine for more than two centuries. Digoxin is the most frequently used cardiac glycoside because of its several routes of administration, intermediate duration of action and rapid assays of serum level. Digoxin is useful in the managements of congestive heart failure and supraventricular tachyarrhythmias. We will limit our discussion of the current status of digoxin for cardiac arrhythmias. Mechanism of action, pharmacokinetics, dosages, therapeutic serum levels, efficacy, and side effects will be discussed.

Digoxin has direct and indirect dose-dependent effects on the electrical properties of the intact heart. The dominant effects are indirect and mediated by the autonomic nervous system.[54] This vagomimetic action results in decreased conduction velocity and increased refractoriness of AV node. This reduction of the capability of the AV node to transmit atrial impulses to the ventricles is the most common use of digoxin. In higher doses, digoxin increases sympathetic outflow from the central nervous system. This may be an important factor in digoxin proarrhythmic effects.

Digoxin may be administered intravenously, orally (tablet or elixir), or intramuscularly (IM). The IM route is not recommended due to variable absorption. Absorption from the gastrointestinal (GI) tract is 60%–80% compared to an identical intravenous dose. Many drug interactions may increase or decrease GI absorption.[55] Common agents decreasing GI absorption include antacids, neomycin, and metoclopramide. Administering digoxin 2 hours before these agents can minimize this interaction. Renal excretion is exponential with an average half-life of 1.5 days.[56] When needed for a prompt onset of action, digoxin is given in a loading dose followed by a daily maintenance dose. In an undigitalized patient an intravenous dose of 0.5 mg usually produces an effect in 5–30 minutes. This effect becomes maximal in 1–4 hours. Additional doses of 0.1–0.3 mg may be given at 4-hour intervals until a clinical effect is seen.

The usual amount for a 70 kg patients is 0.6 to 1.0 mg. Maintenance digoxin dosing is once per day and should be reduced in the elderly or patients with renal insufficiency. Excretion is proportional to glomerular filtration rate and in anuric patients the excretory half-life increases to 4–6 days.[56,57] Digoxin is not removed from the body by dialysis or during cardiopulmonary bypass. This is because most of the drug is bound by tissue and not in circulation.

Digoxin reduces ventricular rate and can improve hemodynamic parameters in supraventricular tachyarrhythmias. Although digoxin still plays an important role in treatment of arrhythmias, its use has been modified because of the availability of verapamil. We will discuss the current role of digoxin in atrial fibrillation, atrial flutter, and supraventricular tachycardias.

Treatment of chronic atrial fibrillation seeks to control the ventricular rate. For acute atrial fibrillation in addition to controlling the ventricular rate, it is desirable to terminate the atrial fibrillation and suppress recurrences. Through its vagomimetic effects on the AV node, digoxin decreases ventricular response to atrial fibrillation. However, because these effects are easily overcome by exercise, verapamil, or β-blockers are useful adjuncts for chronic arrhythmia control.[58] Digoxin is not efficacious for converting atrial fibrillation to sinus rhythm. Restoration of sinus rhythm following digoxin is usually a spontaneous event. A recent study demonstrated that the incidence of conversion to sinus rate was virtually identical in placebo and digoxin treated patients, who had atrial fibrillation for less than 1 week.[59] Digoxin is also not effective for suppressing recurrences of atrial fibrillation.

Digoxin plays an adjunctive role in the treatment of atrial flutter. Restoration of sinus rhythm in atrial flutter is best treated with a synchronized countershock or rapid atrial pacing.[60,61] Maintenance treatment with quinidine or procainamide infrequently restores sinus rhythm, but will control ventricular rate. These agents slow atrial conduction velocity. Occasionally this atrial slowing will allow more frequent AV nodal conduction (i.e., convert a 3:1 block to a 2:1 block) and increase ventricular rate. For this reason pretreatment with agents that reduced AV node transmission is important prior to treatment of atrial tachyarrhythmias with quinidine or procainamide. Digoxin, β-blockers, or verapamil are effective pretreatments.

Paroxysmal supraventricular tachycardia (PSVT) has multiple etiologies and may originate in any anatomical structure of the supraventricular area. The SA node, atrial muscle, AV node, or abnormal accessory AV connections are the four etiological structures of PSVT (Fig. 6). Atrioventricular nodal reentry is the most common electrophysiologic mechanism in about 60% of unselected patients with PSVT.[62] Digoxin treatment is effective in blocking the reentrant circuit in the AV node and terminating this arrhythmia. Digoxin should be used in refractory episodes unresponsive to verapamil. Long-term maintenance with verapamil, digoxin, or a β-blocker is commonly used.

Accessory AV connections are the second most common cause of PSVT, occurring in 30% of patients.[62] These connections along with the AV node form a reentry pathway that can initiate PSVT. Most commonly, the accessory AV connections conduct in a retrograde fashion from ventricle to atrium. While digoxin may be useful for its AV nodal depression, Class II or IV agents are most suitable because they also retard conduction in concealed bypass tracts.[58]

Anterograde conduction over accessory pathways may occur in patient with the Wolff-Parkinson-White (WPW) syndrome. Par-

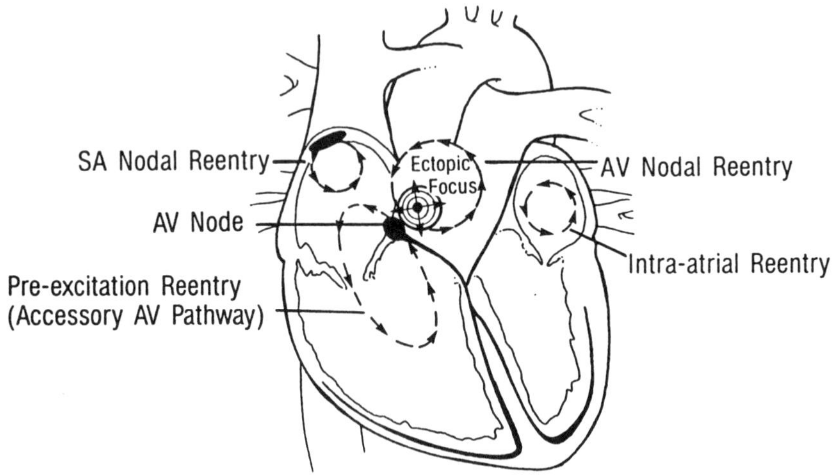

Figure 6. Four anatomic structures of PSVT include the SA and AV nodes, atrial muscle or accessory AV pathways.

oxysmal supraventricular tachycardia is the most common arrhythmia in WPW syndrome, occurring in approximately 80% of symptomatic patients.[63] Less frequently, but more ominously, atrial fibrillation or flutter may develop. Because of the very fast conduction velocity and short refractory period of the accessory pathway, extremely rapid ventricular rates may develop. This can lead to ventricular fibrillation, a well documented cause of sudden death in patients with WPW syndrome.[64] Digoxin's effect on the accessory pathway is variable, and it may accelerate conduction resulting in faster ventricular rates. Thus, digoxin may be hazardous in patients with WPW syndrome and a history of atrial fibrillation or flutter.[65]

Digitalis glycosides have a narrow margin between therapeutic and toxic levels. A variety of neurologic symptoms have been ascribed to digoxin's central nervous system effects. Confusion, delirium, psychoses, seizures, and altered vision perception may occur. Nausea and vomiting appear to be caused by a direct effect on the chemoreceptor trigger zone in the brain. Gastrointestinal symptoms are the most common site of noncardiac toxic effects.

Digitalis toxicity may result in a variety of cardiac arrhythmias. The most common cardiac manifestation of digoxin toxicity are AV junctional rhythm, PVC, bigeminal rhythm, and second-degree AV block.[66] However, it is known that digitalis can cause every variety of arrhythmias. Some of these toxic arrhythmias may be caused by digitalis-induced delayed afterdepolarizations (DAD) that are sufficient to reach threshold.[67] For example, ventricular bigeminy would result from the regular production of DAD that reached threshold potential.

Several drugs that can increase serum digoxin levels have been summarized elsewhere.[69–70] Of particular note are the antiarrhythmic agents quinidine, verapamil, and amiodarone. Careful clinical monitoring and serum digoxin levels should be determined when these agents are administered concurrently with maintenance digoxin therapy. When quinidine therapy is initiated, the dose of digoxin should be decreased by half since the serum digoxin is increased by twofold and the myocardial-to-serum digoxin concentration ratio remains constant.[71–72]

In many patients, no specific plasma level can be identified that can clearly separate toxic and nontoxic states. There is much individual variation and many causes for digoxin enhanced sensitivity. Electrolyte abnormalities are common precipitants of digitalis toxicity. Diuretic-induced hypokalemia, hypomagnesemia, or hypercalcemia can precipitate toxicity even when serum digoxin levels are in the "therapeutic range".[73] Hypomagnesemia is a frequent, but often occult precipitant of digitalis toxicity.

After discontinuing further digoxin administration, the treatment of bradyarrhythmias utilizes atropine and if necessary a pacemaker. Isoproterenol should usually be avoided because it may provoke more serious arrhythmias. Tachyarrhythmias require normalization of serum potassium concentrations followed by lidocaine or diphenylhydantoin.

Immunologic treatment with digitalis antibodies is approved for the treatment of advanced life-threatening toxicity that does not respond to conventional measures. Digoxin affinity for the antibodies is about tenfold higher than for cell membranes, and reversal of toxicity is clinically evident within 30 minutes to 1 hour. Previously, antidigoxin IgG antibodies were utilized, but recently Fab fragments have been shown to have several advantages over the entire IgG molecule. Fab fragments result in a more rapid reversal and evoke less immunogenicity. A multicenter trial of digoxin-specific Fab antibody fragments reported dramatic resolution of advanced life-threatening digoxin toxicity in 52 of 56 patients treated.[74] Until further safety information is available, current indications for digoxin-specific Fab antibodies include life-threatening arrhythmias unresponsive to conventional therapy, refractory hyperkalemia, and acute massive digoxin overdose.

Pharmacologic Antiarrhythmic Agents

Agents are classified according to the drugs' dominant effect on a single myocardial cell's action potential. The Vaughan-Williams classification arranges antiarrhythmic agents into four groups as depicted in Table III.[75] We will initially discuss the common electrophysiologic mechanisms distinguishing these four classes. Then, agents from each class are reviewed in terms of their mechanism of action, efficacy, and side effects.

Table III
Vaugh-Williams Classification of Antiarrhythmic Agents

Class 1	*Class 2*	*Class 3*	*Class 4*
Depress phase 0 sodium entry	block myocardial Beta receptors	Prolong phase 3 repolarization. Elevate fibrillation threshold	Block nodal phase 0 calcium entry
1A: Prolong repolarization Quinidine Procainamide Disopyramide 1B: Accelerate repolarization Lidocaine Diphenylhydantoin Mexiletine	Propranolol Metroprolol Esmolol	Bretylium Amiodarone NAPA	Verapamil
1C: No repolarization effect Flecainide Encainide			

NAPA = N-acetyl-procainamide.

Class I

These "membrane-stabilizing" drugs block membrane bound sodium (Na^+) channels thereby depressing the rapid inward sodium current. With this Na^+ channel blocking, $\mathring{V}_{max}$ and AP amplitude are diminished. This ability to reduce conduction velocity ($\dot{V}_{max}$) makes them useful for terminating reentrant arrhythmias. In addition automaticity of fast response cells (Purkinje fibers) is suppressed because it is also dependent on Na^+ inward currents for spontaneous phase 4 depolarization.

Class I is further subdivided by effect on repolarization. Class IA drugs prolong repolarization while IB drugs increase the potassium repolarization current, thereby decreasing refractorization. While Class IB agents shorten the effective refractory period (ERP), they also more profoundly shorten AP duration (APD). Overall, the ratio of ERP/ARD is increased resulting in increased refractoriness. Class IC has minimal effects on repolarization and are currently only available as oral preparations.[76] Previously, this paper discussed the present status of Class IC agents, which include flecanide and encainide. These subclasses also differ in their speed of attachment to and detachment from sodium channels.[77]

Procainamide

Procainamide increases the effective refractory period and reduces conduction velocity in the atria, ventricles and Purkinje fibers. It has variable nodal effects because of a direct slowing offset by an indirect vagolytic effect.[78]

Procainamide is metabolized by the liver and excreted by the kidney. The metabolite N-acetyl-procainamide (NAPA) is an active compound and may contribute to toxicity. This can occur despite apparently therapeutic procainamide doses. This is particularly true in patients who have renal insufficiency. These patients are at risk for toxicity and need to have serum levels monitored. Both procainamide and NAPA are proarrhythmic and produce additive side effects. Therefore in assessing serum concentrations, both procainamide and NAPA must be assayed.[79] Therapeutic blood levels (procainamide plus NAPA) range from 4 to 8 μg per mL.

Procainamide is commonly used to treat or prevent recurrences of PSVT, atrial fibrillation or flutter. It is efficacious for converting atrial fibrillation or sinus rhythm.[80] However, as conduction is slowed in the atrium, more atrial impulses may get conducted to the ventricles. This may result in an increased ventricular response beyond tolerable limits. For this reason, patients are frequently treated with digoxin, verapamil, or propranolol prior to procainamide (or quinidine) for suppression of atrial fibrillation. Procainamide, unlike quinidine, will not elevate plasma digoxin levels.

Procainamide may be useful for ventricular arrhythmias and may be used to prevent recurrences of VT or ventricular fibrillation (VF) in patients who have survived cardiac arrest. Its efficacy can be assessed by EPS testing. Administered intravenously, procainamide is an effective emergency treatment for ventricular tachyarrhythmias that are unresponsive to lidocaine. It may be useful for recurrent or refractory ventricular tachycardia. Procainamide is rarely used for acute VF because it requires a prolonged time to achieve adequate levels. Intramyocardial distribution of procainamide during ischemia is believed to be an important component of its therapeutic effect. In a canine infarction model, higher concentrations of procainamide were present in ischemic areas.[81]

Procainamide is effective for treating supraventricular arrhythmias associated with the Wolf-Parkinson-White (WPW) syndrome. Prolongation of repolarization and increased refractoriness in accessory AV pathways terminate reentrant arrhythmias in these patients.

In high doses, procainamide may depress myocardial contractility. It may also produce peripheral arterial vasodilation via a mild ganglionic blocking action. Cautious intravenous administration of 100 mg every 5 minutes at a rate of 20 mg/min is advised, and should be temporarily discontinued if hypotension occurs, QRS complex widens by 50% or a total of 1 g has been given. If the arrhythmia is suppressed a maintenance infusion of 1–4 mg/min is started.

A very high incidence of adverse side effects frequently limits chronic therapy. Within the first 6 months, 40% of patients will discontinue the drug.[82] Almost all patients on chronic treatment develop antinuclear antibodies. This alone is not sufficient to discontinue therapy. Approximately 15% develop signs or symptoms of a lupus-like syndrome. These patients are at risk for pleural effusions or even a possibly lethal cardiac tamponade.[83] Symptoms disappear with discontinuation of drug. The aromatic amino group on the procainamide molecule appears important for the induction of this syndrome (Fig. 7). Acetylating this amino group to form NAPA removes this side effect.

An interaction with cimetidine results in elevated plasma levels due to decreased tubular secretion of procainamide.[84] Cimetidine therapy given to patients taking procainamide can cause concentrations of procainamide to rise to toxic levels. Procainamide toxicity may be characterized by a variety of cardiac proarrhythmias. Rarely do lethal ventricular arrhythmias due to QT interval prolongation, including torsade de pointes occur.[85–86] Torsade de pointes is an atypical ventricular tachycardia associated with QT interval prolongation. The electrocardiographic pattern is characterized by

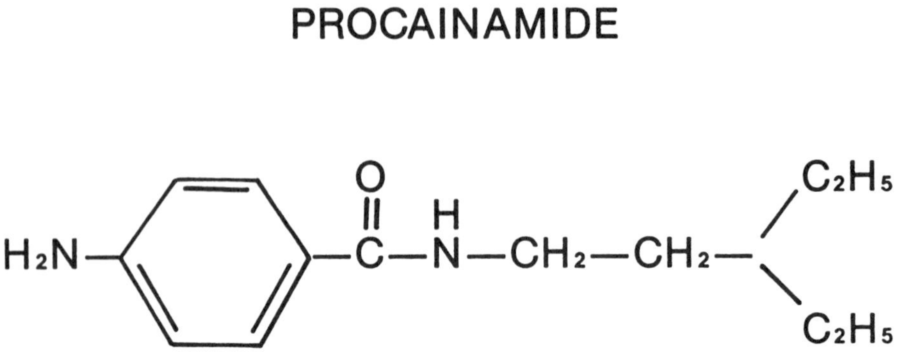

Figure 7. Structure of procainamide. The aromatic amine group is believed to cause lupus-like side effects.

an irregular, wide QRS complex that twists around the isoelectric line (Fig. 8). Torsade usually terminates spontaneously, hence it is termed a nonsustained polymorphic ventricular tachycardia. However, torsade may degenerate into ventricular fibrillation. It is essential to identify this rhythm correctly to its unique therapeutic approach. The goals of therapy are to normalize the QT interval to abolish reentry. This is best accomplished with rapid cardiac pacing. The pacing rate is increased until the arrhythmia is terminated. If pacing is not available, cardioversion can be used. Isoproterenol is the drug of choice, however, this is a very arrhythmogenic agent. Because electrolyte imbalances can be associated with this condition, they should be assayed. Beside procainamide, all other class

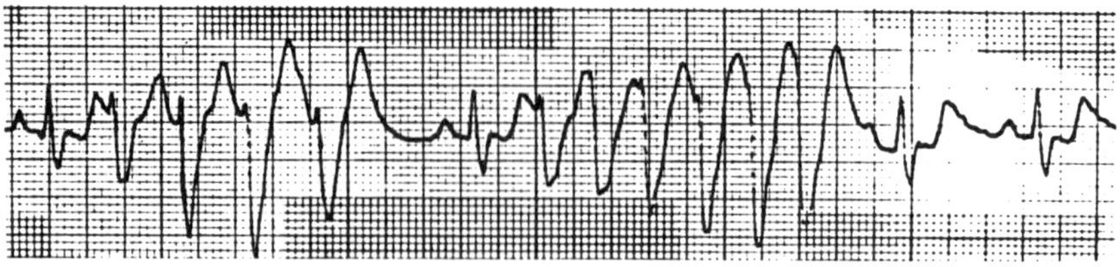

Figure 8. Two brief episodes of torsade de pointes with spontaneous conversion to sinus rhythm. This nonsustained polymorphic ventricular tachycardia is an adverse side effect of all group 1A antiarrhythmic agents.

IA agents are associated with QT interval prolongation and torsade de pointes.[87]

Elevation of pacing thresholds accompanies procainamide toxicity and may occur resulting in loss of pacemaker capture.[88] Complete blood counts should also be performed at regular intervals in patients taking this agent because of the remote possibility of agranulocytosis.[89]

Quinidine

Quinidine's electrophysical properties and mechanism of arrhythmia termination are similar to procainamide.[90] The choice between them for maintenance therapy is usually based on side-effect profiles. Prolongation of the QRS complex, QT interval, SA node, or AV node slowing are electrophysiologic effects of quinidine as well as other Class IA agents.

Quinidine is primarily hydroxylated by the liver and excreted in the urine. An α-adrenergic blocking effect may cause significant hypotension and is the principal limitation to intravenous administration. Oral administration is preferred with virtually 100% absorption and peak serum levels achieved in 2 hours. Drugs that induce hepatic enzymes may shorten the duration of action of quinidine.

Like procainamide, quinidine is effective for both supraventricular and ventricular arrhythmias. Either drug may suppress an arrhythmia that is refractory to the other drug. Quinidine, like other Class IA agents, is utilized for suppression of atrial and ventricular premature contractions. Quinidine can be used for chronic suppression of recurrent VT or VF in patients who have had cardiac arrest.[91] Quinidine successfully converts atrial flutter or atrial fibrillation to sinus rhythm in about 10% to 20% of patients.[91] Better rates are achieved if the arrythmia is of more recent onset and if the left atrium is not enlarged. However, like procainamide, quinidine may accelerate the ventricular rate in atrial fibrillation or flutter and should be preceded by AV nodal suppression with propranolol, digitalis, or verapamil. Like other Class IA agents, by increasing the refractoriness of accessory pathways, quinidine can be used effectively to treat or prevent ventricular tachyarrhythmias in the Wolf-Parkinson-White syndrome.

In patients with sick sinus syndrome, or other SA node dysfunction, quinidine can decrease SA node discharge. However, in normal hearts, significant anticholinergic efects and α-adrenergic blockade with reflex sympathetic stimulation, may increase SA node discharge rate and also increase AV nodal conduction.[92,93]

Adverse effects associated with chronic oral quinidine, may result in discontinuation in 30% to 40% of patients. The most common adverse effect is due to gastrointestinal disturbances that may be minimized by concomittant food ingestion. Central nervous system toxicity or cinchonism may be manifest as tinnitus, hearing, or visual disturbances, confusion, delirium, or psychosis. Mild cinchonism does not usually require quinidine withdrawal.

Quinidine has a well-described interaction with digoxin.[94] Clinical digitalis toxicity occurs in 20%–40% of patients receiving both agents. Serum digoxin levels increase about twofold with therapeutic doses of quinidine. Individual dosing varies widely and digitalis toxicity may occur when quinidine dosage is increased. This interaction can be potentiated by the addition of cimetadine.[95]

Quinidine may produce syncope in 0.5%–10% of patients during the first days of treatment.[96–98] This is likely the result of a nonsustained polymorphic ventricular tachyarrhythmia of a specific variety: torsades de pointes (Fig. 8). This syncope does not correlate with serum quinidine levels and may be more prone to occur with hypokalemia and a slow heart rate, producing early afterdepolarizations.

Allergic thrombocytopenia may develop due to antibodies to quinidine-platelet complexes. This may cause bleeding in patients on oral anticoagulants. Other rare allergic reactions include: rash, fever, hemolytic anemia, and anaphylaxis.

Disopyramide

Like other Class IA agents, disopyramide produces depression of $\dot{V}_{max}$ of phase 0 and increases refractoriness of atrial and ventricular muscle. Like procainamide, it also reduces the disparity in conduction between normal and ischemic cardiac tissue thus terminating reentry. Disopyramide causes little or no prolongation of the PR interval or QRS complex, but like all Class IA agents may prolong the QT interval or further depress preexisting nodal disease.[99–101]

Disopyramide is approved in the United States for oral administration only. Disopyramide has an efficacy profile similar to quinidine and procainamide. However, most clinicians consider disopyramide as second-line therapy. This is probably due to concerns for its negative inotropic action and anticholinergic side effects. Reduced myocardial contractility is a predictable effect. In normal patients cardiac output usually decreases 10%–15%. Half of the patients with a history of CHF may have recurrence of symptoms.[102] Avoidance of a loading dose may attenuate this myocardial depression.

Most commonly, disopyramide produced dose-related anticholinergic side effects and should be avoided in patients with obstructive uropathy or closed angle glaucoma. Anticholinergic symptoms may be minimized by concomittant administration of anticholinesterase agents.[103] Similar to other IA agents, proarrhythmic activity in the form of ventricular tachyarrhythmias associated with QT prolongation and torsade de pointes may occur.[104,105] Disopyramide has not been reported to elevate digoxin levels.

Lidocaine

Lidocaine's primary antiarrhythmic effect is to decrease the slope of (phase 4) Purkinje fibers thus depressing their automaticity. It also reduces the refractory period in Purkinje fibers that may eliminate the unidirectional block necessary for reentrant arrhythmias. Conduction velocity is not affected by lidocaine in normal tissue but it is significantly decreased in ischemic tissue.[106] Lidocaine has little if any effect on atrial fibers, accessory pathways, SA, or AV nodes. However, if there is preexisting nodal disease lidocaine may further depress nodal activity.[107]

Due to its minimal effect on supraventricular activity lidocaine is indicated only for ventricular ectopy. Lidocaine is the standard drug of choice used for the acute treatment of ventricular arrhythmias of almost all types. A major advantage of lidocaine is its lack of effect on cardiac output or sinus rate. Lidocaine is useful for life-threatening VT or VF that has not responded to electrical countershock. Lidocaine is also indicated for prophylaxis against recurrence after the successful emergency electrical conversion of VF or VT.[108] The use of lidocaine for prophylaxis against ventricular arrhythmias in patients with acute MI is controversial. Studies have shown a decreased incidence of post-MI arrhythmias after the prophylactic administration of lidocaine.[109,110] Other investigators have shown this not to be so.[111,112] Additionally, no investigations have shown that suppressing arrhythmias occurring in the early post-MI period improves survival. Classically, lidocaine has also been indicated for the treatment of premalignant ventricular ectopy. Ectopy believed to lead to malignant arrhythmias (VT or VF) includes PVC that occur more frequently than 5 per minute, occur during the T wave (R on T phenomenon), are multiform or grouped. However these classic indications are now controversial because investigation has shown persons with PVC without associated heart disease are not at increased risk of sudden death.[23]

For the treatment of acute VF or pulseless VT lidocaine is given as a bolus of 1 mg/kg, with additional bolus injections of 0.5 mg/kg every 2–10 minutes if needed to a total dose of 3 mg/kg. For nonimmediately life-threatening arrhythmias lidocaine is administered as an initial intravenous bolus followed by a continuous infusion. The initial bolus dose is 1 mg/kg. An infusion of 2–4 mg/min is started if clinical response is observed. If the initial bolus does not produce the desired response, a second similar dose can be given after 5 minutes. Lidocaine undergoes extensive first pass metabolism in the liver. The rate of clearance is extremely sensitive to hepatic blood flow. Clearance is decreased in patients with liver disease, congestive heart failure, and the elderly. These conditions necessitate reducing the initial bolus by 50%. Therapeutic plasma concentrations range from 1.5–6 μg/ml.[113]

The most commonly observed adverse effects of lidocaine are dose-related manifestations of central nervous system toxicity that include: dizziness, paresthesia, confusion, delirium, stupor, coma, and seizures.

Diphenylhydantoin

Like lidocaine, diphenylhydantoin (DPH) shortens repolarization and AP duration. However, refractoriness is increased because the ERP:APD ratio is increased. In addition to class IB properties, DPH's action also includes a central sympatholytic effect that decreases cardiac sympathetic efferent nerve activity.[114] The antiarrhythmic effects of DPH are enhanced in partially depolarized cells that occur from hypoxia or digitalis toxicity.[115,116]

Elimination half-life is about 24 hours and may be slowed in the presence of liver disease. Elimination of DPH is also prolonged when administered concomitantly with drugs such as phenylbutazone, dicumarol, isoniazid, chloramphenicol, and phenothiazines. These drugs compete with DPH for hepatic enzymes. Because of the large number of medications that alter phenytoin plasma concentrations, plasma levels should be determined when changes are made in other medications.

Diphenylhydantoin's value as an antiarrhythmic agent is limited to atrial and ventricular arrhythmia caused by digitalis toxicity.[116] This is accomplished by abolishing delayed afterpotentials responsible for automatic arrhythmias induced by digitalis preparations. Diphenylhydantoin is not effective in treating ventricular arrhythmias in patients with ischemic heart disease. To achieve therapeutic plasma concentrations rapidly, 100 mg of DPH may be given intravenously every 5 minutes, up to a maximum dose of 1 g. However, vital signs must be closely monitored because intravenous DPH produces decreased left ventricular (LV) contractility and a corresponding increase of LV end diastolic pressure.[117] These potentially adverse hemodynamic effects are evident at rapid administration rates and can result in cardiovascular collapse.[118]

Diphenylhydantoin toxicity most commonly manifests as CNS signs (nystagmus, nausea, vertigo, ataxia and cerebellar dysfunction) and sometimes hypotension and respiratory arrest. Thrombophlebitis, due to acidity of the parenteral preparation, may occur and can be minimized by administration into a central intravenous line. Chronic use is not routinely utilized for arrhythmia control.

Tocainide

Tocainide has a chemical structure, mechanism of action and a spectrum of antiarrhythmic activity similar to lidocaine. Both mexiletine and tocainide were developed specifically for oral administration. Although intravenous preparations exist there is as yet no additional clinical effect or advantage over lidocaine. By removing two ethyl groups from lidocaine, tocainide avoids first-pass hepatic metabolism and is effective orally.[119,120]

Tocainide can be used in the prophylaxis or treatment of complex ventricular arrhythmias after myocardial infarction and in preventing recurrence of cardiac arrest in patients with malignant ventricular arrhythmias.[121,122] A double-blind study of intravenous tocainide for suppression of ventricular arrhythmias after cardiac surgery showed similar efficacy with lidocaine.[123] In patients responsive to lidocaine therapy, lidocaine should be discontinued 1–2 hours before initiating tocainide because side effects will be additive.

Proarrhythmias can occur and are reported to occur in 1%–8%.[124] One percent incidence of SA nodal depression also has been reported.[123–125] The combination of propranolol and tocainide may cause paranoia and confusion.[125] Oral administration in patients after MI does not affect hemodynamic compensation adversely. In patients with compensated left ventricular dysfunction there is no change in cardiac output. However a slight negative inotropic effect may cause worsening of congestive heart failure in patients with poor cardiac reserve.[126]

Tocainide is associated with adverse side effects that are of sufficient severity to require discontinuation in 10–30% of patients.[123,124,127] Neurologic symptoms of tremor or nausea are common and nondose related paresthesias are also reported. Gastrointestinal side effects occur in approximately 15% of patients and may be partially alleviated by concomitant food or antacid ingestion. Dermatologic reactions occur in 7%–12% of patients. An associated lupus-like syndrome is rare. One to two patients per thousand may develop catastrophic pulmonary fibrosis or agranulocytosis.[127] Because of these potentially fatal side effects, any patient taking tocainide should be monitored with periodic chest radiographs and complete blood counts.

Mexiletine

Mexiletine, like tocainide, is similar to lidocaine in its chemical structure, electrophysiologic properties, spectrum of antiarrhythmic activity, and toxicity.

Mexiletine is effective in reducing the frequency of ventricular premature beat and decreasing symptomatic arrhythmias in patients not responding to other therapy.[128] Mexiletine has also been used in the prophylactic treatment of arrhythmias after acute myocardial infarction.[129] Fifty to 60% of patients studied using ambulatory Holter monitoring showed an 80% decrease in frequency of PVC.[119,129,130] It has been suggested that mexiletine in combination with quinidine and other Class IA agents has synergistic effects on ventricular arrhythmias. This however, has been challenged.[131]

Minimal myocardial depressant effects warrant cautious administration in patients with advanced heart failure. Sinus node depression may occur in patients with preexisting SA node dysfunction. Other cardiac toxicities include: proarrhythmia 10%, CHF 2%, heart block 1%. The margin between therapeutic (0.75–2 mcg/mL) and toxic (greater than 2 mcg/mL) concentration is narrow and side effects are reported to occur in 47%–65% of patients.[132–134] This requires discontinuation in up to 10%–40% of patients.[133–136] Nausea or vomiting is common and anorexia or epigastric burning may occur. Neurologic toxicity is manifest as a fine intention tremor, dizziness, ataxia and paresthesia, dysarthria or a menthol taste. Some recommend avoidance of mexiletine in patients with seizure disorders.[137]

Similar to tocainide, cumulative toxicity may be observed with lidocaine, and this necessitates discontinuation of lidocaine 1–2 hours prior to initiation of mexiletine. Mexiletine has several drug interactions because it is extensively metabolized by the liver. Drugs such as phenobarbital, rifampin, and phenytoin, which cause hepatic enzyme induction, will shorten the serum half-life.[138] In contrast, cimetidine, isoniazid, chloramphenicol, and dicumarol will prolong the half-life. Congestive heart failure, end stage renal disease, and cirrhosis decrease the clearance of mexiletine and necessitate a reduction in the dosage.

Class II

These β-receptor blocking drugs terminate arrhythmias by their competitive antagonism on β-adrenergic receptors. Catecholamines stimulate β-receptors and increase automaticity and conduction velocity in the sinus node, AV node, and His-Purkinje fibers. Catecholamines may also induce delayed afterdepolarizations in atrial, ventricular, and Purkinje fibers.[139] The β-adrenergic blockers exert their antiarrhythmic effect indirectly by inhibiting catecholamine stimulation of β-receptors. It has been suggested that the antagonism of β_{-2} mediated hypokalemia may contribute to the β-blockers mechanism of action.[140] β-Blockade produces a decrease in sinus rate, AV conduction, and an increase in AV node refractoriness. In high doses, β-blockers depress the fast sodium current and have class I-like actions. However, this direct "membrane stabilizing" effect is evident in doses much higher than would be achieved clinically.[141] Hence, the major antiarrhythmic mechanism of this class of drugs comes from their indirect effects. Propranolol is the prototype agent in this class.

Propranolol

Propranolol nonselectively blocks beta-$_1$ and beta-$_2$ adrenergic receptors. This property is therapeutic for sinus tachycardias and paroxysmal supraventricular tachyarrhythmias (PSVT), in which the AV node is part of the reentry circuit. Propranolol's increase in AV node refractoriness is also useful for slowing the ventricular response to atrial fibrillation and flutter. Propranolol reduces the amplitude of digitalis-induced DAD, thereby suppressing arrhythmias due to digitalis toxicity.

Although not as effective as Class IA antiarrhythmic agents for suppression of PVC, the use of β-blockers is successful in approximately half of the patients studied.[142–144] Importantly they are usually better tolerated than Class I agents and less likely to produce a proarrhythmic effect. In addition, they are the treatment of choice for symptomatic mitral valve prolapse, and idiopathic hypertrophic subaortic stenosis (IHSS). When more than one agent is needed for control of an arrhythmia, β-blockers are used as adjunctive agents in combination with Class IA drugs. Propranolol has also been shown to be useful intraoperatively to reestablish sinus rhythm during accelerated AV junctional rhythm and isorhythmic dissociation.[145]

β-Blockers are the only group of drugs shown to prolong survival of patients after an MI. Investigations have shown the correlation between ventricular ectopic activity post-MI is independently correlated with mortality.[24–27] In postinfarction patients β-blockers reduce the incidence of reinfarction, postinfarction ventricular arrhythmias, and ventricular fibrillation.[146–148] However, studies have failed to demonstrate that propranolol can alter the relation between post-MI ventricular arrhythmias and mortality.[149,150] Hence, the mechanism by which propranolol improves post-MI survival remains unclarified.

There is no simple correlation between dose and therapeutic effect. Clinical response varies widely principally because sympathetic tone varies widely among individuals. Oral administration undergoes extensive first pass hepatic metabolism of about two thirds of the administered dose. The degree of metabolism is highly variable between individuals and this also contributes to the lack of correlation between dose and response. Oral administration results in substantially different pharmacokinetics than intravenous administration.[151] Intravenous propranolol may be given up to a dose of 0.1–0.15 mg/kg. This should be administered cautiously and titrated in 0.2–0.5 mg aliquots. Frequent monitoring of the blood pressure, heart rate and rhythm is required to observe clinical response.

β-Blockers depress cardiac contractility and may precipitate or worsen heart failure. Bradycardia or AV nodal block are potential side effects. Propranolol should not be given to patients who have preexisting significant AV block. These adverse cardiac effects may be synergistic of those of other agents. For example, the negative inotropic effects of verapamil are synergistic with propranolol. Bronchospasm, in suspectible individuals, is another serious side effect of propranolol. Propranolol should not be administered to patients with bronchospastic disease since blocking of β-$_2$ receptors may precipitate bronchoconstriction.

The use of β-$_1$ selective agents such as esmolol is advantageous in patients with obstructive pulmonary disease. Additional benefits of esmolol include its rapid onset and brief duration of action. Esmolol's half-life is 9 minutes and is therefore administered as an initial bolus and maintenance infusion. Esmolol is currently finding widespread application in the perioperative period, when a titratable and brief β-blockade is desirable.

Class III

The Class III drugs primarily prolong repolarization and prolong the effective refractory period (ERP) of the AP (Fig. 9). A

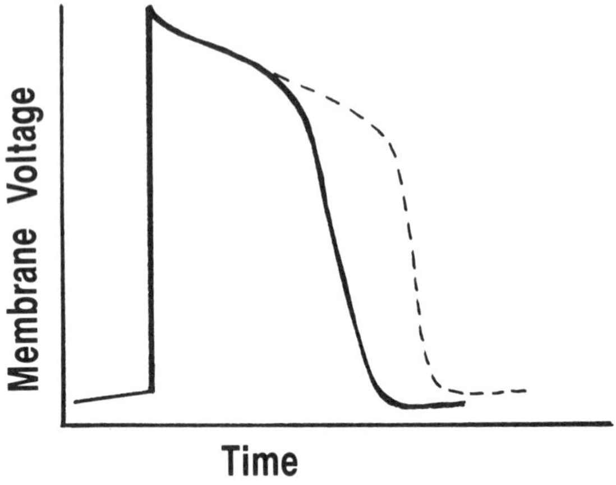

Figure 9. Effect of class III agents (----) on the action potential.

mechanism of this class of drugs may be their ability to homogeneously prolong ERP, thereby decreasing the dispersion of refractoriness required for reentry.[152] Class III agents also produce an increase in fibrillatory threshold.[153] The two prototype drugs in Class III, bretylium and amiodarone, are commonly referred to as the "antifibrillatory agents".

Bretylium

Bretylium has both indirect adrenergic effect and direct myocardial effects. The antiarrhythmic and antifibrillatory mechanisms of bretylium are poorly understood and may be different. Bretylium's adrenergic effects are triphasic. After initial release of norepinephrine, bretylium accumulates in pre- and postganglionic sympathetic neurons and prevents norepinephrine release. The subsequent chemical sympathectomy has an onset about 15 minutes after injection and results in prolongation of action potential duration (APD) and a refractory period (ERP) for atrial and ventricular muscle and Purkinje fibers. Prolonging refractoriness without a change in APD/ERP may help prevent reentry. In canine hearts with infarcted areas, bretylium has been shown to reduce disparity between impulse conduction in regions of normal and ischemic or infarcted myocardium.[154] The restoration of ischemic myocardial cell electrophysiology toward normal as well as sympatholytic effects may be factors in suppressing reentrant arrhythmias. Bretylium also elevates the ventricular fibrillation threshold in normal and infarcted hearts within minutes of injection.[153,155]

Bretylium has been effective in treating patients with refractory ventricular tachyarrhythmias. Bretylium is as efficacious as lidocaine for the treatment of VF. No difference in clinical outcome and survival has been found in studies that have compared the use of lidocaine and bretylium for treating patients with out-of-hospital VF.[156,157] However, because bretylium is associated with adverse hemodynamic side effects it is not recommended as a first line treatment.

Bretylium is indicated in patients with VF or unstable VT that are refractory to electrical countershock and lidocaine. In refractory VF 5 mg/kg of bretylium is given. If the VF persists, electrical defibrillation is attempted prior to increasing the dose of bretylium to 10 mg/kg. This later dose can be repeated at 15-minute intervals until a maximum of 30 mg/kg. The antifibrillatory effects of bretylium are evident in minutes.[153]

A significant hypotension frequently develops due to sympatholysis. With the vasoconstriction reflex diminished, orthostatic hypotension is common, although even when supine, up to 50% of patients may also become hypotensive. Orthostatic hypotension may persist for several days after drug discontinuation. Bretylium is not a myocardial depressant.

Amiodarone

Amiodarone prolongs repolarization and refractoriness in the SA and AV nodes, atrial and ventricular myocardium, and Purkinje fibers.[158] It has also been shown to block sodium channels, thus depressing conduction during phase 0 (Class I actions). The repolarization effects of this drug are reversed by thyroid hormone administration. This has caused some to propose that an additional mechanism of amiodarone is blockade of the cardiac effects of circulating tri-iodothyronine (T3).[152]

Amiodarone has been used to suppress a wide spectrum of supraventricular and ventricular tachyarrhythmias, and its efficacy exceeds or equals that of all other antiarrhythmic agents.[159–161] However, because of its extremely long and variable half-life (13–107 days) and multiple adverse side effects, the use of amiodarone is very limited. Amiodarone is only used for therapy for suppression of recurrence of life-threatening ventricular arrhythmias (VF or VT). It should be among the last antiarrhythmic agents to be tried and should be used only by experienced cardiologists. Amiodarone is commonly the final drug utilized in an attempt to prevent recurrences of VT or VF. Electrophysiologic induction of ventricular tachyarrhythmias in the presence of amiodarone therapy results in the need for AICD implantation. After cessation of amiodarone therapy, antiarrhythmic action may persist for 30 to 45 days.[152,162] This persistence may prolong intraoperative testing of the AICD.

Adverse effects occur in about 75% of patients treated after 4 years of treatment and require discontinuation in up to 20%.[163,164] Also, a correlation exists between total dose and number of side effects. Amiodarone has a cumulative toxicity that depends on total dose rather than daily dose. Of the noncardiac adverse reactions, diffuse pulmonary fibrosis is the most serious with a reported mortality up to 10%.[165] The incidence of pulmonary side effects is quite common, 15%, 23% at 1 and 2 years, respectively. The initial pulmonary inflammation can occur within 2 weeks of initiation of therapy. Usually, however, this complication occurs within the first 30 months of the treatment. The mechanism is not obvious but may be caused by a hypersensitivity reaction.[166]

Clinically, this pulmonary inflammation complication may mimic deteriorating heart disease or pneumonia. Signs of dyspnea, nonproductive cough, fever, and pulmonary infiltrates on chest X-ray suggest of this problem. Chest radiographs every 3 months are recommended. Amiodarone must be discontinued if such changes develop. The slow breakdown of amiodarone in plasma and tissue makes such adverse reactions possible for up to a year or more after drug withdrawal.

Other noted side effects include: dermal and corneal accumulation of the drug resulting in a photosensitive dermatitis (20%) and corneal microdeposits (9%), respectively. Thyroid toxicity with hyperthyroidism with elevated T3 (1%–2%) or hypothyroidism (1%–5%) may occur.

Amiodarone completely binds cytochrome P450 hepatic enzymes and thus alters the metabolism of several drugs. There are increased plasma concentrations of antiarrhythmic drugs of classes IA, IB, IC, II, and III. It is therefore difficult to use another antiarrhythmic drug in combination with amiodarone. Torsade de pointes, heart block, and atropine-resistant bradycardia have been reported when amiodarone is used in combination with class I antiarrhythmic agents.[109,167]

Class 4

These agents block the slow calcium channels responsible for depolarization (phase 0) in cardiac nodal tissue. Hence, they exert their antiarrhythmic influence primarily in the AV and SA nodes. They slow the discharge rate in the SA node and prolong the AV node refractory period. There is no effect on the sodium-dependent phase 0 or RMP in cardiac muscle or Purkinje fibers (fast-response cells).[168] These agents also lower intracellular calcium in vascular beds and cause vasodilation of coronary and peripheral vascular beds. These effects make these drugs efficacious as antihypertensive and antianginal agents. Despite a direct depressant effect on SA node depolarization, the sinus rate usually does not change significantly in vivo. This is because verapamil's peripheral vasodilation elicits a reflex sympathetic stimulation that maintains heart rate. Although Class IV agents are useful in supraventricular arrhythmias, they are not effective for ventricular arrhythmias.

Verapamil

Verapamil is the treatment of choice for the emergent treatment of paroxysmal supraventricular tachyarrhythmias that do not require cardioversion. Verapamil terminates 60%–80% of episodes of paroxysmal supraventricular tachycardia within minutes.[169,170] Verapamil is contraindicated for ventricular arrhythmias but is used to decrease the ventricular response over the AV node in the presence of atrial fibrillation or atrial flutter.[171,172] Verapamil is most successful with atrial fibrillation of recent onset and when the atria are not enlarged.

In atrial fibrillation in the WPW syndrome, verapamil may decrease normal nodal conduction and accelerate conduction over the anomalous AV pathway.[173] This results in more rapid excitation of the ventricles and may cause VF in these patients.[174–176] It is therefore contraindicated in atrial fibrillation or flutter associated with the WPW syndrome.

In patients with acute cardiac failure precipitated by PSVT, therapy with verapamil is beneficial because termination of the PSVT results in hemodynamic improvement. However, cardiovascular collapse may occur if intravenous verapamil is given to patients with ventricular tachycardia. Therefore, differentiation of PSVT and VT is important. A general rule of thumb is not to give intravenous verapamil to any patients with a wide QRS tachycardia.

For PSVT, verapamil dosage in adults is usually given in 2.5 mg aliquots up to 10 mg (0.15 mg/kg) over a 3–5 minute period. Effects are seen within minutes. A transient decrease in arterial pressure due to peripheral vasodilation is common in response to verapamil and necessitates slow administration. Verapamil's peripheral vasodilatation elicits a reflex sympathetic stimulation that maintains cardiac output and heart rate. Verapamil directly depresses myocardial contraction as well as conduction and may result in severe adverse hemodynamic effects in patients with impaired left ventricular function or preexisting conduction disturbances. Congestive heart failure with severe hypotension or asystole may occur in patients with preexisting disease. In patients with normal left ventricular function, combined therapy with propranolol and verapamil may be tolerated. However, cautious administration is required because hypotension, bradycardia, AV block, and asystole are more likely to occur when verapamil is given to patients who are already receiving β-blocking agents.[177,178] Isoproterenol may be effective for treating verapamil-induced bradyarrhythmias. Intravenous calcium can reverse the hypotensive effect of verapamil without reversing its electrophysiologic actions.[179] However, reversal of hypotension from the combination of calcium channel and β-receptor blockade is uncertain. Digoxin levels may also be increased by concomitant verapamil. Up to a 70% increase in steady-state serum digoxin concentrations can be seen when verapamil is added to digoxin.

The Automatic Implantable Cardioverter Defibrillator

An automatic internal cardioverter-defibrillator (AICD) is capable of detecting either VT or VF and delivering a 25–30 J, defibrillating or R wave synchronous countershock. It has been estimated that 300,000 people die annually from sudden cardiac arrest in the United States.[180] The AICD has dramatically changed the treatment of patients at risk for sudden death from ventricular fibrillation. By 1990, 10 years after Mirowski and colleagues[181] performed the first human implantation, the AICD system has been implanted in many thousands of patients. The results from several series of tests on adult patients with AICDs show an approximately 2% 1-year sudden cardiac death rate.[182–185] Application of AICD has extended to pediatric patients. Initial data in 38 pediatric patients at a mean follow-up period of 2.5 years, have reported survival and complication rates similar to those in adult studies.[186]

The AICD device consists of a pulse generator and three electrodes. The generator is in a hemetically sealed case containing the electronic circuitry and power source and weighs approximately 300 g. The three electrodes include two defibrillating leads that deliver shocks. The third or rate sensing electrode inputs the myocardial electrogram to the internal circuitry and is usually attached to the epicardium of the left ventricle. A patch electrode on the LV to deliver the shock and an intravascular spring electrode at the SVC/RA junction acting as an anode form a common defibrillating lead configuration (Fig. 10).

In very large dilated hearts or hearts that have high defibrillation thresholds, a second right ventricular patch lead can be substituted for the SVC spring electrode (Fig. 11). This second patch lead enables higher energy shocks to be delivered. A recent echocardiographic study showed that the patch lead does not alter left ventricle (LV) systolic or diastolic function.[187] Because children, have a smaller heart, a spring-patch configuration is usually preferred to the patch-patch configuration.

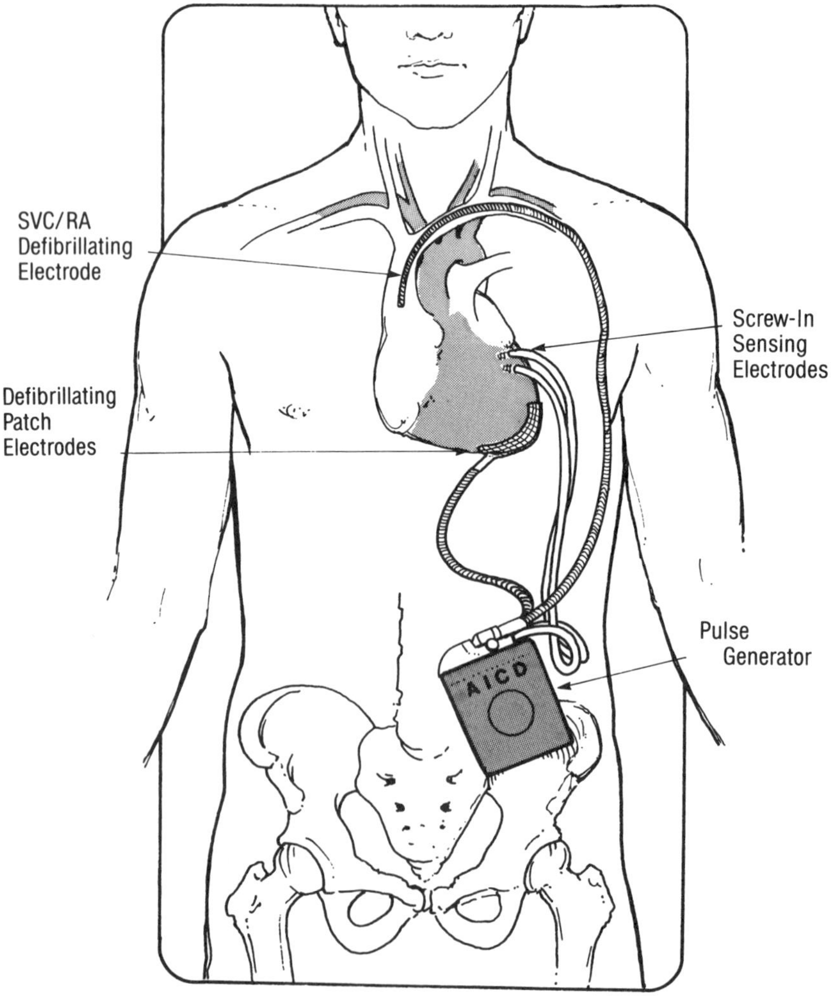

Figure 10. The intravascular spring electrode–LV patch defibrillating configuration.

The sensing lead has either two screw-in left ventricular epicardial electrodes (Figs. 10 and 11) or an endocardial bipolar lead usually placed into the right ventricular apex. This lead senses and counts the heart rate and contains synchronizing circuits for shock delivery with R wave synchronization. Upon placement of the elec-

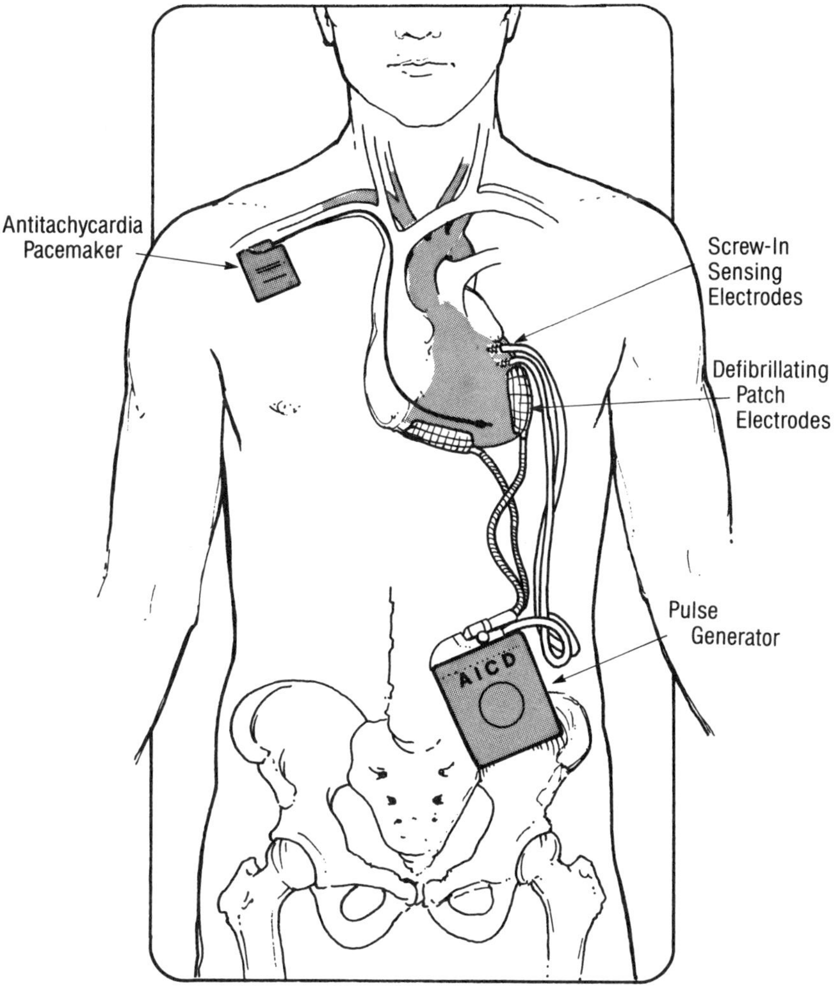

Figure 11. Patch-patch defibrillating configuration of the AICD. Recently treatment of stable VT with both an antitachycardia pacemaker and AICD has been reported.

trodes, VT or VF are induced by programmed stimulation. The energy threshold required to defibrillate (or cardiovert) the heart is determined by a series of shocks delivered by the AICD. Testing is continued until optimal defibrillating lead positions are determined by minimal energy requirements. The time interval tolerated between fibrillations has been determined by return of phasic arterial pressure to baseline. Recently it has been shown that this is a poor indictor of tissue recovery. Mixed venous oxygen saturation is a more sensitive indicator of tissue recovery and should be utilized to determine proper recovery and fibrillatory intervals.[188] The sensing and defibrillating leads are subcutaneously tunneled to a pocket in the upper quadrant of the abdomen where the pulse generator is located.

The sensing electrode was originally designed to detect both rate and rhythm and the AICD to deliver a countershock when criteria were met for both rate and rhythm. Cardiac rhythm was analyzed by circuits that sense the time the electrogram spends away from a straight (isoelectric) line. These circuits provide input to a mathematical formula called the probability density function (PDF). During rhythms with much time away from the PDF isoelectric template (i.e., VT or VF), the rhythm criteria for shock initiation were satisfied. Problems with the PDF arrhythmia detection lead to many spurious shocks, especially with lead faults, or rapid wide complex SVT. Hence, the use of rate (sensing) only AICD has gained much popularity. This rate-only device is preferred by some investigators because it reduces spurious discharges and detects arrhythmias the PDF would miss, e.g., a VT with a narrow QRS complex.[189,190]

However, false-positive discharges may become problematic in patients who develop SVT that are faster than the preset rate. Setting this device at a rate just above the patient's maximum rate SVT reduces false-positive discharges. Present development is directed toward combining AICD with pacemaker capabilities to treat postdefibrillation bradycardias. Another area of active research is in the development of devices with memory capabilities that can display the rhythm that triggered shocks. This will demonstrate appropriateness of shocks that is presently ascertained only by a patient's symptoms.

Initial AICD implants were approved only in patients with at least two cardiac arrests and who had failed all antiarrhythmic regimens. Because its safety and efficacy have been proven, the indications for implantation have broadened. The device is now indicated for several groups of patients including:[89,191]

(1) Patients with recurrent ventricular tachyarrhythmias who have inducible VT or VF despite drug therapy;
(2) Patients who have had a cardiac arrest presumably due to a hemodynamically unstable ventricular arrhythmia not associated with an acute MI; and
(3) Patients with a history of cardiac arrest who are not taking antiarrhythmics and have no inducible ventricular arrhythmias at initial EPS study.

Because they are uninducible, this latter group of patients cannot be adequately tested by EPS studies. Furthermore, recent data have identified patients with cardiac arrest (without reversible factors) and not EPS inducible as being at high risk of sudden death. Hence, these patients are candidates for an AICD.[192]

Poor left ventricular function is not a contraindication to AICD implantation. Although overall survival in AICD patients is closely correlated with LV ejection fraction (LVEF), investigation supports that survival is enhanced in patients with LVEF less than or equal to 15%.[193] In patients with severe LV dysfunction, cardiac transplantation would be the preferred antiarrhythmic treatment. However at the authors' institution, AICD is utilized for selected patients with severely depressed LV function and frequent ventricular arrhythmias who are awaiting a donor heart for transplantation.

Hemodynamically stable sustained VT has not been an indication for AICD. However, the combination of an antitachycardia pacemaker with an AICD back-up in case of pacemaker-induced arrhythmia acceleration has been reported as satisfactory (Fig. 11).[194] Due to the well-documented success of the AICD, compared to pharmacologic agents, it is also being advocated as an initial therapy of choice after an episode of VF or unstable VT.

Patients who do not tolerate, or have recurrence during oral amiodarone therapy are candidates for AICD implantation. No randomized trials comparing amiodarone with the AICD have been performed. The major contraindication to use of AICD is the occurrence of VT or VF during transient reversible conditions unlikely to recur. Examples of these would include electrolyte disturbances, rapid ventricular response to atrial fibrillation, arrhythmias during the first 48 hours of an MI, and proarrhythmias from antiarrhythmia agents. Another contraindiction is poorly controlled ventricular tachyarrhythmias of sufficient frequency to cause the AICD battery to rapidly deplete.[191]

Surgeons have utilized a number of surgical approaches for AICD implantation including median sternotomy, left thoracotomy, subxiphoid, and subcostal approaches. The AICD is commonly implanted with additional antiarrhythmic cardiac surgery. The AICD can be implanted at the time of cardiac surgery because 20% to 30% of the survivors of endocardial resection for VT will have recurrent dysarrhythmias with 2 years.[195–197] Recently, cardiac surgeons have increasingly obviated the need for repeated thoracotomy by placing prophylactic AICD patches in patients at high risk for postoperative ventricular tachyarrhythmias. In a series of 34 patients, undergoing endocaridal resection (22 patients) or coronary artery bypass grafting (12 patients), subsequent thoracotomy was avoided in 20% of patients eventually needing the AICD.[198] Routine placement of AICD leads for coronary artery bypass grafting is not indicated. This is because of the risk of infection, and the extreme fibrotic reaction that is generated by the patch electrodes, which may preclude future coronary artery bypass grafting.[199]

REFERENCES

1. Hoffman BF, Cranefield PF. *Electrophysiology of the Heart.* Mt. Kisco, NY: Futura Publishing Co; 1960.
2. Chung EK. *Principles of Cardiac Arrhythmias.* 2 ed. Baltimore, MD: Williams and Wilkins; 1977.
3. Baumgarten CM, Fozzard HA. The resting and pacemaker potentials. In: Fozzard HA, Haber E, Jennings RB, et al., eds. *The Heart and Cardiovascular System.* New York, NY: Raven Press; 1986: 601-626.
4. Marriott HJ, Conner MH. *Advanced Concepts in Arrhythmias.* St. Louis, MO: CV Mosby, 1983.
5. Hoffman BF, Rosen MR. Cellular mechanism for cardiac arrhythmias. *Circ Res* 49:1, 1981.
6. Noble D. Cardiac action potentials and pacemaker activity. In: Linden RJ ed. *Recent Advances in Physiology.* London, Churchill; 1974: 25.
7. Cranefield PF. *The Conduction of the Cardiac Impulse.* Mt. Kisco, NY: Futura Publishing Co; 1975: 199–265.
8. Attlee JL, Bosnjak ZJ. Mechanisms for cardiac dysrrhythmias during anesthesia. *Anesthesiology* 72:347, 1990.
9. Wit AL, Rosen MR. After depolarizations and triggered activity. In: Fozzard HA, Haber E, Jennings RB, et al., eds. *The Heart and Cardiovascular System.* New York, NY: Raven Press; 1986: 1449–1490.

10. Ferrier GR. Digitalis arrhythmias: role of oscillatory afterpotentials. *Prog Cardiovasc Dis* 19:459, 1977.
11. Janse MJ. Reentry rhythms. In: Fozzard HA, Haber E, Jennings RB, et al., eds. *The Heart and Cardiovascular System.* New York, NY: Raven Press; 1986: 1203–1238.
12. Gallagher JJ. Mechanisms of arrhythmias and conduction abnormalities. In: Hurst JW, Rackley CE, Shlant RC, et al. eds. *The Heart.* 5 ed. New York, NY: MacGraw-Hill Books, 1982.
13. Rozamski GJ, Jalife J, Moe GK. Reflected reentry in nonhomogeneous ventricular muscle as a mechanism of cardiac arrhythmias. *Circulation* 69:163, 1984.
14. Antzelevitch C, Moe GK. Electronically mediated delayed conduction and reentry in relation to "slow responses" in mammalian ventricular conduction tissue. *Circ Res* 49:1129, 1981.
15. Bigger JT Jr. Definition of benign versus malignant ventricular arrhythmias: targets for treatment. *Am J Cardiol* 52:47C–54C, 1983.
16. Bigger JT Jr. Antiarrhythmic treatment. An overview. *Am J Cardiol* 53:8B, 1984.
17. Brodsky M, Wu D, Denes P, et al. Arrhythmias documented by 24 hour continuous electrocardiographic monitoring in 50 male medical students without apparent heart disease. *Am J Cardiol* 39:390, 1977.
18. Sobotka PA, Mayer JH, Bauerfeind RA, et al. Arrhythmias documented by 24-hour continuous ambulatory electrocardiographic monitoring in young women without apparent heart disease. *Am Heart J* 101:753, 1981.
19. Clarke JM, Shelton JR, Hammer J, et al. The rhythm of the normal human heart. *Lancet* 2:508, 1976.
20. Kostis JB, McCrone K, Moreyra AE, et al. Premature ventricular complexes in the absence of identifiable heart disease. *Circulation* 163:1351, 1981.
21. Faris JV, McHenry PL, Jordan JW, et al. Prevalence and reproducibility of exercise-induced ventricular arrhythmias during maximal exercise testing in normal men. *Am J Cardiol* 37:616, 1976.
22. Podrid PJ, Graboys TB, Lampert S, et al. Exercise stress testing for exposure of arrhythmias. *Circulation* 23:299, 1987.
23. Barret PA, Peter CT, Swan JHC, et al. The frequency and prognostic significance of electrocardiographic abnormalities in clinically normal individuals. *Prog Cardiovasc Dis* 23:299, 1981.
24. Bigger JT Jr, Fleiss JL, Kleiger R, et al. The relationship between ventricular arrhythmias, left ventricular dysfunction and mortality in the 2 year after myocardial infarction. *Circulation* 69:250, 1984.
25. Lavie CJ, Gersh BJ. Acute myocardial infarction: initial manifestations, management and prognosis. *Mayo Clin Proc* 65:531, 1990.
26. Mukharji J, Rude RE, Poole WK, et al. Risk factors for sudden death after acute myocardial infarction: two Year follow-up. *Am J Cardiol* 54:31–36, 1984.

27. Ruberman W, Weinblatt E, Goldberg JD, et al. Ventricular premature beats and mortality after myocardial infarction. *N Engl J Med* 297:750, 1977.
28. Cardiac Arrhythmia Pilot Study (CAPS) Investigators. Effect of encainide, flecainide, imipramine and moricizne on ventricular arrhythmias during the year after acute myocardial infarction: the CAPS. *Am J Cardiol* 61:501, 1988.
29. The Cardiac Arrhythmia Suppression Trial (CAST) Investigators. Preliminary report: effect of encainide and flecainide on mortality in a randomized trial of arrhythmia suppression after myocardial infarction. *N Engl J Med* 321:406, 1989.
30. Morganroth J, Bigger JT Jr, Anderson JL. Treatment of ventricular arrhythmias by United States cardiologists: a survey before the Cardiac Arrhythmia Suppression Trial results were available. *Am J Cardiol* 65:40, 1990.
31. The ESVEM Investigators. The ESVEM trial: electrophysiologic study versus electrocardiographic monitoring for selection of antiarrhythmic therapy of ventricular tachyarrhythmias. *Circulation* 79:1354, 1989.
32. Mason JW, Winkle RA. Accuracy of the ventricular tachycardia induction study for predicting long-term efficacy and inefficacy of antiarrhythmic drugs. *N Engl J Med* 303:1077, 1980.
33. Opie LH, Nathan D, Lubbe WF. Biochemical aspects of arrhythmogensis and ventricular fibrillation. *Am J Cardiol* 43:284, 1979.
34. Hulting J. In-hospital ventricular fibrillation and its relation to serum potassium. *Acta Med Scand* 647:109, 1981.
35. Nordrehaug JE. Malignant arrhythmias in relation to serum potassium values in patients with an acute myocardial infarction. *Acta Med Scand* 647:101, 1981.
36. Lown B, Block H, Moore FD. Digitalis, electrodes and the surgical patient. *Am J Cardiol* 6:309, 1960.
37. Levine SR, Crowley JJ, Hai HA. Hypomagnesemia and ventricular tachycardia: a complication of ulcerative colitis and parenteral hyperalimentation in the nondigitalized noncardiac patient. *Chest* 81:244, 1982.
38. Dyckner T. Serum magnesium in acute myocardial infarction. Relation to arrhythmias. *Acta Med Scand* 207:59, 1980.
39. DiCarolo LA Jr, Moady F, DeBuitleir M, et al. Effects of magnesium sulfate on cardiac conduction and refractoriness in humans. *J Am Coll Cardiol* 7:1356, 1986.
40. Rasmussen HS, Thomsen PE. The electrophysiological effects of intravenous magnesium on human sinus node, atrioventricular node, atrium, and ventricle. *Clin Cardiol* 12:85, 1989.
41. Kulick DL, Hong R, Ryzen E, et al. Electrophysiologic effects of intravenous magnesium in patients with normal conduction systems and no clinical evidence of significant cardiac disease. *Am Heart J* 115:367, 1988.

42. Shils ME. Experimental human magnesium depletion. *Medicare (Baltimore)* 48:61–85, 1969.
43. Whang R, Flink E, Dyckner MD, et al. Magnesium depletion as a cause of refractory potassium repletion. *Arch Intern Med* 145:1686, 1985.
44. Ryzen E, Ethayam U, Rude R. Low blood mononuclear cell magnesium in intensive cardiac care unit patients. *Am Heart J* 111:475–480, 1986.
45. Whang R, Oci T, Aikawa J, et al. Predictors of clinical hypomagnesemia. *Arch Intern Med* 144:1794–1796, 1984.
46. Cohen L, Kitzes R. Magnesium sulfate and digitalis—toxic arrhythmias. *J Am Med Assoc* 249(20):2808–2810, 1983.
47. Keren A, Tzivoni D. Magnesium therapy in ventricular arrhythmias. *PACE* 13:937, 1990.
48. Perticone F, Adinolfi L, Bonaduce D. Efficacy of magnesium sulfate in the treatment of torsade de pointes. *Am Heart J* 112:847–849, 1986.
49. Sager PT, Widerhorn J, Petersen R, et al. Prospective evaluation of parenteral magnesium sulfate in the treatment of patients with reentrant AV supraventricular tachycardia. *Am Heart J* 119:308, 1990.
50. Wesley JC Jr, Haines DE, Lerman BB, et al. Effect of intravenous magnesium sulfate on supraventricular tachycardia. *Am J Cardiol* 63:1129, 1989.
51. Rasmussen H, Worregand P, Lindenego O, et al. Intravenous magnesium in acute myocardial infarction. *Lancet* 1:234–236, 1986.
52. Crampton R, Clark C. Varying extracellular magnesium alters ischemic and reperfusion ventricular tachyarrhythmias. *Circulation* 68(Suppl):146, 1983.
53. Iseri LT, Chung P, Tolus J. Magnesium therapy for intractable ventricular tachyarrhythmia in normomagnesmic patients. *West J Med* 138:823, 1983.
54. Giles RA, Quest JA. The role of the central nervous system in the cardiovascular effects of digitalis. *Pharmacol Rev* 31:19–97, 1980.
55. Marcus FL. Pharmacokinetic interactions between digoxin and other drugs. *J Am Coll Cardiol* 5:82A, 1985.
56. Steiness E. Renal tubular secretion of digoxin. *Circulation* 50:103–107, 1974.
57. Bissett JK, Doherty JE, Glanigan WJ, et al. Tritiated digoxin: XIX. Turnover studies in diabetes insipidus. *Am J Cardiol* 31:327–330, 1973.
58. Antman EM, Friedman PL. Use of digitalis glycosides in the management of cardiac arrhythmias. In: Smith TW, ed. *Digitalis Glycosides.* New York, NY: Grune & Stratton; 1986: 127–151.
59. Falk RH, Knowlton AA, Bernard SA, et al. Digoxin for converting recent-onset atrial fibrillation to sinus rhythm. *Ann Intern Med* 106:503–506, 1987.
60. De Silva RA, Graybvoys TB, Podrid PJ, et al. Cardioversion and defibrillation. *Am Heart J* 100:881, 1980.
61. Waldo AL, MacLean WAH. *Diagnosis and Treatment of Cardiac Arrhythmias Following Open Heart Surgery: Emphasis on the Use of*

Atrial and Ventricular Epicardial Wire Electrodes. Mt Kisco, NY: Futura Publishing Co.; 1980: 65–70.
62. Josephson ME, Kastor JA. Supraventricular tachycardia: mechanisms and management. *Ann Intern Med* 87:346–358, 1977.
63. Richardson JM. Ventricular preexcitation: practical considerations. *Arch Intern Med* 143:760, 1983.
64. Dreifus LS, Haiat R, Watanabe Y, et al. Ventricular fibrillation: a possible mechanism of sudden death in patients with Wolff-Parkinson-White syndrome. *Circulation* 43:520–527, 1971.
65. Sellers TD Jr. Brashore TM, Gallagher JJ. Digitalis in the preexcitation syndrome: analysis during atrial fibrillation. *Circulation* 56:260–267, 1977.
66. Shapiro W. Correlative studies of serum digitalis levels and the arrhythmias of digitalis intoxication. *Am J Cardiol* 41:852, 1978.
67. Rosen MR. Cellular electrophysiology of digitalis toxicity. *J Am Coll Cardiol* 5:22A, 1985.
68. Johnson BF. Drug interactions with digoxin. *Drugs* 20:198–206, 1980.
69. Bigger JT Jr, Stranuss HC. Digitalis toxicity: drug interactions promoting toxicity and the management of toxicity. *Semin Drug Treat* 2:147, 1972.
70. Brown DD, Spector R, Juhl RP. Drug interactions with digoxin. *Drugs* 20:198–206, 1980.
71. Warner NJ, Barnard JJ, Bigger JN Jr. Tissue digoxin concentrations and digoxin effect during the quinidine-digoxin interactions. *J Am Coll Cardiol* 5:680, 1985.
72. Bigger JT Jr, Leakey EB. Quinidine and digoxin—an important interaction. *Drugs* 24:229, 1982.
73. Smith TW, Antman EM, Friedman PC, et al. Digitalis glycosides: mechanism and management. *Prog Cardiovasc Dis* 26:437, 1984.
74. Wenger TL, Butler VP Jr, Haber E, et al. Treatment of 63 severely digitalis-toxic patients with digoxin-specific antibody fragments. *J Am Coll Cardiol* 5:118A, 1985.
75. Vaughan-Williams EM. Some factors that influence the activity of antiarrhythmic drugs. *Br Heart J* 40(Suppl):52, 1978.
76. Harrison DC. Antiarrhythmic drug classification: new science and practical applications. *Am J Cardiol* 56:185–187, 1985.
77. Campbell TJ. Kinetics of onset of rate-dependent effects of Class I antiarrhythmic drugs are important in determining their effects on refractoriness in guinea pig ventricle and provide a theoretical basis for subclassification. *Cardiovasc Res* 17:344, 1983.
78. Josephson M, Caracta A, Riccuitti M. Electrophysiologic properties of procainamide in man. *Am J Cardiol* 33:596, 1974.
79. Roden DM, Reele JB, Higgins JB, et al. Antiarrhythmic efficacy, pharmacokinetics, and safety of N-acetylprocainamide in human subjects: comparison with procainamide. *Am J Cardiol* 46:463–468, 1980.
80. Fenster PE, Comess KA, Marsh R, et al. Conversion of atrial fibrillation to sinus rhythm by acute intravenous procainamide infusion. *Am Heart J* 106:501, 1983.

81. Wenber TL, Browning DL, Masterton E, et al. Procainamide delivery to ischemic canine myocardium following rapid intravenous administration. *Circ Res* 46:789, 1983.
82. Kosausky BD, Taylor J, Lorin B, et al. Long-term use of procainamide following acute myocardial infarction. *Circulation* 47:1204, 1973.
83. Anderson RJ, Gentsin E. Procainamide-induced pericardial effusion. *Am Heart J* 83:798–800, 1972.
84. Bauer LA, Black D, Gensler A. Procainamide-cimetadine drug interaction in elderly male patients. *J Am Geriatric Soc* 38:467, 1981.
85. Strasberg B, Schlarasky S, Erdberg A, et al. Procainamide-induced polymorphous ventricular tachycardia. *Am J Cardiol* 47:1309, 1981.
86. Swartz PJ. Idiopathic long Q-T syndrome progress and questions. *Am Heart J* 109:399, 1985.
87. Moss AJ, Schwartz PJ. Delayed repolarization (QT or QTV prolongation) and malignant ventricular arrhythmias. *Mod Conc Cardiovasc Dis* 51:58, 1982.
88. Gay RJ, Brown OF. Pacemaker failure due to procainamide toxicity. *Am J Cardiol* 34:728, 1974.
89. Ellrodt AG, Murata GH, Reidinger MS, et al. Severe neutropenia associated with sustained release procainamide. *Ann Intern Med* 100:197–201, 1984.
90. Hoffman BF, Rosen MR, Wit AL. Electrophysiology and pharmacology of cardiac arrhythmias. VII. Cardiac effects of quinidine and procainamide. *Am Heart J* 90:117, 1975.
91. DeMarco JP, Garan H, Ruskin JN. Quinidine for ventricular arrhythmias: value of electrophysiologic testing. *Am J Cardiol* 51:90, 1983.
92. Maston JW, Hondeghen LM. Quinidine. *Ann NY Acad Sci* 432:162, 1984.
93. Mirro MJ, Manalan AM, Bailey JC, et al. Anticholinergic effects of disopyramide and quinidine on guinea pig myocardium: medication by direct muscarinic receptor blockade. *Circ Res* 47:855, 1980.
94. Leakey EB Jr, Reiffel JA, Drusin RE, et al. Interaction between quinidine and digoxin. *J Am Med Assoc* 240:533, 1978.
95. Polish LB, Branch RA, Fitzgerald KA. Digitoxin-quinidine interaction: potential during administration of cimetadine. *South Med J* 74:633, 1981.
96. Seltzer WM, Wray HW. Quinidine syncope: paroxysmal ventricular fibrillation occurring during treatment of chronic atrial arrhythmias. *Circulation* 30:17, 1964.
97. Smith WM, Gallagher JJ. "Les torsades de pointes": An unusual ventricular arrhythmia. *Ann Intern Med* 93:578, 1980.
98. Roden DM, Woosley RL, Primm K. Incidence and clinical features of the quinidine-associated long QT syndrome: implications for patient care. *Am Heart J* 111:1088–1093, 1986.
99. Vaughan-Williams EM. Disopyramide. *Ann NY Acad Sci* 432:189, 1984.

100. Wilkson PR, Desai J, Hollister J, et al. Electrophysiologic effects of disopyramide in patients with atrioventricular nodal dysfunction. *Circulation* 66:1211, 1982.
101. Sasyniuki BI, Kirs T. Cellular electrophysiologic changes induced by disopyramide phosphate in normal and infarcted hearts. *J Ont Med* 4:20, 1976.
102. Podrid PG, Schoenenberger A, Lown B. Congestive heart failure caused by oral disopyramide. *N Engl J Med* 302:614, 1980.
103. Teichman SL, Fisher JD, Matso JA, et al. Disopyramide-pyridostigmine: report of beneficial drug interaction. *J Cardiovasc Pharmacol* 7:108, 1985.
104. Morady F, Scheinmann MM, Desai J. Disopyramide. *Ann Intern Med* 96:337, 1982.
105. Tzironi D, Kerin A, Stern S, et al. Disopyramide-induced torsades de pointes. *Arch Intern Med* 141:946, 1981.
106. Collinsworth KA, Kalman SM, Harrison DC. The clinical pharmacology of lidocaine as an anti-arrhythmic drug. *Circulation* 50:1217, 1974.
107. Kupersmith J. Electrophysiological and antiarrhythmic effects of lidocaine in canine acute myocardial ischemia. *Am Heart J* 97:360–366, 1979.
108. Haynes RE, Chinn TL, Copass MK, et al. Comparison of bretylium tosylate and lidocaine in management of out-of-hospital ventricular fibrillation. A randomized clinical trial. *Am J Cardiol* 48:353, 1981.
109. Lie KI, Wellens HJ, Van Capelle FJ. Lidocaine in the prevention of primary ventricular fibrillation. A double-blind, randomized study of 212 consecutive patients. *N Engl J Med* 291:1324–1326, 1974.
110. DeSilva RA, Hennekens CH, Lown B, et al. Lignocaine prophylaxis in acute myocardial infarction. An evaluation of randomized trials. *Lancet* 2:855, 1981.
111. Carruth SE, Silverman ME. Ventricular fibrillation complicating acute myocardial infarction: reasons against the routine use of lidocaine. *Am Heart J* 104:545, 1982.
112. Dunn HM, McComb JM, Kenney CD, et al. Prophylactic lidocaine in the early phase of suspected myocardial infarction. *Am Heart J* 110:353, 1985.
113. White RD. Cardiovascular pharmacology: Part I. In: McIntyre KM, Lerins, AJ, eds. *Textbook of Advanced Clinical Life Support.* Dallas, TX: American Heart Association; 1983: 104–107.
114. Gillis RA, McCellan JR, Sanes TS, et al. Depression of cardiac sympathetic nerve activity by diphenylhydantoin. *J Pharmacol Exp Ther* 173:599, 1971.
115. Ferrier GR. Digitalis arrhythmias: role of oscillatory after potentials. *Prog Cardiovasc Dis* 19:459, 1977.
116. Rosen MR, Danilo P Jr, Alonso MB, et al. Effects of therapeutic concentrations of diphenylhydantoin on transmembrane potentials of normal and depressed Purkinje fibers. *J Pharmacol Exp Ther* 197:594–604, 1976.

117. Konn RD, Kennedy JW, Blackman JR. The hemodynamic effects of diphenylhydantoin. *Am Heart J* 73:500, 1967.
118. Unger AH, Sklaroff HJ. Fatalities following intravenous use of sodium diphenylhydantoin of cardiac arrhythmias. *J Am Med Assoc* 200:335, 1967.
119. Siddoway LA, Roden CM, Woosley RL. Clinical pharmacology of old and new antiarrhythmic drugs. *Cardiovasc Clin* 15:199–248, 1985.
120. Winkle RA, Meffin PJ, Fitzgerald JW, et al. Clinical efficacy and pharmacokinetics of a new orally effective antiarrhythmic, tocainide. *Circulation* 54:884–889, 1976.
121. Anderson JL, Mason JW, Winkle RA, et al. Clinical electrophysiologic effects of tocaimide. *Circulation* 57:685–691, 1978.
122. Maloney JD, Nissen RG, McClogan JM. Open clinical studies at a referral center: chronic maintenance tocainide therapy in patients with recurrent sustained ventricular tachycardia refractory to conventional antiarrhythmic agents. *Am Heart J* 100:1023–1030, 1980.
123. Maroganroth J, Panidis IP, Harley S, et al. Efficacy and safety of intravenous tocainide compared with intravenous lidocaine for acute ventricular arrhythmias-immediately after cardiac surgery. *Am J Cardiol* 54:1253, 1984.
124. Denaro CP, Benowitz NL. Poisoning due to class 1B antiarrhythmic drugs: lignocaine, mexilitine and tocainide. *Med. Toxicol Adverse Drug Exp* 4:412, 1989.
125. Hasegama GR. Tocainide: a new oral antiarrhythmic. *Drug Intell Clin Pharm* 19:514–517, 1985.
126. Kaplan HR, Mertz TE, Steffe TJ. New class I antiarrhythmic agents. In: Luccese BR, Single JV, Schwartz RP Jr, eds. *Clinical Pharmacology of Antiarrhythmic Therapy.* New York NY: Raven Press; 1984: 77–94.
127. Hohnloser SH, Lange HW, Raeder EA, et al. Short and long-term therapy with tocainide for malignant ventricular tachyarrhythmias. *Circulation* 73:143–149, 1986.
128. Waspe LE, Waxman HL, Buxton AE, et al. Mexiletine for control of drug-resistant ventricular tachyarrythmias and electrophysiologic results in 44 patients. *Am J Cardiol* 51:1175–1181, 1983.
129. Campbell RW, Talbot RG, Dolder MA, et al. Comparison of procainamide and mexiletine in prevention of ventricular arrhythmias after acute myocardial infarction. *Lancet* 1:1257–1260, 1975.
130. Greenspan AM, Spielman SR, Webb CR, et al. Efficacy of combination therapy with mexiletine and a type 1A agent for inducible ventricular tachyarrhythmias secondary to coronary artery disease. *Am J Cardiol* 56:277–284, 1985.
131. Duff HJ, Roden D, Prinam RK. Mexiletine in the treatment of resistant ventricular arrhythmias: enhancement of efficacy and reduction of dose-related side effects by combination with quinidine. *Circulation* 67:1124, 1983.
132. Poole JE, Werner JA, Bardy GH, et al. Intolerance and ineffectiveness of mexiletine in patients with serious ventricular arrhythmias. *Am Heart J* 112:322–326, 1986.

133. Mygaard TW, Sellers TD, Cook TS, et al. Adverse reactions to antiarrhythmic drugs during therapy for ventricular arrhythmias. *J Am Med Assoc* 256:55, 1986.
134. Cetnanowski AB, Rihn TL. A review of adverse reactions to mexiletine and tocainide. *Cardiovasc Rev Rep* 6:1335–1342, 1985.
135. Roden DM. Tocainide and mexilitine. Orally effective lidocaine analogues. *Arch Intern Med* 145:417, 1985.
136. Mead RH, Harrison DC. Therapy with investigational antiarrhythmic drugs. *Med Clin North Am* 68:1321, 1984.
137. Akhtar M. Practical considerations in the treatment of ventricular arrhythmias with mexiletine. *Am Heart J* 107:1086–1090, 1984.
138. Pentikainen PJ, Koivula IH, Hiltunen HA. Effects of rifampicin in treatment of kinetics of mexiletine. *Eur J Clin Pharmacol* 23:261–266, 1982.
139. Hewett KW, Rosen MR. Alpha and beta adrenergic interactions with ouabain induced delayed after depolarization. *J Pharmacol Exp Ther* 229:188, 1984.
140. Brown MJ, Brown DC, Murphy MD. Hypokalemia from beta-2 receptor stimulation by circulating epinephrine. *N Engl J Med* 309:1414, 1983.
141. Singh BN. Clinical aspects of the anti-arrhythmic actions of beta-receptor blocking drugs. *NZ Med J* 178:529, 1973.
142. Winkle RA, Lopes MG, Goodman DJ, et al. Propranolol for patients with mitral valve prolapse. *Am Heart J* 93:422–427, 1977.
143. De Soyza N, Kane JJ, Murphy ML, et al. The long-term suppression of ventricular arrhythmia by oral acebutolol in patients with coronary artery disease. *Am Heart J* 100:631, 1980.
144. Morganroth J. Short-term evaluation of atenolol in hospitalized patients with chronic ventricular arrhythmias. *Drugs* 25(Suppl 2):181–185, 1983.
145. Hill RF. Treatment of isorhythmic A-V dissociation during general anesthesia with propranolol. *Anesthesiology* 70:141, 1989.
146. β-Blocker Heart Attack Research Group. A randomized trial of propranolol in patients with acute myocardial infarction. I. Mortality results. *J Am Med Assoc* 247:1708–14, 1982.
147. Pederson TR. Six-year follow-up of the Norwegian Multicenter Study on timolol after acute myocardial infarction. *N Engl J Med* 313:1055–1058, 1985.
148. Braunwald E, Muller JE, Klones RA, et al. Role of beta-adrenergic blockade in the therapy of patients with myocardial infarction. *Am J Med* 74:113, 1983.
149. Kostis JB, Wilson AC, Sanders MR, et al. Prognostic significance of ventricular ectopic activity in survivors of acute myocardial infarction who receive propranolol. *Am J Cardiol* 61:975–978, 1988.
150. Friedman L, Byington RP, Capone RJ, et al. Effect of propranolol in patients with myocardial infarction and ventricular arrhythmia. *J Am Coll Cardiol* 7:1–8, 1986.

151. Frishman WH. Drug therapy: beta-adrenergic antagonists-new drug new indications. *N Engl J Med* 305:500, 1981.
152. Zipes DP, Prystowsky EN, Heger JJ. Amiodarone: electrophysiologic actions, pharmacokinetics, and clinical effects. *J Am Coll Cardiol* 3:1059, 1984.
153. Koch-Wesser J. Drug therapy. Bretylium. *N Engl J Med* 300:473, 1979.
154. Wenger TK, Lederman S, Starmer CF, et al. A method for quantitating antifibrillatory effects of drugs after coronary reperfusion in dogs: improved outcome with bretylium. *Circulation* 69:142, 1984.
155. Kerber RE, Pandian NF, Jensen SR, et al. Effect of lidocaine and bretylium on energy requirement for transthoracic defibrillation. Experimental studies. *J Am Coll Cardiol* 7:397–405, 1986.
156. Haynes RE, Chinn RL, Copass MK, et al. Comparison of bretylium tosylate and lidocaine in management of out-of-hospital ventricular fibrillation: a randomized clinical trial. *Am J Cardiol* 48:353, 1981.
157. Olson DW, Thompson BM, Darin JC, et al. A randomized comparison study of bretylium tosylate and lidocaine in resuscitation of patients from out-of-hospital ventricular fibrillation in a paramedic system. *Ann Emerg Med* 13:807, 1984.
158. Rosen MR, Wit AL. Electrophysiology of the antiarrhythmic drugs. *Am Heart J* 106:829, 1983.
159. Greene HL, Graham EL, Werner JA, et al. Toxic and therapeutic effects of amiodarone in the treatment of cardiac arrhythmias. *J Am Coll Cardiol* 2:1114, 1983.
160. Haedo AH, Chiale PA, Bandieri JD, et al. Comparative antiarrhythmic efficacy of verapamil, 17-monochloroacetyl-cymaline, mexiletine, and amiodarone in patients with severe chagostic myocarditis: relation with the underlying arrhythmogenic mechanisms. *J Am Coll Cardiol* 7:114, 1986.
161. McKenna WJ, Harris L, Rowland E, et al. Amiodarone for long-term management of patients with hypertrophic cardiomyopathy. *Am J Cardiol* 54:802, 1984.
162. Podrid PJ. The new antiarrhythmic drugs. *Resident Staff Phys* 31:23–33, 1985.
163. Raeder EA, Podrid PJ, Loun B. Side effects and complications of amiodarone therapy. *Am Heart J* 109:975, 1985.
164. Herre JM, Sauve MJ, Malone P, et al. Long-term results of amiodarone therapy in patients with recurrent sustained ventricular tachycardia or ventricular fibrillation. *J Am Coll Cardiol* 13:422–449, 1989.
165. Sobel SM, Rakita L. Pneumonitis and pulmonary fibrosis associated with amiodarone treatment: a possible complication of a new antiarrhythmic drug. *Circulation* 65:819, 1982.
166. Mason JW. Amiodarone. *N Engl J Med* 316:455, 1987.
167. Marcus FI, Fontaine GH, Frank R, et al. Clinical pharmacology and therapeutic applications of the antiarrhythmic agents, amiodarone. *Am Heart J* 101:480, 1981.

168. Gilmorin RF, Zipes DP. Basic electrophysiology of the slow inward current. In: Antman EM, Stone PH, eds. *Cardiac Arrhythmias.* Mt. Kisco, NY: Futura Publishing Co. 1983: 25–30.
169. Rickenberger RL, Prystowsky EN, Heger JJ, et al. Effects of intravenous and chronic oral verapamil administration in patients with supraventricular tachyarrhythmias. *Circulation* 62:996, 1980.
170. Sung RJ, Elser B, McAllister RG Jr. Intravenous verapamil for termination of reentrant supraventricular tachycardia. Intracardiac studies correlated with plasma verapamil concentrations. *Ann Intern Med* 93:682, 1980.
171. Waxman HL, Myerburg RJ, Appel R, et al. Verapamil for control of ventricular rate in paroxysmal supraventricular tachycardia and atrial fibrillation or flutter: a double-blind, randomized, cross-over study. *Ann Intern Med* 94:1, 1981.
172. Plumb VJ, Karp RB, Kouchoukos NT, et al. Verapamil therapy of atrial fibrillation and atrial flutter following cardiac operation. *J Thorac Cardiovasc* 83:590–596, 1982.
173. Spurrell RA, Kirkler DM, Sowton E. Effects of verapamil on electrophysiological properties of anomalous atrioventricular connexion in Wolff-Parkson-White syndrome. *Br Heart J* 36:348–354, 1982.
174. Gulamhusein SK, Ko P, Carruthers SG, et al. Acceleration of the ventricular response during atrial fibrillation in the Wolff-Parkinson-White syndrome after verapamil. *Circulation* 65:348, 1982.
175. McGovern B, Garan H, Ruskin JN. Precipitation of cardiac arrest by verapamil in patients with Wolff-Parkinson-White syndrome. *Ann Intern Med* 104:791, 1986.
176. Jacob AS, Nielsen DH, Gianelly RE. Fatal ventricular fibrillation following verapamil in Wolff-Parkinson-White syndrome with atrial fibrillation. *Ann Emerg Med* 14:159, 1985.
177. Pacer M, Mellen J, Medina N, et al. Hemodynamic consequences of combined beta-adrenergic and slow calcium channel blockade in man. *Circulation* 65:660, 1982.
178. Kiervial J, Kristen EB, Kessler KM, et al. The effects of intravenous verapamil on hemodynamic status of patients with coronary artery disease receiving propranolol. *Circulation* 65:653, 1982.
179. Haft JI, Habbab MA. Treatment of atrial arrhythmias: effectiveness of verapamil when preceded by calcium infusion. *Arch Intern Med* 106:501–504, 1983.
180. Oppenheim EB. Sudden cardiac death: what primary care providers need to know. *Res & Staff Physician* 35:97, 1989.
181. Mirowski M, Reid PR, Mower MM, et al. Termination of malignant ventricular arrhythmias with an implanted automatic defibrillator in human beings. *N Engl J Med* 303(6):322–324, 1980.
182. Winkle RA, Hardwin M, Ruder M, et al. Long term outcome with automatic implantable cardioverter-defibrillator. *J Am Coll Cardiol* 13:1353, 1989.
183. Mirowski M, Reid RR, Mover MM, et al. Clinical performance of the implantable cardioverter-defibrillator. *PACE* 7:1345, 1984.

184. Barbola J, Denes P, Ezri MD, et al. The automatic implantable cardioverter-defibrillator. Clinical experience, complications and follow up in 25 patients. *Arch Intern Med* 148:71, 1988.
185. Gabry MD, Brodman R, Johnson D, et al. Automatic implantable cardioverter defibrillator: patient survival, battery longevity and shock delivery analysis. *J Am Coll Cardiol 9:1349–1356, 1987.*
186. Kron J, Oliver RP, Norsted S, et al. The automatic implantable cardioverter defibrillator (AICD) in young patients (abstract). *Circulation* 80:II-389, 1989.
187. Trappe HJ, Daneiel WG, Klein H, et al. Evaluation of global and regional left ventricular function using two-dimensional and M-mode echocardiography in patients with an automatic implantable cardioverter defibrillator. *PACE* 11:1070–76, 1988.
188. Riper DF, Horrow JC, Kutalek SP, et al. Mixed venous oximetry during automatic implantable cardioverter-defibrillator placement. *Cardiothorac Anesth* 4:453–457, 1990.
189. Winkle RA, Stinson EB, Echt DS, et al. Practical aspects of automatic cardioverter-defibrillator implantation. *Am Heart J* 108:1335, 1984.
190. Echt DS, Armstrong K, Schmidt P, et al. Clinical experience, complications, and survival in 70 patients with the automatic implantable cardioverter defibrillator. *Circulation* 71:289–296, 1985.
191. Reid PR, Griffith SC, Mower MM, et al. Implantable cardioverter-defibrillator: Patient selection and implantable protocol. *PACE* 7:1338, 1984.
192. Kay GN, Plumb VJ, Dailey SM, et al. Current role of the AICD in the treatment of life-threatening ventricular arrhythmias. *Am J Med* 88:25N–34N, 1990.
193. Levine JH, Richards A, Mellitis D, et al. Does poor cardiac function preclude benefit from an AICD? *Am J Cardiol* 13:65A, 1989.
194. Epstein AE, Kay GN, Plumb VJ, et al. Combined AICD and pacemaker systems: implantation techniques and follow-up. *J Am Coll Cardiol* 13:121, 1989.
195. Josephson ME, Harken AH, Horowitz LN. Long-term results of endocardial resection for sustained ventricular tachycardia in coronary disease patients. *Am Heart J* 104:51, 1982.
196. Page PL, Arciniegas JG, Plumb VJ, et al. Value of early posteroperative epicardial programmed ventricular stimulation studies after surgery for ventricular tachyarrhythmias. *J Am Coll Cardiol* 6:1046–52, 1983.
197. Moran JM, Kehoe RH, Loeb JM, et al. Extended endocardial resection for the treatment of ventricular tachycardia and ventricular fibrillation. *Ann Thorac Surg* 34:538–50, 1982.
198. Mamolis AS, Dastegan H, Estes NA. Prophylactic automatic implantable cardioverter-defibrillator patches in patients at high risk for postoperative ventricular tachyarrhythmias. *J Am Coll Cardiol* 13:1367, 1989.
199. Olinger GN, Chapman PD, Troup PJ, et al. Stratified application of the AICD. *J Thorac Cardiovasc Surg* 96:141, 1988.

Chapter 14

Mechanical Support of the Failing Heart

Michael Kesselbrenner, MD,
David Bregman, MD,
and Jeffrey Sack, MD

The intra-aortic balloon pump is currently the most widely used temporary circulatory assist device. Since its inception in 1962 by Moulopoulous et al.[1] intra-aortic balloon pumping has represented a simple and practical approach to support the failing circulation. The principles of counterpulsation arose from the pioneering work of Harken[2] and Kantrowitz[3,4] who surmised that poor left ventricle indices could possibly be influenced by retarding the diastolic pressure. Counterpulsation, as used by the intra-aortic balloon pump, is accomplished when the intra-aortic balloon is positioned in the descending aorta; the balloon is rapidly inflated in diastole concurrent with closure of the aortic valve (Fig. 1).

Mechanism of Balloon Action

Our classic device is a unidirectional dual-chambered intra-aortic balloon (Fig. 1). The balloon has a spherical distal chamber

From Casthely PA, Bregman D, (eds): *Cardiopulmonary Bypass: Physiology, Related Complications, and Pharmacology.* Mount Kisco, NY, Futura Publishing Company, Inc., © 1991.

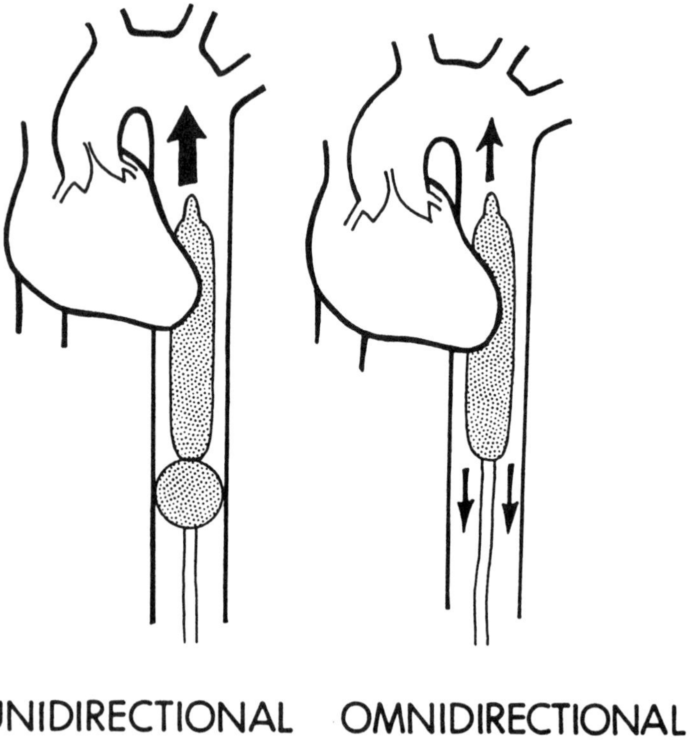

Figure 1. Mechanism of action of the intra-aortic balloon. Tip of catheter is positioned just beyond origin of left subclavian artery. Balloon is inflated in diastole and deflated during systole.

that inflates early in diastole and occludes the aorta. This is followed sequentially by the inflation of a narrower, cylindrical proximal pumping chamber in the same diastolic interval, which displaces intra-aortic blood entirely (unidirectional) towards the aortic root. Both chambers are completely deflated by an active vacuum just prior to ventricular ejection.

The action of the dual-chambered balloon in a patient is illustrated in Figure 2. With the onset of ventricular systole, the balloon is rapidly deflated. The inflation of the balloon displaces blood in the aorta (by an amount equal to the volume of the balloon) towards the coronary tree, thereby augmenting coronary perfusion

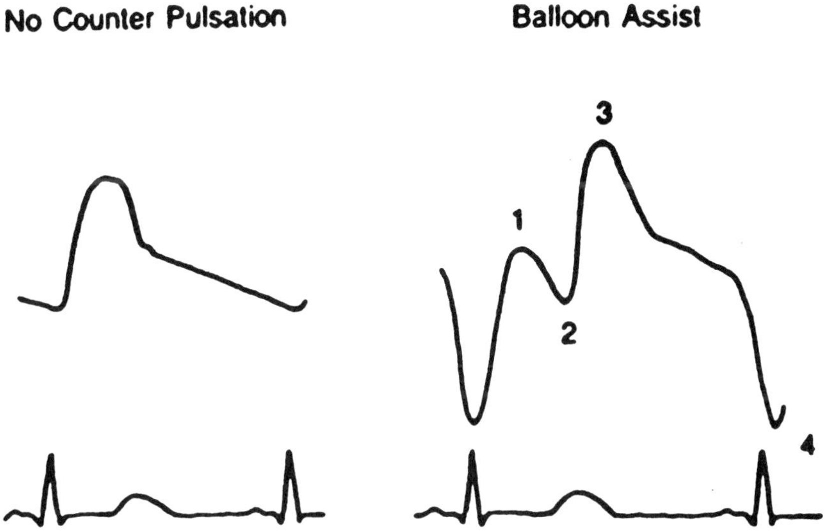

Figure 2. Shown here is a comparison in the arterial pressure waveform without counterpulsation and during balloon assist. Note (1) the sharp angle (point 2) between the fall in systolic arterial pressure and augmented diastolic pressure. (2) An augmented diastolic pressure (point 3) greater than the peak systolic pressure (point 1). (3) An end diastolic pressure during augmentation less than the end diastolic pressure without augmentation (point 4).

pressure and blood flow (Fig. 3). The collapse of the balloon creates a reduction in impedance to left ventricular ejection (i.e. decreased afterload), and consequently reduces left ventricular work.[5]

In 1968, Adrian Kantrowitz introduced the intra-aortic balloon pump to the clinical setting of cardiogenic shock.[6] Careful follow-up of such patients showed that mortality remained largely unaltered.[7] However, the findings that counterpulsation decreases the extent and severity of ischemic injury[8-12] and opens dormant coronary vessels,[12] suggested that perhaps counterpulsation ought to be applied in patients sustaining uncomplicated myocardial infarction. This then could minimize the quantity of myocardium that ultimately became necrotic,[13] theoretically preserving left ventricular function.

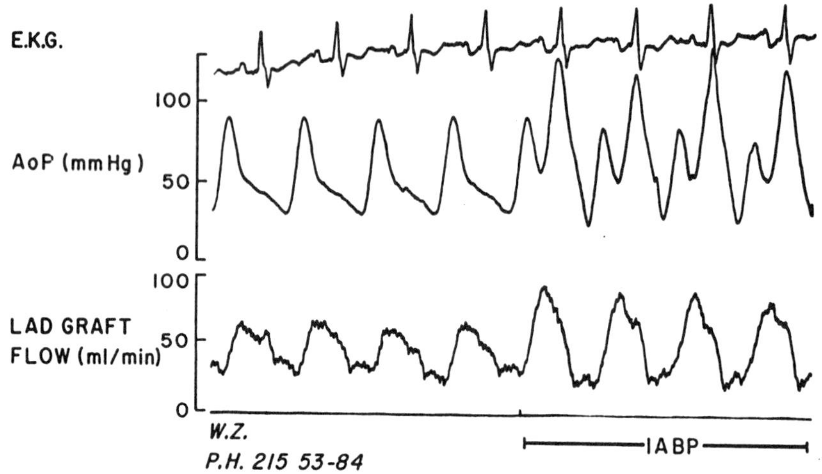

Figure 3. Shown here is the increase in coronary blood flow during diastole produced by the intra-aortic balloon pump.

The applications and indications for intra-aortic balloon pumping have come a long way since the early days of counterpulsation. At present, the intra-aortic balloon pump is widely used for circulatory support in patients with postoperative left ventricular failure, unstable angina pectoris refractory to medical treatment, recurring myocardial ischemia in the setting of acute myocardial infarction, as well as refractory congestive heart failure and recurrent ventricular arrhythmia. We have seen increasing use of intra-aortic balloon counterpulsation in the pediatric population, as a bridge to cardiac transplantation, and for prophylactic use during high-risk percutaneous transluminal coronary angioplasty. The intra-aortic balloon is now also used at times once thought relatively contraindicated, such as patients with acute myocardial infarction who have received thrombolytic therapy.

Principles

The principle of counterpulsation is based upon the assumption that the reduction of end diastolic pressure will improve left ventricular function. This is accomplished with improved stroke volume as created by the balloon. The balloon is positioned in the proximal descending thoracic aorta.[4] During diastole, it is rapidly inflated concurrent with closure of the aortic valve. At the onset of systole, initiated via a sensing electrocardiogram, the balloon is then rapidly deflated. This creates a "vacuum" effect, decreasing the afterload, thereby augmenting ventricular outflow (Fig. 4).

The mechanism of improved hemodynamics is therefore twofold. First, by raising diasolic pressures within the proximal aorta at balloon expansion, coronary perfusion pressure is increased, generating an increased myocardial oxygen supply, with concomitant bolstering of myocardial contractility. Then, with rapid balloon deflation, there is a sudden volume loss within the aorta (proportional to the volume of the balloon), effectively reducing the afterload by which the left ventricle must work against. This decreases myocardial oxygen demand, and at the same time, increases cardiac output at any given level of filling pressure.[14]

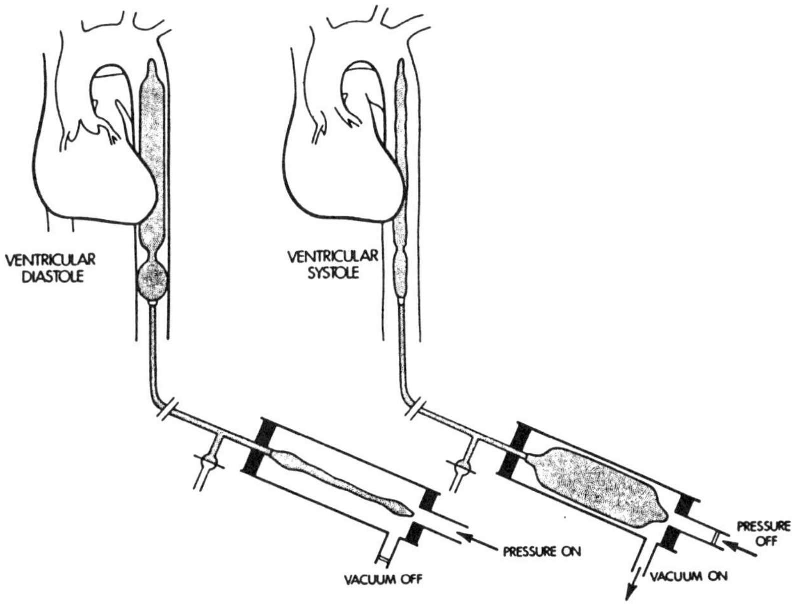

Figure 4. The balloon is inflated when the vacuum is off and deflated when the vacuum is on.

The main advantages of the intra-aortic balloon pump over conventional arterio-arterial counterpulsation are: (1) circulatory assistance may be maintained at prolonged periods of time without clinically significant hemolysis; (2) a single arterial puncture is required; (3) coronary blood flow is augmented even in the hypotensive state.[15]

Two additional advantages result from the use of either counterpulsation or intra-aortic balloon pumping: (1) it has been demonstrated by Jacoby et al.[16] that after a short period of counterpulsation, dormant intercoronary collateral beds are opened; and these channels remain open after termination of counterpulsation; (2) it has been demonstrated by several investigators[17-20] that early institution of intra-aortic balloon pumping decreases the size of the potential myocardial infarction after coronary occlusion.

There is clinical and experimental evidence to demonstrate that the critical factor that improves the performance of the heart suffering from an acute myocardial infarction and power failure is an increase in coronary blood flow.[21-25] It has also been shown that a major determinant of improved retrograde coronary blood flow is an elevation in the mean aortic diastolic pressure.[26-30] Under conditions of hypoxemia, cardiac performance is coronary flow dependent, and unloading of the left ventricle does not in itself improve myocardial efficiency. Therefore, any method of mechanical assistance should be aimed at maximally increasing coronary blood flow. Years of early work confirmed that this assistance to circulatory performance would decrease the extent and severity of ischemic injury[31,32] as well as perfuse dormant coronary vessels[33] during left ventricular power failure.

The description of intra-aortic balloon pump insertion was first described by Kantrowitz et al.[34] The common femoral artery is exposed through a ventricular incision beginning high in the groin over the inguinal ligament. The vessel is then encircled by tapes for control (Fig. 5).

A 10-mm woven Dacron sidearm graft is sutured onto the arterial site. Using bulldog clamps to control the blood flow above and below the arteriotomy site, the balloon catheter is inserted through the graft into the artery. An umbilical snare is used to secure the balloon catheter within the graft. The balloon catheter can now be advanced up into the descending aorta.[35,36]

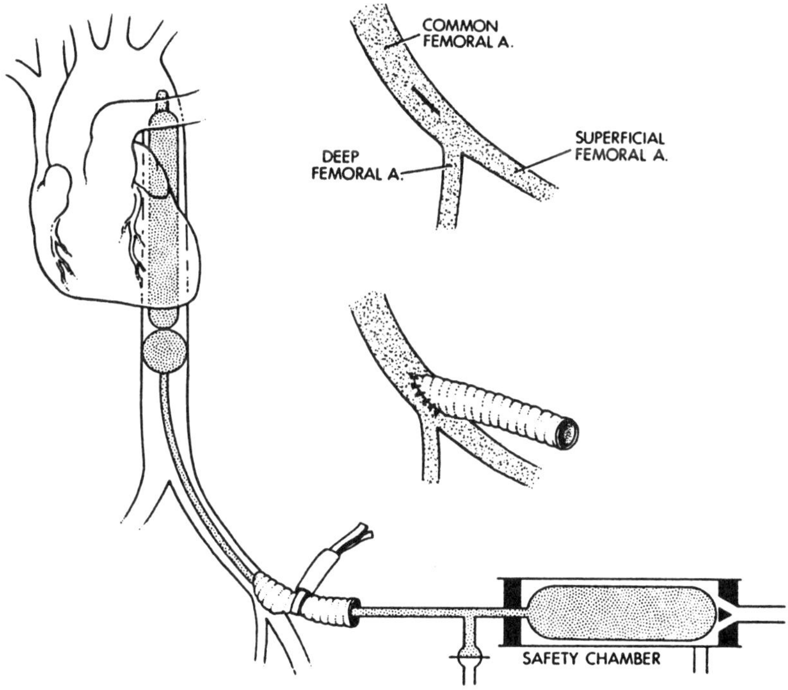

Figure 5. Mechanism of insertion of the intra-aortic balloon pump using a Dacron[R] graft.

Transiliac Artery Insertion

Using the same surgical procedure, the balloon can be inserted into the common iliac artery if passage through the femoral arteries is too narrow. The iliac artery is exposed by a retroperitoneal approach through an oblique incision above the left inguinal ligament.[37]

Transaxillary Insertion

In situations in which femoral insertion is not possible, owing either to severe diffuse aorto-iliac atherosclerotic disease, tortuosity, or some other contraindication, the intra-aortic balloon catheter can be inserted through the left subclavian artery[38,39] through surgical exposure of the vessels and the attachment of a sidearm graft. The balloon is then advanced antegrade into the descending thoracic aorta. This technique is used very rarely.

Transthoracic Intra-Aortic Balloon Insertion

The technique of transthoracic intra-aortic balloon insertion can be used when either the balloon cannot be advanced through the femoral artery or when the previous surgical exposure of the aortic arch makes this technique more expedient.[40-42]

Percutaneous Intra-Aortic Balloon Insertion

In 1979, a single-chambered 40-ml percutaneous intra-aortic balloon was constructed around a central wire.[43-46] The intra-aortic balloon was wrapped manually about the wire, and was then appropriate for percutaneous insertion into the femoral artery (Fig. 6).[47] Percutaneous insertion difficulties were sometimes encountered during the following circumstances: (1) tortuous vessels preventing intra-aortic balloon insertion; (2) a diminished femoral pulse; (3) balloons failing to unfurl because of overwrapping; and (4) dislodging of atherosclerotic plaques or thombus. Isner et al.[48] found that most complications appeared related to the balloon catheter insertion. This information coupled with the clinical experience gained through the use of the first percutaneous balloons[49] resulted in a redesign of the percutaneous balloons.

In 1981, the second-generation percutaneous intra-aortic balloons were introduced, featuring a dual-lumen catheter.[50,51] This dual-lumen intra-aortic balloon has a flexible lumen incorporated inside the catheter that allows the balloon to be advanced over the

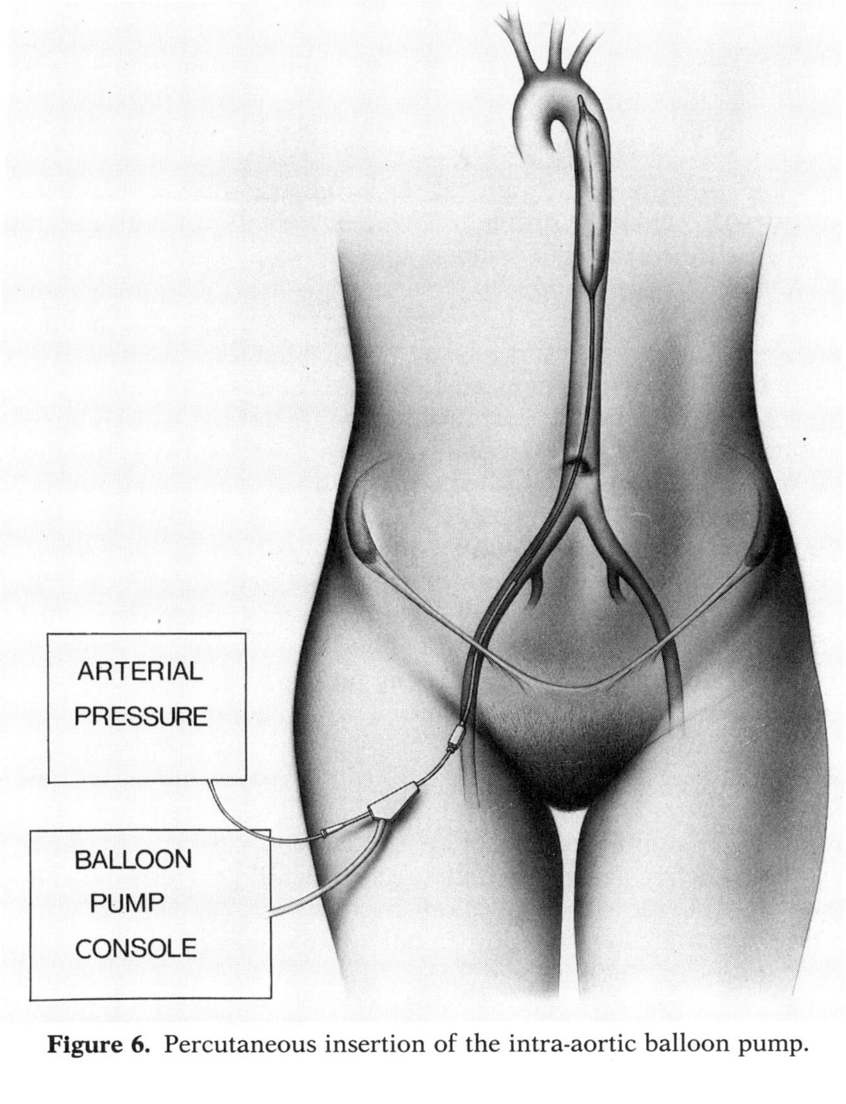

Figure 6. Percutaneous insertion of the intra-aortic balloon pump.

0.038-inch J-tip guidewire, which has been already advanced into the descending thoracic aorta. Access to this central lumen is achieved by removing the central stylet attached to the "wrapping knob" assembly. After the balloon has been advanced over the 0.038-inch J-tip guidewire, the wire is removed, and the central lumen can be closed with a male Luer-Lok cap or it can be used to monitor the aortic arch pressure.[52] The ability to establish an arterial line quickly along with the rapid insertion of the balloon makes the percutaneous dual-lumen intra-aortic balloon a powerful adjunct in the emergency setting.

The wrapping procedure of the original percutaneous intra-aortic balloon posed a problem. To ameliorate the difficulties with wrapping the intra-aortic balloon, the Datascope Percor Stat intra-aortic balloon was introduced. This specially designed package contains a prewrapped dual-lumen intra-aortic balloon. The balloon does not leave the sterile package until after the sheath-dilator assembly has been introduced into the femoral artery. Once the intra-aortic balloon has advanced into the aorta, the balloon is unfurled by rotating the wrapping knob counterclockwise. Because the balloon is prewrapped, the problems associated with improper wrapping are now eliminated.

There are four new adult balloons included in the second-generation intra-aortic balloon. All four balloons incorporate the "wrapping knob" assembly into the catheter's base. The 50-mL dual-lumen balloon was especially developed for the patient with a large diameter aorta. By increasing the cross-sectional diameter of the 40-mL balloon (a 1.25-mm increase), balloon volume is enlarged to 50 cm and blood volume displacement is increased by 25%. The Percor stat 9.5 D > L > (double lumen) that can be inserted through a 10F sheath has effectively resulted in an 18% decrease in luminal diameter of the sheath, thereby mitigating against ischemic peripheral balloon complications. This is now the balloon of choice in most hospital circumstances. The more supple 8.5F Pecor Stat is a single-lumen balloon best suited for transthoracic insertion. The 8.5F and 9.5F intra-aortic balloons are ideally suited for women who have smaller aortoiliac arteries.[52]

In addition, the newest balloon pumps are the System 90 and the 90T (Data Scope, Paramus, NJ, USA), its more portable counterpart adaptable for transplant. The System 90 is a semicomputerized mobile pump with unique capabilities of monitoring arrhythmias and an ability to handle AV sequential pacing more reliably. The 90T is similar in design but has two components in order to facilitate transport for helicopter or ambulances.

Ideal Balloon Function

The primary goals of intra-aortic balloon pumping are to implement the maximal increase in coronary blood flow during diastole and at the same time effect a decrease in left ventricular work.[53] Realization that these two beneficial effects are dependent upon one another permits maximal benefit to be obtained from each factor in the following fashion: the diastolic augmentation ordinarily begins at the dicrotic notch (Fig. 3), using an initial timing sequence of 1:3, whereby every third ventricular beat is augmented by the intra-aortic balloon. One can encroach upon the dicrotic notch to begin balloon inflation slightly earlier in diastole. Provided the patient does not have premature ventricular contractions from this manipulation, it can be performed in patients who appear to be responding poorly to intra-aortic balloon pumping to give them additional benefit. The right-hand side or downslope of the augmentation is the part most intimately involved with the ventricular unloading aspect of intra-aortic balloon pumping. If the fall in left ventricular end diastolic pressure is too great, the following sequence of events occurs: excessive fall in left ventricular end diastolic pressure essentially means that the balloon has collapsed too soon before the aortic valve has opened. Because blood must flow to occupy the space of the formerly expanded balloon, it flows retrograde from all branches of the aorta, including the coronary arteries (if the fall in left ventricular end diastolic pressure is excessive).[54] Therefore, one must effect a compromise and have some fall in left ventricular end diastolic pressure, but not an excessive decrease. Recent experimental and clinical work has indicated that this fall in left ventricular end diastolic pressure should not exceed 10 mm Hg.

As far as the position of the balloon is concerned, initially we place the balloon as far proximally in the aorta as possible (that is, with the tip of the balloon just distal to the left subclavian artery). Be sure to feel the pulse in the left arm so that the tip of the balloon is not in the subclavian orifice and is not occluding the left subclavian inflow.

At rapid heart rates, there is more dead space in the safety chamber balloon. Therefore, one could increase the volume of carbon dioxide in the safety chamber balloon (e.g., to 45 mL with a 30-mL balloon) at heart rates over 120 beats/min. This will improve intra-aortic balloon function.[55]

In this clinical setting, heart rates of up to 140 beats/min can usually be followed with the smaller size balloon. If the rate is higher, it may be necessary to assist on 1:2 (every other beat) in order to achieve effective diastolic augmentation, until the rate slows, when 1:1 assistance can be instituted.

If weaning a patient from intra-aortic balloon assistance is undertaken by changing from a 1:1 to a 1:2 or 1:3 assisting sequence, additional time will be present for the vacuum to build up, and augmentation may demonstrate a deep "sink"; the end diastolic point may need elevation by a minor adjustment on the console.

Paramount for effective counterpulsation is the timing of balloon inflation and deflation. A pulse contour recorder within the central lumen, or radial arterial monitor, will display pressure waveform onto the console screen. An electronic signal, which may be manually maneuvered within the cardiac cycle, then indicates balloon inflation and deflation.

For optimal augmentation of hemodynamics, the balloon should be deflated just prior to left ventricular ejection (i.e., at the QRS complex.) Delay would present the ventricle with an obstruction to outflow. If deflated too early, the "vacuum" effect to enhance cardiac output is not only compromised, but may actually hinder left ventricular ejection, thereby markedly decreasing cardiac output.

Inflation should take place during the dicrotic notch of the arterial pressure wave, corresponding to the peak of the T-wave on the electrocardiogram. Early expansion creates increased afterload for the contracting ventricle. Delayed expansion will decrease coronary perfusion and create less diastolic augmentation. Most consoles will automatically collapse the balloon in case of timing errors.

Obviously, cardiac arrhythmias will also alter the efficiency of intra-aortic balloon counterpulsation, owing to the reliance of timing of balloon inflation and deflation on the surface electrocardiogram. Therefore, every effort should be made to suppress cardiac arrhythmias while the patient is on intra-aortic balloon support. Atrial arrhythmias, especially atrial fibrillation with a rapid ventricular response may also lead to inadequate augmentation.

Metabolic Effects of Intra-Aortic Balloon Pumping

The metabolic effects of intra-aortic balloon pumping are now well described. Feola et al.[56] have examined myocardial lactate metabolism with pacing induced tachycardia in seven patients. They found that lactate production changed from 0.24 ± 0.07 extraction at rest to 0.94 ± 0.01 production after pacing ($P \leq 0.001$) without and from 0.10 ± 0.003 extraction at rest to 0.57 ± 0.001 production after $P \leq 0.001$) with intra-aortic balloon pumping. The difference between the lactate production levels occurring with and without ($P < 0.005$) counterpulsation was statistically significant.

Previous studies have demonstrated that intra-aortic balloon pumping or arterial counterpulsation reduces MVO_2 in the normal circulation by diminishing heart rate, peak left ventricular systolic wall stress, and possibly, contractility.[57,58] Wall stress in the left ventricle, the major determinant of myocardial oxygen demand, can be decreased through a reduction of either peak systolic pressure or a reduction in left ventricular end diastolic pressure and heart size.[59] Decreases in heart rate and a reduction in the frequency of ventricular ectopic beats suggest that intra-aortic balloon counterpulsation may reduce sympathetic tone and cardiac contractility through baroreceptor-mediated reflexes. This impression has been strengthened by observations of peripheral vasodilation[60] and increased frequency of discharge of the carotid sinus nerve[61] during intra-aortic balloon pumping. The postulated reduction of sympathetic tone during intra-aortic balloon pumping is further supported in the present study by observation of a decrease in circulating arterial epinephrine and norepinephrine during intra-aortic balloon counterpulsion.

Effect of Intra-Aortic Balloon Pumping on Right Heart Hemodynamics

The hemodynamic effect of intra-aortic balloon pumping on left ventricular performance is well known. Intra-aortic balloon pump support immediately decreases heart rate, left ventricular end diastolic pressure, and mean left atrial pressure and improves endocardial viability ratio (EVR) (Fig. 7). It also causes a moderate increase in cardiac output. Johnson et al.[62] have looked at the effects of intra-aortic balloon pumping on right heart hemodynamics. Implementation of intra-aortic balloon pumping was consistently found to produce an instantaneous decrease in right atrial pressure averaging 11%, reflecting a decrease in preload. In addition, the major determinants of right ventricular afterload were found to decrease significantly. Pulmonary artery pressure decreased 12% on average, and pulmonary vascular resistance decreased 19%. These hemodynamic changes all occurred without a significant change in mean aortic pressure.

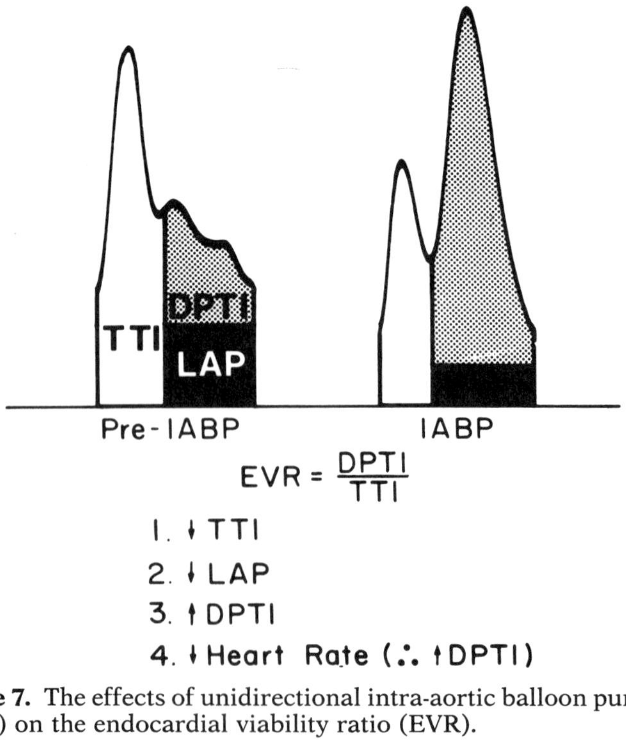

Figure 7. The effects of unidirectional intra-aortic balloon pumping (IABP) on the endocardial viability ratio (EVR).

Preoperative Intra-Aortic Balloon Pumping in High-Risk Cardiac Patients

The risks of early infarction and death in patients with acute coronary insufficiency undergoing cardiac surgery are generally considered greater than in patients with stable angina pectoris. The most appropriate therapy, however, and the timing of that therapy, are points of controversy. Cooper et al.[126] reported on 63 high-risk myocardial revascularization patients who had preoperative intra-aortic balloon pumping. Only six patients required rapid institution of cardiopulmonary bypass after anesthetic induction despite a marked drop in blood pressure in 50% of the patients. There were two instances of postpump power failure, with two deaths in this series. The author concluded from this experience that preoperative intra-aortic balloon pumping is a valid method of limiting morbidity associated with coronary surgery in high-risk patients. Scully et al.[127] have recently studied the effects of preoperative intra-aortic balloon pumping in 42 patients with acute coronary insufficiency complicated by abnormal left ventricular hemodynamics and refractory chest pain. Aggressive medical therapy had previously failed in all cases.

The perioperative mortality rate, when compared to that of similar patients treated before and after the use of the intra-aortic balloon pump, was lowered from 25% to 8%. Similar results have been achieved by Weintraub et al. Langon et al., and McEnany et al.[65-67] In addition, inotropic support and duration of stay, both in the intensive care unit and in the hospital, were significantly decreased in the patients treated preoperatively with the intra-aortic balloon pump. Bolooki et al.[68] also reported a shorter time on cardiopulmonary bypass, and Feola et al.[69] have noted an improvement in metabolic status as measured by decreased cardiac lactate production.

Others[70-72] have applied the intra-aortic balloon pump preoperatively in cases of decreased left ventricular function, but the interpretation of the data is not as clear-cut as in the case of acute coronary insufficiency.

Use in Noncardiac Surgery

An indication that ultimately may prove to be very practical is the prophylactic use of intra-aortic balloon counterpulsation in major noncardiac surgery. Perloth and Haltgren[73] reported a 6% to 7% risk of perioperative myocardial infarction in patients with prior myocardial infarction. That number may be as high as 37%

in patients undergoing major noncardiac surgery within 3 months of a previous infarction with an associated mortality of 54%.[74] Grotz and Yeston[75] recently presented three case reports supporting the thinking that prophylactic intra-aortic balloon pumping in high-risk patients may improve myocardial perfusion and overall hemodynamics, thereby reducing the risk of perioperative myocardial infarction and mortality.

Tachyarrhythmia and Ventricular Irritability

The increase in coronary blood flow associated with the use of the intra-aortic balloon pump as well as the decrease in myocardial wall tension as a result of the acute reduction in left ventricular afterload is ideally suited for the treatment of refractory ventricular tachyarrhythmia, both in the setting of the coronary care unit and in the postoperative surgical patient.[76] Unfortunately, while the treatment of tachyarrhythmia after open heart surgery with the intra-aortic balloon pump can frequently be definitive,[77] it is underutilized in this setting. Likewise, in the coronary care unit, many patients with ventricular irritability can be stabilized, and the frequency of their arrhythmias decreased significantly. It is the policy of these authors to catheterize every medical patient on an intra-aortic balloon pump whose indication for insertion has been ventricular tachyarrhythmia so that the patient's anatomy can be defined; and surgical intervention can proceed if indicated.

Mundth et al.[78,79] have indicated that in the medical setting life-threatening, recurrent ventricular tachyarrhythmia in the acute postinfarction phase and in chronic coronary disease can be controlled initially with intra-aortic balloon pumping as a prelude to cardiac catheterization and cardiac surgery. Ten patients with recurrent ventricular tachyarrhythmia underwent cardiac surgery, and seven of those patients survived.

Williams et al.[80] have reported success with intra-aortic balloon pumping therapy even when no surgically correctable lesion is present, and recommend the use of the intra-aortic balloon pump for all patients who develop ventricular arrhythmias and low nodal bradyarrhythmia that are refractory to standard medical therapy.

Controversial indications include "prophylactic" support for high-risk patients undergoing cardiac catheterization, or percutaneous coronary angioplasty (PTCA), cardiac, or major noncardiac surgery, septic shock, and limitation of infarct size in patients without cardiogenic shock.

Weaning Feature

After the patient has become hemodynamically stable during balloon pumping, it may be desirable to wean him from the assist device. This can be easily accomplished with the System 82, 90 and 90T, because not only can the balloon volume be gradually decreased, but the assist can also operate in the 1:1, 1:2, and 1:3 modes so that the patient is assisted with every beat, every other beat and every third beat respectively (Fig. 8). Hence, by a combination of these features, the balloon volume and assist frequency can be gradually and synchronously[81] decreased until assist has been discontinued.

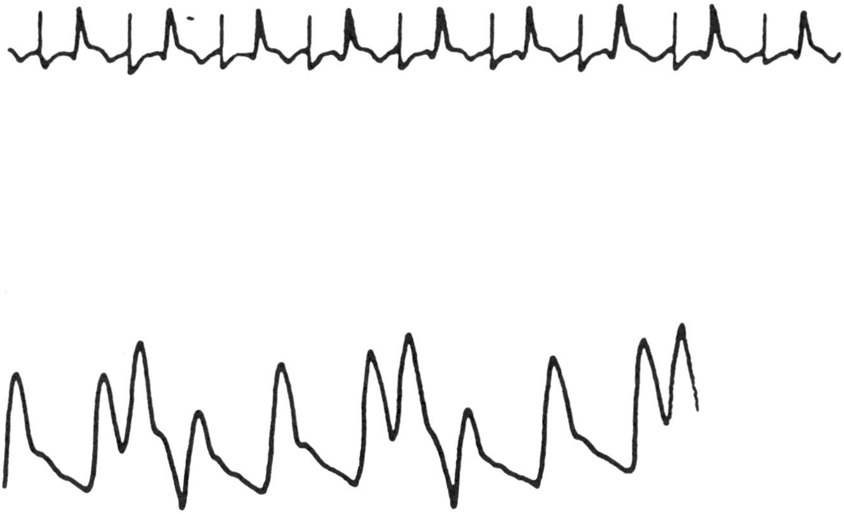

Figure 8. Shown here is balloon assistance on every third cycle.

Complications Associated with Intra-Aortic Balloons

The nature of intra-aortic balloon insertion and function, as well as the critical status of those patients requiring its use, presents potential for major complications. Alcan et al.[82] collected data on 321 patients from 1974–1982 requiring intra-aortic balloon counterpulsation for a variety of reasons, under both emergent and controlled situations. They reported major complications in 9% of patients who had undergone intra-aortic balloon counterpulsation. Complications ranged from thrombosis and embolization for greater than half of these, to aortic dissection in one case. If the contingency exists, however, it is felt that risk factors include severity of peripheral vascular disease, extent of myocardial failure, significant long-standing hypertension, female, and duration of use.

The principle complications associated with intra-aortic balloon pumping fall into three main categories:

1. Trauma to the arterial wall incurred while inserting and advancing the guidewire or balloon.
2. Limb ischemia associated with the position of the balloon catheter, which disappears with catheter removal.
3. Dislodged thrombus created during balloon removal resulting in distal embolization.

Isner and associates[48] found that 60% of the complications of the intra-aortic balloon appear to result from trauma associated with insertion of the catheter. These included aortoiliac dissection, arterial perforation, and dislodged atherosclerotic plaque. In addition, it was noted that the older the patient, the more likely that atherosclerotic disease will diminish the arterial lumen diameter, resulting in a greater potential for insertion damage. Along with these more common types of complications, several notable ones have appeared including, a patient with an improperly positioned intra-aortic balloon which intermittently occluded the origin of the superior mesentric artery. The resulting abdominal pain was relieved upon advancing the balloon to its correct position.[83] A splenic infarction precipitated by intra-aortic balloon placement was reported by Busch.[84]

Removal of the Percutaneous Intra-Aortic Balloon Pump

The principal problem associated with removal of the percutaneous balloon catheter is release of thrombi as the sheath-catheter assembly is withdrawn. These thrombi form around the catheter at the insertion site where blood flow is reduced.[85] Complications associated with distal embolization have been well documented.[86-88] The initial experience with the use of the percutaneous intra-aortic balloon at the Columbia University-Presbyterian Medical Center has resulted in a protocol that greatly reduces the likelihood of distal embolization.[89]

Before removal of the balloon catheter, completely collapse the balloon by aspiration with a 50-mL syringe and a stopcock. Pull the balloon down to (but not into) the sheath. Compress the femoral artery distal to the insertion site and remove the balloon and sheath as a single unit. Blood is allowed to spurt from the artery for a few seconds so that any thrombus material is removed. Now, shift compression of the femoral artery over the puncture site for 30 minutes. Distal pulses are monitored with Doppler apparatus, and manual compression is adjusted so that an audible pulse is registered. A compression dressing is applied to the puncture site for a 24-hour period.

Rodigas and Finnegan[90] reported good results with a variation of this procedure; after flushing out any proximal thrombi from the artery, the pressure applied to the insertion site was reversed to allow backbleeding and the removal of any distal thrombi.

Investigators in the TAMI trials similarly applied pressure above the insertion site while subsequently "milking" the thigh to extrude distal clots. Again, the safety record was not adversely affected by the use of thrombolysis.[91]

Long-Term Survival of Intra-Aortic Balloon Pump Patients

The ability of the intra-aortic balloon pump to support and stabilize hemodynamically the failing circulation is well established. However, does the short-term stabilization by the intra-aortic balloon pump result in long-term survival for any group of patients? Several investigators have addressed this question.

The first study on the long-term effect of balloon pumping was initiated by Bolooki et al.[46] Of 43 patients who required intra-aortic balloon pump support to be weaned off the cardiopulmonary bypass circuit, they reported that 23 (53%) patients were discharged from the hospital and were living four months longer. Golding and associates[92] studied 197 patients who underwent intra-aortic balloon pump either pre-, peri-, or postoperatively. Of these 197 patients, 143 (72.6%) were discharged from the hospital. The 2-year survival was 96%. Golding's group also reported that the survival statistics for patients who require intra-aortic balloon pump in conjunction with myocardial revascularization were similar to the patients who did not require the intra-aortic balloon pump assistance. Saneflippo et al.[9] reported their experiences with 283 patients discharged from the hospital after cardiac and balloon support. Of these 283 patients, 181 (64%) survived 3 or more years.

Kucher et al.[94] inserted intra-aortic balloon pump in 225 patients for left ventricle failure refractory to medical therapy following myocardial infarction and cardiac surgery. Ninety-seven (43%) were discharged from the hospital. Patients were followed an average of 5.8 years.

Long-Term Support by Intra-Aortic Balloon Pump

Several instances have been reported where patients have remained on the balloon pump for an extended period.[95] Except for the patient's discomfort associated with a lengthy immobolization of the limb with the catheter, no toxicity has been associated with long-term balloon pumping. Brantigan et al.[96] reported on a woman with peripartum cardiomyopathy who was balloon-dependent for 7 weeks and improved during this period; she subsequently expired 3 weeks after the balloon's removal.

The majority of patients on long-term balloon support cannot be weaned off and are in fact balloon-dependent. Most often, these are patients with end-stage coronary artery disease and cardiomyopathy, although several instances of septicemia have been reported.[94]

Thrombolysis and Intra-Aortic Balloon Pumping

The use of the intra-aortic balloon pump in conjunction with thrombolytic therapy has proved to be not only effective but safe.

In the nearly 15% of TAMI study patients who required the balloon in helping to restore hemodynamic stability, only minor bleeding problems occurred. (Although more blood transfusions were required in intra-aortic balloon pump patients, the majority of these patients had by-pass surgery during their hospitalization necessitating increase transfusion requirement.[97-100]

In the TAMI trials, patients who were hypotensive 20 minutes after the start of a thrombolytic agent were randomized to intra-aortic balloon pump theraphy, often in the emergency room. The patients who failed to respond adequately to thrombolysis were frequently in the greatest need of the balloon pump.[97-100]

Appropriate intra-aortic balloon pump technique in the treatment of this large study population clearly played an important role in the results achieved.

Use of the "single wall needle", rather than the classical Seldinger approach, puncturing only the anterior arterial wall of the common femoral artery followed by careful insertion of the guidewire and sheath has resulted in far fewer bleeding complications.[100]

Several recent reports address these variables while comparing the surgical and percutaneous approaches to balloon pumping. The data suggest an overall increase risk of vascular complications with the percutaneous approach.[101-103] However, the increased risks have been diminishing with the newest generations of balloons, consequently most balloons are now inserted percutaneously.

Intra-Aortic Balloon Pump in the Pediatric Population

Not long after the introduction of the intra-aortic balloon in clinical use, Pollock et al.,[104] in 1979, reported on the use of the intra-aortic balloon pump in a series of infants and children undergoing open heart surgery. The patients ranged in age from 1½ years to 18 years. There were six long-term survivors; however, all the patients under 5 years of age died. Insertion was via the common femoral artery using a side arm Dacron^{R} graft. Eight-millimeter and 10 mm adult balloons were inserted through the graft up into the thoracic aorta. It was noted that effective augmentation was difficult to achieve. This was felt to be related to the relatively compliant aortic walls in children. Although no bleeding or thrombocytopenia was seen, there were several serious complications noted, including superior mesenteric artery occlusion, renal artery occlusion, and severe limb ischemia. The use of the adult size balloons allowed a large segment of the pumping chamber to lie below the level of the diaphragm, thereby accounting for most of the ischemic related complications.

In an effort to overcome these problems, Veasy[105] has sought to adapt the intra-aortic balloon pump for use in the pediatric population. The major obstacles, however, are balloon and catheter size. Unlike adults, there is much concern over varying aortic diameters and length, as well as femoral artery length. Veasy developed balloons ranging from 0.75 mL to 5 mL attached to 4F. and 5F catheters. These were then tested in vitro in animal models using the Utah heart driver and three other pumping systems. All the balloons were introduced percutaneously. In small animals with reduced cardiac output from acutely produced mitral regurgitation, the newly developed intra-aortic balloon effectely reduced aortic peak systolic pressure (afterload), lowered aortic end diastolic pressure and reduced left atrial pressure. In addition, the Datascope 80 system most effectively augmented diastolic pressure and increased aortic forward and negative flow as compared with the AVCO^R and UHS^R systems.

A balloon catheter should be selected with a volume equal to at least 50% of the stroke volume.

The following formula has been suggested with a larger size balloon being used should the calculation fall between available sizes:[106]

$$\frac{2000 \times (\text{cardiac index}) \times (\text{body surface area})}{\text{Heart Rate}} \times 0.5 = \text{Balloon Volume}$$

One concern with the use of intra-aortic balloon pumping in pediatric patients is poor augmentation. This is due to several reasons: (1) the pediatric aortic wall displays increased elasticity and compliance compared with the adult aorta. Since the balloon inflates against a relatively distensible lumen, the degree of augmentation seen in children may not match that of adults; (2) the increased heart rates seen in the pediatric population at any given level of cardiac output can present a timing challenge, even to the experienced operator. Therefore, it has been recommended (Dunn 1988; unpublished data) that larger balloons than expected be used to overcome the distensibility problem, and that at heart rates greater than 160, 1:2 intra-aortic balloon assistance may afford better diastolic augmentation than at every beat assistance. Other difficulties include designing catheters capable of permitting rapid exchange of gas to match the faster heart rates of infants and children.

Through 1985, the clinical experience of Veasy et al. included patients from age 5 to 12 years, with weight ranging from 3.2 kg to 33.2 kg. Of their first 18 patient, 9 survived over the short-term, tolerating weaning from the intra-aortic balloon pump; and of these, 5 left the hospital and were surviving 6 months after discharge. The inherent complications were few. Only one patient required discontinuation because of lower limb ischemic injury.

Del Nido[107] in 1988, reported the successful circulatory support of a low-cardiac output state in a 2 kg, 3-week old infant.

As with adults, diligent monitoring of balloon position, respiratory support, inotropic support, renal function, infection control, anticoagulation, and more specifically for this population, of abdominal girths and gastrointestinal function is paramount.

Contraindications to Intra-Aortic Balloon Pump

There is an ever-expanding list of uses for the intra-aortic balloon pump. However, there remain only two absolute contraindications to its implementation. These include gross aortic insufficiency and acute aortic dissection. Minor aortic insufficiency should not be a deterrent.[108] The presence of an aortic aneurysm or the history of prior aortic surgery are only relative contraindications, their significance to be judged in light of the entire clinical picture.

The use of the intra-aortic balloon pump with cardiac standstill, especially in the setting of open heart surgery, remains controversial,[109] however, never impairs survival when continued with closed chest cardiopulmonary resuscitation.

Conclusion

Since the intra-aortic balloon pump was first introduced in the early 1960s, there has been a dramatic increase in its use. Currently more than a million have been inserted worldwide. Since the transition to the percutaneous method of insertion, it is now relatively easy to initiate intra-aortic balloon pumping in patients who require its use. No longer is the only indication cardiogenic shock. Recently, its applications have been substantially broadened; the intra-aortic balloon pump is used not only as an aid to the failing heart and as a last resort antiarrhythmic device but during thrombolytic therapy, and as an adjunct to percutaneous transluminal angioplasty in patients with marginal hemodynamics to salvage ischemic myocardium. The intra-aortic balloon pump is now used easily during transportation of patients, and in smaller community hospitals with relative safety. The intra-aortic balloon has been adapted efficiently for use in infants and small children. Further advances in hardware and software will no doubt continue to maintain the intra-aortic balloon pump as the most widely used temporary circulatory assist device.

Ventricular Assist Devices

The clinical use of ventricular assist devices (VAD) in the treatment of low-cardiac output syndrome is an outgrowth of early experience showing that optimal cardiac performance could be gradually improved by prolonging partial or complete cardiopulmonary bypass. A variety of assist devices have been used both experimentally and clinically. Unlike the intra-aortic balloon pump, which augments existing circulation, VAD (specifically, the left ventricular assist device) pump large flows of blood independently of inherent cardiac activity and intact ECG signals (Fig. 9).

The first successful attempts at circulatory assistance with VAD were published by Spencer et al. in 1965[110] and Debakey in 1971.[111] With the growth of cardiac transplantation over the ensuing years accompanied by a shortage of donor organs, there has been an increasing use of assist and replacement devices in bridging patients to transplantation.[112] Much work on the design of ventricular assist devices has been done by several investigators and biomedical researchers. Currently, there are several different devices in use at various centers.

There are two main goals of ventricular assistance. The first is the reestablishment of satisfactory levels of blood flow so that

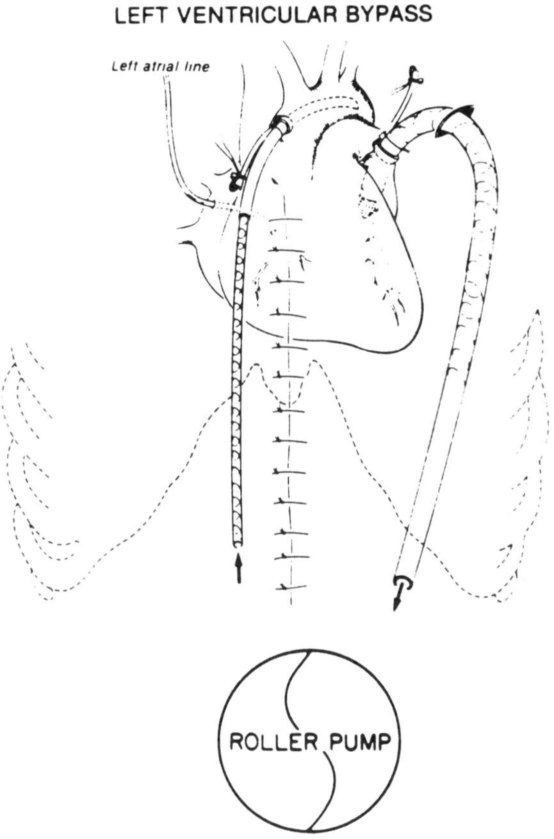

Figure 9. Left ventricular bypass. Blood is extracted from the left atrium and reinfused into the aorta by a roller pump.

adequate perfusion of all organ systems is maintained at a time when the myocardium can not deliver a sufficient level of cardiac output. The second main goal is the reduction in work of the myocardium, thereby decreasing myocardial oxygen demand ($M\dot{V}O_2$). The ideal left ventricular assist device (LVAD) will maximally reduce myocardial oxygen demand, decrease afterload of the left ventricle by means of sequenced counterpulsation, and deliver blood to the aorta or one of its branches during diastole. It should be easily placed, and not require sternal reentry for cannula removal upon termation of its use.

There have been many critical appraisals over the last several years concerning the type of pump employed. Pump roller, centrifugal, pneumatic, and electrical pumps are all in use today. There are no conclusive studies regarding the superiority of one type over another. Regardless of the specific system used, it has been found that survival is improved when left heart cannulation is performed via the left atrium rather than through the left ventricle directly (Fig. 10).[123] This has been shown with the evidence to date even though there is a theoretical advantage to directly cannulating the left ventricle. One would expect that direct cannulation of the left ventricle would provide optimum unloading. However, the added mortality of traumatizing the left ventricle via direct cannulation outweighs any added benefit. Two important points should be noted, however. While most of the available data supports cannulation of the left atrium, the newest electromechanical pump is available for direct left ventricular cannulation only. So far, the results have been good. Also, while we have limited our discussion to left heart assist, the majority of devices available today can be used for right heart assist of biventricular assist as well. Clearly, more work with use of these devices is needed.

The majority of patients can be managed with conventional therapy consisting of adequate volume loading, inotropic support, and the intra-aortic balloon pump. However, a small percentage of patients will fail to respond adequately to the above measures. Hemodynamic criteria indicating the consideration of a left ventricular assist device is a cardiac index of less than 1.7 $L/min/m^2$, a systolic aortic pressure of less than 90 mm Hg, a left atrial pressure of greater than 25 mm Hg, or other evidence of continued end organ hypoperfusion, after conventional therapy as outlined above has failed.

The basic design of most of the available ventricular systems uses a pneumatic sac-type device with segmented polyurethane that is flexible and seam-free. The sac is encased in a polycarbonate housing. The most notable of these is the Pierce-Donachy ventricular assist device. The Pierce-Donachy device utilizes Bjork-Shiley valves at both the inlet and outlet ports. The device has a stroke volume of 65 mL with a dynamic ejection fraction of 75%, and allows direct cannulation of the left ventricle, the left or right atrium, the aorta, or pulmonary artery.[124-128]

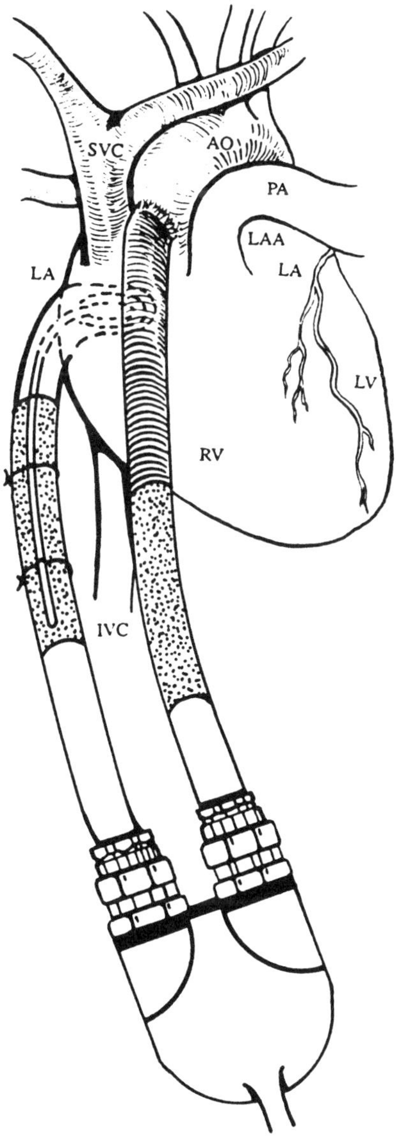

Figure 10. Completed cannulation for left ventricular support using the interarterial groove location for inflow cannulation. SVC = superior vena cava; LAA = left atrial appendage; IVC = inferior vena cava; AO = aorta; PA = pulmonary artery.

The pneumatic power control unit is generally capable of functioning in three different modes: a manual set rate mode; a synchronized mode that detects the R-wave of the electrocardiogram; or a fill-to-empty mode that operates by activating a Hall effect switch when the sac is full, thus initiating the emptying cycle. When the VAD is operating in the fill-to-empty mode, the rate times the stroke volume (65 mL) equals the VAD flow. In general, heparinization is not necessary with this device until the weaning process is begun and the flow rates through the VAD are thereby sufficiently low to allow clotting within the device, however, antiplated therapy with low-molecular weight dextran is used throughout the period of ventricular assistance. An infusion of 10% low-molecular weight dextran is begun postoperatively when chest tube drainage is less than 50 mL/hr and adequate platelet numbers (> 50,000 mm^3) are demonstrated. This continuous infusion is maintained throughout the period to assist pumping and discontinued approximately 6 hours prior to removal of the device. Other devices incorporate variations on the Pierce-Donachy system. Extracorporeal roller-pumps are available. These utilize specifically designed, silicone-elastomer cannulas with double polyester skirts that allow bypass flows of up to 5 L/min.[129-131] This design allows easy removal of the devices. When left ventricular support is terminated, the distal cannula tips are exposed and a snug-fitting, silicone elastomer obturator is inserted into each cannula to obliterate its lumen. The advantage of this method is that it doesn't require reentry of the thorax for discontinuation, therefore, decreasing the incidence of sternal infections.

An intracorporeal abdominal left VAD is still in the initial stages of clinical use. However, of 22 reported clinical trials, only 3 cases demonstrated sufficient ventricular recovery to allow weaning and removal of the device.[132]

Implanted Electromechanical Pump

All of the currently available artificial left ventricular assist devices are inherently unsuitable for permanent circulatory support. The Novacor^{R} (Novacor Medical Corp., Oakland, CA, USA) device is totally implantable left ventricular assist system designed for long-term circulatory support. Unlike the pneumatically driven systems, the Novacor device is an electromechanical pump. It is an advanced stage of development, and currently in use at several centers around the country. The electromechanical pump system makes the Novacor system unique to date.

The Novacor system is comprised of two major components: an implanted pump/drive unit, and an external console (Fig. 11). The pump/drive unit is positioned in the anterior abdominal wall of the left upper quadrant, posterior to the rectus abdomini muscle. It is connected to the console by power and control leads contained within a percutaneous vent tube. Traversing the diaphragm, externally reinforced low-porosity Dacron inflow and outflow conduits connect the pump between the left ventricular apex and the ascending aorta. The Novacor left VAD is designed for implantation to the left ventricular apex only. It cannot be used with left atrial cannulation or right ventricular assistance.

The pump geometry is designed for optimal flow patterns without areas of stasis, flow separation, or turbulence. Symmetrical

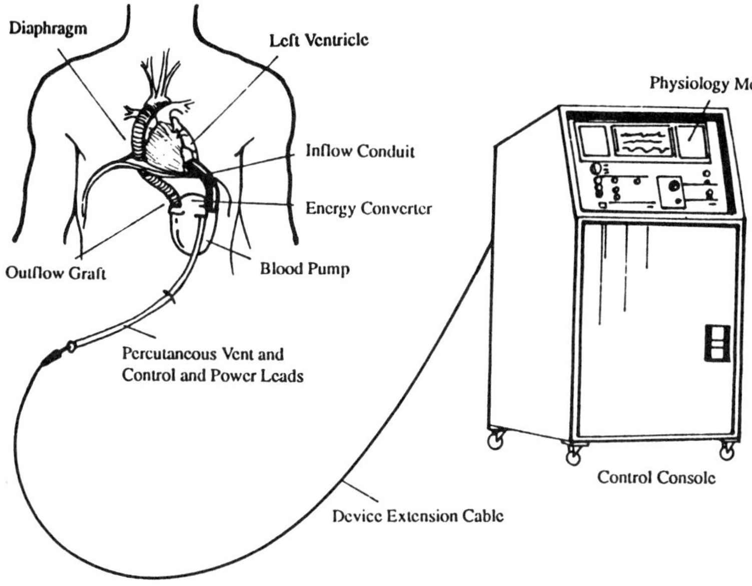

Figure 11. Configuration of Novacor left ventricular assist device illustrating implanted pump/drive and external control console.

sac deformation maintains optimal flow throughout the pumping cycle. Normal operation is synchronous counterpulsation based on interval sensors responsive to pump filling. Electrocardiogram-triggered synchronous and fixed rate operation are also available. The Novacor LVAD has a nominal maximum stroke volume of 70 mL and can pump in excess of 10 L/min. It is extremely responsive and can operate synchronously at cardiac rates as high as 240 beats/min.

In one series of 20 patients undergoing left ventricular assistance with the Novacor device, patients with terminal refractory heart failure were stabilized hemodynamically with marked improvement in end-organ perfusion.[118]

In half, severe multiorgan dysfunction resolved, and orthotopic cardiac transplantation was achieved after 2–90 days of synchronous circulatory support. Hematological variables were within normal limits over extended periods of time, with normal platelet function and no clinically significant hemolysis over extended periods.

Weaning

In general, ventricular assist pumping is discontinued for short periods (30–60 seconds) every 24 hours to assess the patient's ventricular function. Initially, atrial pressures are allowed to transiently rise to 30 mm HG. However, weaning is not begun until the patient's ventricular function has recovered sufficiently to maintain systolic pressures greater than 100 mm Hg in the presence of filling pressures below 20 mm Hg. A cardiac output determination is made with the VAD off. Weaning is initiated when the unassisted cardiac output index exceeds 2.0 L/min/m^2. Patients should require little or no inotropic support at all during this time. Weaning of the VAD down to a rate of 30 beats/min is the ultimate goal prior to removal of the VAD. Lower rates are generally not used because of the problem of stasis and thrombus formation within the device. The patient should be fully anticoagulated with intravenous heparin prior to the start of the weaning process as previously described. The patient is generally taken to the operating room for pump removal.

Results

The use of these devices over the last decade has allowed preliminary observations regarding the efficacy of ventricular assistance. Short-term survival of patients who require ventricular assist pumping for postcardiotomy cardiogenic shock has been encouraging. In one study of an initial group of 25 patients who required ventricular assist pumping,[127] 18 of them (72%) required the left ventricular assist pump, 10 of 18 (55.6%) were weaned, and 7 (39%) of this group survived. One third of these patients had right ventricular failure which was responsive to drug therapy. A right ventricular assist pump and an intra-aortic balloon pump were used in 3 patients; all were weaned and two survived (66.7%). Biventricular assist pumping was used in 4 patients, none of whom were weaned from support. In the 9 long-term survivors, peak device flows ranged from 2.7 to 4.0 L/min (mean = 3.3 L/min) and the total ventricular assist perfusion times ranged from 72 to 288 hours (mean = 158 hours). Other studies by different investigators have also yielded encouraging results.[117,126,129,131,133]

Complications of Left Ventricular Assist Devices

Infection remains a major cause of morbidity and mortality in patients who have undergone implantation of the ventricular assist device. Other complications include respiratory failure, postoperative bleeding requiring reexploration of the thorax, renal failure, and neurological impairment. Some are endogenous to the setting of the intensive care unit; others are related specifically to the use of the device itself.

Complications related solely to the device itself include hemolysis and thrombosis, with resultant thromboembolic phenomenon. Pathological studies have revealed pulmonary embolism in several patients who required the VAD but did not survive.[127] In one postmortem study of patients who had undergone implantation of the VAD, it was found that death was mostly due to extensive myocardial necrosis, followed by hemorrhage, cerebrovascular accident, infection, and other causes.[134] Also, in this particular study, it was noted that no pump-related thromboemboli, foreign material emboli, or other significant pump-related injury was detected in any patient. It would appear inuitively, that a strong predictor of survival then is myocardial function.

Two very strongly negative predictors of survival have been found to be: perioperative myocardial infarction[134] and renal failure.[135] In one recent series that reported the effect of perioperative myocardial infarction on survival of patients who had undergone implantation of the VAD, only 1 of 11 survivors had sustained a perioperative myocardial infarction, whereas, 11 of the 19 nonsurvivors had acute myocardial injuries severe enough to preclude survival.[126] Other investigators have reported on the negatively predictive value of both perioperative myocardial infarction, and the development of renal failure while undergoing support with the VAD.

Total Artificial Heart

Replacement of the heart in an animal with a mechanical prosthesis was first reported by Akutsu and Kolff in 1958.[136] Denton Cooley, in 1969, implanted a pneumatically driven right and left ventricle in a 47-year-old man who had a ventricular aneurysm resected, but could not be weaned from cardiopulmonary bypass.[122] This was the first artificial heart implantation in a human being, Between 1969 and 1987, there were 79 implants of orthotopic biventricular pneumatic pulsatile artificial hearts. Over the last decade, several orthotopic devices have been designed at various centers. The most notable of these devices is the JARVIK-7^{R} from the University of Utah. The majority of the devices in use at present are based on the same construction design as the ventricular assist device. The pneumatically driven JARVIK artificial heart consists of two separate ventricles with air chamber (Fig. 12). Air is intermittently pulsed in and out of the air chambers at adjustable rates, activating the diaphragm. The ventricles are fashioned so that the blood surface is attached to the housing in a continuous layer. The two ventricles have a total displacement of 680 mL, and each ventricle has a stroke volume of 100 mL. Four clinical grade pyrolytic carbon disc valves ensure unidirectional flow. Atrial cuffs

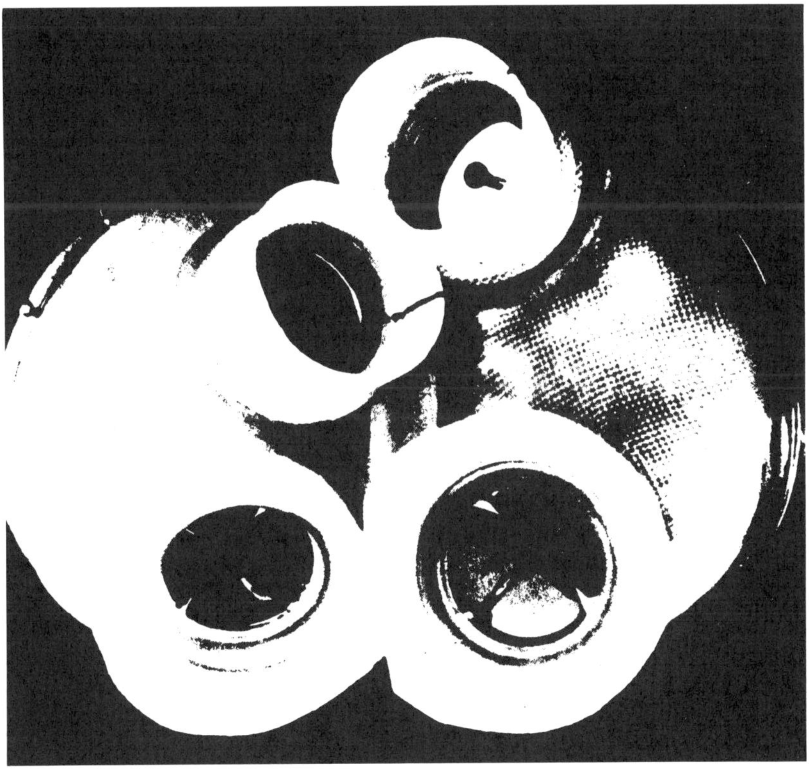

Figure 12. The Jarvik-7.

fabricated of Dacron felt provide the connections to the natural atria. Dacron vascular grafts provide the connection to the great vessels. Special drive lines link the artificial heart with its external power source. The maximal stroke volume of the JARVIK-7 is approximately 100 mL on each side, but varies with the inflow pressure, thereby simulating a physiologic response according to the Frank-Starling law. The device is exquisitely sensitive to preload and afterload. Inflow pressures of 5–7 mm Hg generate a cardiac output of 4–5 L/min, while inflow pressures of 10–15 mm Hg result in a cardiac output of 12–13 L/min without a change in heart rate.

In 1982, the JARVIK-7 total artificial heart was approved for a limited clinical trial. A 61-year-old dentist, who had been experiencing progressive congestive heart failure for several years, had become unresponsive to intensive medical therapy. He was referred to the University of Utah for implantation of the total artificial heart. Because of the age of the patient, and his pulmonary hypertension, the patient was not considered a candidate for the heart transplantation program in the United States. He underwent several operations and lived a total of 112 days. He ultimately experienced severe complications and death.

Most of the patients who have since undergone implantation of the total artificial heart are now dead. Some have been confined to the hospital after suffering strokes and other complications. These include internal bleeding, respiratory failure, malnutrition, suppression of the immune system, and recurrent infections.

Criteria for patient selection at the present time includes three groups of patients. The first group includes those patients who cannot be weaned from cardiopulmonary bypass following cardiac surgery. The artificial heart can be implanted in these patients after other supportive measures, including the intra-aortic balloon pump, fail to restore cardiac function to a level sufficient to sustain life. The second group of patients are those with terminal cardiomyopathy who are not candidates for heart transplantation. Most importantly though, are the third group of patients, i.e., those that are a candidate for cardiac transplantation, but for whom there is no donor heart available immediately. Perhaps this will be the only viable use in the next several decades. However, this raises the ethical questions concerning the placement of these devices in patients when in reality, there may be no possibility of obtaining a suitable donor heart.

Summary

The ventricular assist device is able to support patients at times when the myocardium can no longer supply sufficient output to sustain organ perfusion. The total artificial heart has the ability to continue this support for much longer periods of time. Unfortunately, our technological advances can take us only so far. There remains a need for much continued research and development of new treatment forms and mechanical intervention. More importantly, is the need to educate the public in the prevention of heart disease, thereby obviating the need for such intervention. Equally important are the ethical questions raised in the use of new forms of life support including both the ventricular assist device and the total artificial heart.

REFERENCES

1. Moulopoulos SD, Topaz SD, Kolff WJ. Diastolic balloon pumping (with carbon dioxide) in the aorta—a mechanical assistance to the failing heart. *Am Heart J.* 63:669, 1962.
2. Harlem DE. Presentation of the International College of Cardiology Meeting, Brussels, Belgium 1958.
3. Kantrowitz A, Kantrowitz A. Experimental augmentation of coronary flow by retardation of arterial pressure pulse. *Surgery* 34:678, 1953.
4. Kantrowitz A, McKinnon WMP. The experimental use of the diaphragm as an auxilliary myocardium. *Surg Forum* 9:226, 1958.
5. Corday E, Swan JC, Lang TW, et al. Physiologic principles in the application of circulatory assist for the failing heart. *Am J Cardiol* 26:595, 1970.
6. Kantrowitz A, Tjonneland S, Freed, PS, et al. Initial clinical experience with intra-aortic balloon pumping in cardiogenic shock. *J Am Med Assoc* 203:113, 1968.
7. Bregman D, Bailin M, Bowman FO Jr. A pulsatile assist device (PAD) for improved myocardial protection during cardiopulmonary bypass. *Ann Thorac Surg* 24:574, ,1977.
8. Nachlas HM, Sieband MP. The influence of diastolic augmentation on infarct size following coronary artery ligation. *J Thorac Cardiovasc Surg* 53:698, 1967.
9. Feola M, Limet RR, Glick G. Direct and reflex vascular effects of intra-aortic balloon counterpulsation in dogs at four levels of aortic pressure (abstract). *Clin Res* 19:313, 1971.
10. Weber KT, Janicki JS. Intra-aortic balloon counterpulsation: a review of physiological principles, clinical results and device safety. *Ann Thorac Surg* 17:601, 1974.
11. Johnson SA, Scanlon PJ, Loeb HS, et al. Treatment of cardiogenic shock in myocardial infarction by intra-aortic balloon counterpulsation and surgery. *Am J Med* 62:687, 1977.
12. Gold HK, Leinbach RC, Buckley MD, et al. Refractory angina pectoris: follow-up after intra-aortic balloon pumping and surgery. Circulation 54(Suppl III):41, 1976.
13. Maroko PN, Bernstein EF, Lippy P, et al. Effects of intra-aortic balloon counterpulsation on the severity of myocardial ischemic injury following acute coronary occlusion. *Circulation* 45:1150, 1972.

14. Berger RL, Saini VK, Long W, et al. The use of diastolic augmentation with the intra-aortic balloon pump in human septic shock with associated coronary artery disease. *Surgery* 74:601, 1973.
15. Talpins NL, Kripke DC, Goetz RH. Counterpulsation and intra-aortic balloon pumping in cardiogenic shock. Circulatory dynamics. *Arch Surg* 97:991, 1968.
16. Jacobey JA, Craddock LD, Wolf PS, et al. Clinical experience with counterpulsation in coronary artery disease. *J Thorac Cardiovasc Surg* 56:846, 1968.
17. Cox JL, McLaughlin VW, Flowers NC, et al. The ischemic zone surrounding acute myocardial infarction. Its morphology as detected by dehydrogenase staining. *Am Heart J* 76:650, 1968.
18. Maroko PR, Berstein EF, Libby P, et al. Effects of intra-aortic balloon counterpulsation on the severity of myocardial ischemic injury following acute coronary occlusion. *Circulation* 45:1150, 1972.
19. Nachlas MM, Sieband MP. The influence of diastolic augmentation on infarct size following coronary artery ligation. *J Thorac Cardiovasc Surg* 53:698, 1968.
20. Sugg WL, Webb WR, Ecker RR. Reduction of extent of myocardial infarction by counterpulsation. *Ann Thorac Surg* 7:311, 1969.
21. Clayman RV, DeLaria GA, Johansen KH. The hypertensive balloon: a beneficial synergism for salvage of ischemic myocardium. *Surg Forum* 24:152, 1973.
22. Kralios AC, Zwart HHJ, Yenching W, et al. Coronary flow supplementation in experimental myocardial infarction with shock. *Chest* 61:365, 1972.
23. Kuhn LA. Shock in myocardial infarction-medical treatment. *Am J Cardiol* 26:578, 1970.
24. Kuhn LA, Unger AH, Novick SA, et al. Hemodynamics and cardiac metabolic effects of diastolic intra-aortic balloon obstruction combined with distal aortic "booster" occlusion in experimental acute myocardial infarction. *Am J Cardiol* 25:111, 1970.
25. Reemtsma K, Parodi EN, Bregman D, et al. Clinical intraoperative coronary artery saphenous vein bypass graft pressure-flow relationship. In: Norman JC, ed. *Coronary Artery Medicine and Surgery: Concepts and Controversies*. New York, NY: Appleton-Centruy-Crofts; 1974:30.
26. Brown BG, Gundel WD, Gott VL, et al. Hemodynamic determinants of retrograde arterial coronary flow following acute coronary occlusion (Abstract). *Circulation* 45:(Suppl II):100, 1972.
27. Gill CC, Weschler AS, Newman GE, et al. Augmentation and redistribution of myocardial blood flow during acute ischemia by intra-aortic balloon pumping. *Ann Thorac Surg* 16:445, 1973.
28. Watson JT, Willerson JT, Fixler DE, et al. Changes in collateral coronary blood flow (CCBF) distal to a coronary occlusion during intra-aortic balloon pumping (IABP). *Trans Am Soc Artif Intern Organs* 19:402, 1973.

29. Weber KT and Janicki JS. Coronary collateral flow and intra-aortic balloon counterpulsation. *Trans Am Soc Artif Intern Org* 19:402, 1973.
30. Weber KT, Janicki JS, Walker AA. An assessment of intra-aortic balloon pumping in hypovolemic and ischemic heart preparations. *J Thorac Cardiovasc Surg* 64:869, 1972.
31. Kantrowitz A, Tjonneland S, Freed PS, et al. Initial clinical experience with intra-aortic balloon pumping in cardiogenic shock. *J Am Med Assoc* 203:135, 1968.
32. Nachlas MM, Sieband MP. The influence of diastolic augmentation on infarct size following coronary artery ligation. *J Thorac Cardiovasc Surg* 53:698, 1980.
33. Feola M, Limet RR, Glick G. Direct and reflex vascular effects of intra-aortic balloon counterpulsation in dogs at four levels of aortic pressure. *Clin Res* 19:313, 1971.
34. Kantrowitz A, Phillips SJ, Butner AN, et al. Technique of femoral artery cannulation for phase shift balloon pumping. *J Thorac Cardiovasc Surg* 56:219, 1968.
35. Bregman D. Mechanical support of the failing heart. In: Ravitch MM, ed. *Current problems in surgery*. Chicago Year Book Medical Publishers; 1976(13):1-84.
36. Bregman D, Bokooki H, Malm JR. A simple method to facilitate difficult intra-aortic balloon insertions. *Ann Thorac Cardiovasc Surg* 15:636, 1973.
37. Lamberti JJ, Cohn LH, Collins JJ Jr. Iliac artery cannulation for intra-aortic balloon counterpulsation. *J Thorac Cardiovasc Surg* 67:976, 1977.
38. Mayer JH. Subclavian artery approach for insertion of intra-aortic balloon. *J Thorac Cardiovasc Surg* 76:61, 1978.
39. Rubin R, Nacht R, Sawyer PN, et al. Intra-aortic phase shift balloon utilizing the transaxillary approach. *J Thorac Cardiovasc Surg* 81:641, 1981.
40. Pappas G. Intrathoracic intra-aortic balloon insertion for pulsatile cardiopulmonary bypass. *Arch Surg* 109:842, 1974.
41. Gueldner TL, Lawrence GH. Intra-aortic balloon assist through cannulation of the ascending aorta. *Ann Thorac Surg* 19:88, 1975.
42. Shirley AL, Loughridge BP, Lain KC. Insertion of the intra-aortic balloon through the aortic arch. *Ann Thorac Surg* 21:560, 1976.
43. Bregman D. A new percutaneous intra-aortic balloon. *Trans Am Soc Artif Intern Organs* 26:8, 1980.
44. Bregman D. Intra-aortic balloon counterpulsation. In: *Circulatory Assistance and the Artificial Heart*. Pierce WS (ed). USSR Joint Symposium, Blilisi, USSR, Sept. 20–22, 1979. US Dept. of Health and Human Services, PHS, NIH, 1980:155-165.
45. Bregman D, Cohen SR. Mechanical techniques of circulatory support: a percutaneous intra-aortic balloon device. *Artif Organs* 7(1):38-48, 1983.
46. Bregman D, Nichols AB, Weiss MB, et al. Percutaneous intra-aortic balloon insertion. *Am J Cardiol* 46:261, 1980.

47. Vignola PA, Swaye PS, Gosselin AJ. Guidelines for effective and safe percutaneous intra-aortic balloon pump insertion and removal. *Am J Cardiol* 48:660, 1981.
48. Isner JM, Cohen SR, Virmani R, et al. Complications of the intra-aortic balloon counterpulsation device: clinical and morphologic observations in 45 necropsy patients. *Am J Cardiol* 45:260, 1980.
49. Bregman D, Casarella WJ. Percutaneous intra-aortic balloon pumping: initial clinical experience. *Ann Thorac Surg* 29:153, 1980.
50. Merav AD, Solomon N, Montefusco CM, et al. A new guidable double lumen percutaneous intra-aortic balloon. *Trans Am Soc Artif Intern Organs* 27:593, 1981.
51. Leinbach RC, Goldstein J, Gold HK, et al. Percutaneous wire-guided balloon pumping. *Am J Cardiol* 49:1707, 1982.
52. Bedderman C, McGee MG, Turner SA, et al. Intra-aortic balloon pumping in women: effect of balloon size on survival. *Thorac Cardiovasc Surg* 28:428, 1980.
53. Burnan SO. Intra-aortic balloon pumping for low cardiac output syndromes. *Surg Clin North Am* 55:101, 1975.
54. Bregman D, Kripke DC, Goetz RH. The effects of synchronous unidirectional intra-aortic balloon pumping on hemodynamics and coronary blood flow in cardiogenic shock. *Trans Am Soc Artif Intern Organs* 16:439, 1970.
55. Bregman D. Mechanical support of the failing heart. In: Ravitch MM, ed. *Current Problems in Surgery.* Chicago, IL: Year Book Medical Publishers; 1976:25-32.
56. Feola M, Wiener L, Walinski P, et al. Improved survival after coronary bypass surgery in patients with poor left ventricular function: role of intra-aortic balloon counterpulsation. *Am J Cardiol* 39:1021, 1977.
57. Spotnitz HM, Covel J, Ross J Jr, et al. Left ventricular mechanics and oxygen consumption during arterial counterpulsation. *Am J Physiol* 217:1352, 1969.
58. Summer DN, Kaplitt M, Morris J, et al. Intra-aortic balloon pumping. Hemodynamic and metabolic effects during cardiogenic shock in patients with triple coronary artery obstructive disease. *Arch Surg* 99:733, 1969.
59. American Heart Association. *Heart Facts.* New York, NY: American Heart Association, 1981.
60. Feola M, Limet RR, Glick G. Direct and reflex vascular effects of intra-aortic balloon counterpulsation in dogs at four levels of aortic pressure. *Clin Res* 19:313, 1971.
61. Norman NA, Kennedy JH. Arterial baroreceptor responses to intra-aortic balloon assistance. *J Surg Res* 11:396, 1971.
62. Johnson MD, Holub DA, Winston DS, et al. Retrospective analysis of 286 patients requiring circulatory support with the intra-aortic balloon pump. *Cardiovasc Dis* 4:428, 1977.

63. Cooper GN Jr, Singh AK, Vargas LL, et al. Preoperative intra-aortic balloon assist in high risk revascularization patients. *Am J Surg* 133:463, 1977.
64. Scully HE, Gunstensen J, Williams WG, et al. Surgical management of complicated acute coronary insufficiency. *Surgery* 80:437, 1976.
65. Langon RA, Geha AS, Hammond GL, et al. Surgical approach for patients with unstable angina pectoris: role of the response to initial medical therapy and intra-aortic balloon pumping in perioperative complications after aortocoronary bypass grafting. *Am J Cardiol* 42:629, 1978.
66. McEnany MT, Kay HR, Buckley, MJ, et al. Clinical experience with intra-aortic balloon pump support in 728 patients. *Circulation* 58(Suppl I):124, 1978.
67. Kuhn LA. Management of shock following acute myocardial infarction part II. Mechanical circulatory assistance. *Am Heart J* 95:789, 1978.
68. Bolooki H, Williams W, Thurer RJ, et al. Clinical and hemodynamic criteria for the use of the intra-aortic balloon pump in patients requiring cardiac surgery. *J Thorac Cardiovasc Surg* 72:756, 1976.
69. Feola M, Weiner L, Walinsky P, et al. Improved survival after coronary bypass surgery in patients with poor left ventricular function: role of intra-aortic balloon counterpulsation. *Am J Cardiol* 39:1021, 1977.
70. Lambert JJ, Resnekov L. Cardiac assist devices. *Ann Rev Med* 29:571, 1978.
71. Lefemine AA, Kosowsky B, Madoff I, et al. Results and complications of intra-aortic balloon pumping in surgical and medical patients. *Am J Cardiol* 40:416, 1977.
72. Sammel N, O'Rouke MF, Chang V. Arterial counterpulsation: review of the first 100 patients. *Med J Aust* 2:802, 1976.
73. Perloth MG, Huftgren HN. The cardiac patient and general surgery. *J Am Med Assoc* 232:1279, 1975.
74. Tarhan S, Moffitt EA, Taylor WF, et al. Myocardial infarction after general anesthesia. *J Am Med Assoc* 220:1451, 1972.
75. Grotz RL, Yeston NS. Intra-aortic balloon counterpulsation in high-risk cardiac patients undergoing non-cardiac surgery. *Surgery* 106:1, 1989.
76. Bregman D. Mechanical support of the failing heart. In: Ravitch MM, ed. *Current Problems in Surgery*. Chicago, IL: Year Book Medical Publishers; 1976:27.
77. Willerson JT, Curry GC, Watson JT, et al. Intra-aortic balloon counterpulsation in patients in cardiogenic shock, medically refractory left ventricular failure and/or recurrent ventricular tachycardias. *Am J Med* 58:183, 1975.
78. Mundth ED. Mechanical and surgical interventions for the reduction of myocardial ischemia. *Circulation* 53(Suppl.I):176, 1976.
79. Mundth ED, Buckley MJ, Daggett WM, et al. Intra-aortic balloon pump assistance and early surgery in cardiogenic shock. Integrated

medical-surgical care in acute coronary artery disease. *Adv Cardiol* 15:159, 1975.
80. Williams EH, Tyers GF, Carter SL, et al. Ventricular arrhythmias following mitral valve replacement: control with intra-aortic balloon counterpulsation. *Chest* 68:641, 1975.
81. Bernstein, EF, Murphy AE. The importance of pulsation in preventing thrombosis from intra-aortic balloons. A note of caution. *J Thorac Cardiovasc Surg* 62:906, 1973.
82. Alcan KE, Stertzer SH, Wallsh E, et al. Current status of intra-aortic balloon counterpulsation in critical care cardiology. *Crit Care Med* 12:489, 1984.
83. Karlson SB, Martin EC, Bregman D, et al. Superior mesenteric artery obstruction by intra-aortic balloon simulating embolism. *Cardiovasc Inter Radiol* 4:236-238, 1981.
84. Busch HM Jr, Cogbill TH, Gunderson AE. Splenic infarction: complication of intra-aortic balloon counterpulsation. *Am Heart J* 109:383-385, 1985.
85. Martin RS III, Moncure AC, Buckley MJ, et al. Complications of percutaneous intra-aortic balloon insertion. *J Thorac Cardiovasc Surg* 85:186, 1983.
86. Inverson LI, Herfindahl G, Ecker R, et al. Vascular complications of intra-aortic balloon counterpulsation. *Am J Surg* 154:99-103, 1978.
87. Rodigas PC, Bridges KG. Occlusion of the left internal mammary artery with intra-aortic balloon: clinical implications. *J Thorac Cardiovasc Surg* 91:142-143, 1986.
88. Busch HN Jr, Cogbill TH, Gunderson AE. Splenic infarction: complication of intra-aortic balloon counterpulsation. *Am Heart J* 109:383-385, 1985.
89. Bregman D. Percutaneous intra-aortic balloon pumping: a time for reflection. *Chest* 82:397, 1982.
90. Rodigas PC, Finnegan JO. Technique for removal of percutaneously placed intra-aortic balloons. *Ann Thorac Surg* 40:80, 1985.
91. George BS. Thrombolysis and intra-aortic balloon pumping following acute myocardial infarction — experience in four TAMI studies. *Cardiac Assists* 4:3, 1988.
92. Golding LAR, Loop FD, Peter M, et al. Later survival following use of intraaortic balloon pump in revascularization operations. *Ann Thorac Surg* 30:48, 1980.
93. Sanfelippo PM, Baker NH, Ewy HG, et al. Experience with intraaortic counterpulsation. *Ann Thorac Surg* 41:36, 1986.
94. Kucher DL, Campbell W, O'Rouke, MF. Long-term survival after counterpulsation for medically refractory heart failure complications, myocardiac infarction, and cardiac surgery. *EVR Heart J* 8(5);490-502, 1987.
95. Madras PN, Laird JD, Iatridis E, et al. Effects of prolonged intraaortic balloon pumping. *Trans Am Soc Artif Intern Organs* 15:400, 1969.

96. Brantigan CO, Grow JR Sr, Schoonmaker FW. Extended use of intra-aortic balloon pumping in peripatum cardiomyopathy. *Ann Surg* 183:1, 1976.
97. Topol EJ, Califf RM, George BS, et al. Coronary arterial thrombolysis with combined infusion of recombinant tissue-type plasminogen activator and urokinase in acute myocardial infarction. *Circulation* 77:1100-1107, 1988.
98. Topol EJ, George BS, Keriakes DJ, et al. A multicenter randomized controlled trial of intravenous tissue plasminogen activator and early intravenous heparin in acute myocardial infarction. *J Am Coll Cardiol* 11:232A, 1988.
99. Topol EJ, George BS, Keriakes DJ, et al. Comparison of two dose regimens of intravenous tissue plasminogen activator for acute myocardial infarction. *Am J Cardiol* 61:723-728, 1988.
100. George BS. Thrombolysis and intra-aortic balloon pumping following acute myocardial infarction—experience in four TAMI studies. *Cardiac Assists* 4:3, 1988.
101. Hauser AM, Gordon S, Gangadharan V, et al. Percutaneous intra-aortic balloon counterpulsation: clinical effectiveness and hazards. *Chest* 82:422, 1982.
102. Goldberg MJ, Rubenfine M, Kantrowitz H, et al. Intraaortic balloon pump insertion: a random study comparing percutaneous and surgical techniques. *J Am Coll Cardiol* 9(3):515-23, 1987.
103. Pelletier LC, Power JR, Bosch X, et al. Complications of circulatory assistance with intra-aortic balloon pumping: a comparison of surgical and percutaneous techniques. *Heart Transplant* 5(2):138-42, 1986.
104. Pollock JC, Charlton MC, Williams WG, et al. Intra-aortic balloon pumping in children. *Ann Thorac Surg* 29:6, 1980.
105. Veasy LG, Blaybock N, Fukumasu H, et al. Preclinical evaluation of intra-aortic balloon pumping for pediatric use. *Trans Am Soc Artif Intern Organs* XXVII:490, 1981.
106. Veasy LG, Webster H. Intra-aortic balloon pumping in infants and children. *Cardiac Assists* 2:1, 1985.
107. Del Nido PJ. Successful use of intra-aortic balloon pumping in a 2-kilogram infant. *Ann Thorac Surg* 46:574, 1988.
108. Yellin E, Levy L, Bregman D. Hemodynamic effects of intra-aortic balloon pumping in dogs with aortic incompetence. *Trans Am Soc Artif Intern Organs* 19:389, 1973.
109. Bregman D. Intra-aortic balloon in open-heart surgery. *New Engl J Med* 284:393, 1971.
110. Spencer FC, Eiseman B, Trinkle JK. Assisted circulation for cardiac failure following intracardiac surgery with cardiopulmonary bypass. *J Thorac Cardiovasc Surg* 49:56, 1965.
111. Debakey ME. Left ventricular bypass pump for cardiac assistance. *Am J Cardiol* 27:3, 1971.
112. Kantor KR, McBride LR, Pennington DG, et al. Bridging to cardiac transplantation with pulsatile ventricular assist devices. *Ann Thorac Surg* 46:134-140, 1988.

113. Pennock JL, Pierce WS, Campell DB, et al. Mechanical support of the circulation followed by cardiac transplantation. *J Thorac Cardiovasc Surg* 92:994-1004, 1986.
114. Zumbri GL, Kitchens WR, Shearer G, et al. Mechanical assistance for cardiogenic shock following cardiac surgery, myocardial infarction, and cardiac transplantation. *Ann Thorac Surg* 44:11-13, 1987.
115. Sivay G, Litwak RS, Griepp RB. Circulatory assist devices. In: *Cardiac Anesthesia* Vol. 2, Saunders, 1987:1021-1036.
116. Kormos RL, Griffith BP, Hardesty RL, et al. The artificial heart: Bridge to cardiac transplantation. *J Am Coll Cardiol (abstracts)* 9(2):28a, 1987.
117. Copeland JG, Smith RG, Icenogle TB, et al. Early experience with the total artificial heart as a bridge to transplantation. *Surg Clinics NA* Vol 68(3):621-634, 1988.
118. Portner PM, Oyer PE, Pennington DG, et al. Implantable electrical left ventricular assist system: bridge to transplantation and the future. *Ann Thorac Surg* 47:142-150, 1989.
119. Bolman RM, Cox JL, Marshall W, et al. Circulatory support with a centrifugal pump as a bridge to cardiac transplantation. *Ann Thorac Surg* 47:108-112, 1989.
120. Magovern G, Panelists. Weaning and bridging. *Ann Thorac Surg* 47:102-107, 1989.
121. Cooley DA, Akutsu T, Norman JC. Total artificial heart in two-staged cardiac transplantation. *Cardiovasc Dis Bull Texas Heart Inst* 8(3):305-319, 1981.
122. Cooley DA, Liotta D, Hallman GL, et al. Orthotopic cardiac prosthesis for two-staged cardiac replacement. *Am J Cardiol* 24:723-730, 1969.
123. Rose DM, Colvin SB, Culliford AT, et al. Late functional and hemodynamic status of surviving patients following insertion of the left heart device. *J Thorac Cardiovasc Surg* 86:639, 1983.
124. Pennington DG, Samuels LD, Palmer D, et al. Experience with the Pierce-Donachy ventricular assist device in postcardiotomy patients with cardiogenic shock. *World J Surg* (9)1:37-46, 1985.
125. Gaines WE, Pierce WS, Donachy JH, et al. The Pennsylvania State University ventricular assist pump: optimal methods of use. *World J Surg* Vol (9)1:47-53, 1985.
126. Pennington DG, McBride LR, Swartz MT, et al. Use of the Pierce-Donachy ventricular assist device in patients with cardiogenic shock after cardiac operations. *Ann Thorac Surg* 47:130-135, 1989.
127. Pae, WE, Pierce WS, Pennock JL, et al. Long-term results of ventricular assist pumping in post-cardiogenic shock. *J Thorac Cardiovasc Surg* 93:434-441, 1987.
128. Jorge E, Pierce WS. Mechanical support or replacement of the heart. *Cardiovasc Clin Cardiac Surg* 361-376, 1987.
129. Litwak RS, Koffsky RM, Jurado RA, et al. A decade of experience with the left heart device in patients undergoing open intracardiac operation. *World J Surg* (9)1:18-24, 1985.

130. Rose DM, Connolly M, Cunningham JN, et al. Techniques and results with a roller pump left and right heart assist device. *Ann Thorac Surg* 47:124-129, 1989.
131. Rose DM, Laschinger J, Grossi E, et al. Experimental and clinical results with a simplified left heart assist device for treatment of profound left ventricular dysfunction. *World J Surg* (9)1:11-17, 1985.
132. Reemtsma, Bregman D, Cohen S. Mechanical circulatory support. In: Shoemaker W, Thompson WL, Holbrook PR, eds. *Textbook of Critical Care.* Philadelphia, PA, Saunders, 1984:482-496.
133. Park SB, Liebler GA, Burkholder JA, et al. Mechanical support of the failing heart. *Ann Thorac Surg* 42:627-631, 1986.
134. Schoen FJ, Palmer DC, Pennington DG, et al. Clinical temporary ventricular assist. *J Thorac Cardiovasc Surg* 92:1071-1081, 1986.
135. Kanter KR, Swartz MT, Pennington DC, et al. Renal failure in patients with ventricular assist devices. *ASAIO Trans* 33:426-428, 1987.
136. Akutsu T, Wolff WJ. Permanent substitutes for valves and hearts. *Trans Am Soc Artif Intern Organs* 4:230-235, 1958.

Chapter 15

Pharmacological Management of Perioperative Right and Left Ventricular Dysfunction

Roberta Hines, MD and Gerard McCloskey, MD

The most appropriate choice of any therapeutic plan used for the treatment of ventricular dysfunction (pharmacological or mechanical) depends upon a complete understanding and evaluation of all factors responsible for the maintenance of overall myocardial performance.

Traditionally, perioperative management of ventricular dysfunction has been directed primarily at the left ventricle. Factors leading to perioperative left ventricular dysfunction include: ischemia, hypertension, valvular heart disease, congestive heart failure, and coronary artery disease.

However, recent evidence demonstrates that in the presence of elevated right ventricular (RV) preload or afterload, coexistent left ventricular dysfunction or right coronary artery disease, changes in right ventricular function become hemodynamically

From Casthely PA, Bregman D, (eds): *Cardiopulmonary Bypass: Physiology, Related Complications, and Pharmacology.* Mount Kisco, NY, Futura Publishing Company, Inc., © 1991.

significant. As a result, the diagnosis and treatment of right ventricular failure presents a challenging clinical problem. The following discussion will focus on the pharmacological management of perioperative right and left ventricular dysfunction.

Determinants of Myocardial Performance

A complete evaluation of the factors influencing myocardial performance, i.e., cardiac output, must include: preload, afterload, heart rate (rhythm), and contractility, (Fig. 1). Although each of these variables may be evaluated and defined independently, clinically the mechanisms that regulates flow, pressure, and resistance are interdependent.[1]

Preload, although strictly defined as the end diastolic volume in either ventricle is monitored by the pressure correlates of that ventricle, i.e., right ventricular end diastolic pressure (RVEDP for the right) and left ventricular end diastolic pressure (LVEDP for the left). These are then further approximated by the central venous pressure (CVP) and pulmonary capillary wedge pressure (PCWP), respectively. In both ventricles, preload is directly dependent upon the venous return and the intravascular volume. Under situations of normal compliance, an increase in preload results in an augmentation of cardiac output defined by the normal Starling relation-

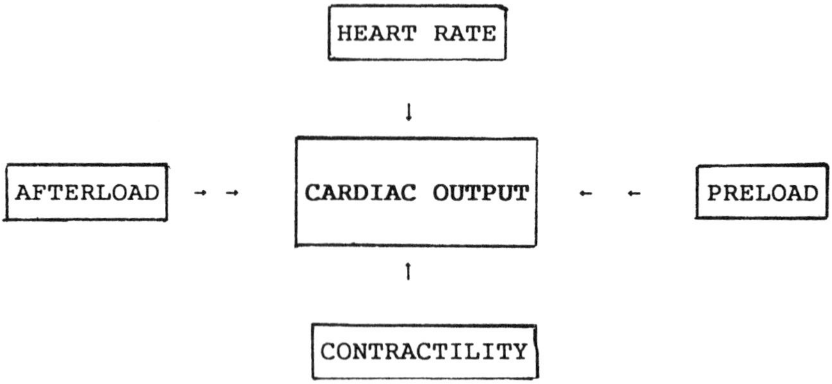

Figure 1. The determinants of cardiac output.

ship.[2] However, it must be remembered that due to the differences in compliance between the right (i.e., the right being more compliant than the left), for a given volume, a greater rise in pressure will occur in the left as compared to the right ventricle.

Afterload, is defined as the tension in the wall of the ventricle during injection (i.e., aortic impedance for the left ventricle and pulmonic impedance for the right ventricle). However, ventricular wall stress does not lend itself to direct clinical measurement. Fortunately, in most clinical situations, it is possible to quantitate the major determinant of the wall tension, impedance to flow. In the absence of outflow tract obstruction, pulmonary or aortic stenosis, the major determinant of this impedance to flow is the vascular resistance. The resistance can be quantitated by the formula.

$$\text{PVR} = \frac{\text{PAP} - \text{CVP}}{\text{CO}} \times 80 \text{ (nl 50-150)}$$

[The units for the above values should be expressed as dynes/sec/cm^{-5}.]

It is important to remember that any changes in afterload will directly impact myocardial performance. Under conditions of normal compliance, the left ventricle can withstand relatively large increases in afterload with only minimal changes in forward ejection.[3] However, in situations where the ventricle has become noncompliant, i.e., congestive heart failure (CHF) or ventricular dysfunction, even small increases in afterload may result in dramatic reductions in forward ejection.[4] However, the effect of increasing impedance to right ventricular ejection is more dramatic. Even small increases in afterload may produce a dramatic reduction in right ventricular (RV) ejection (see section on Right Ventricular Dysfunction) (Fig. 2).

Under normal physiological conditions, heart rate in the ranges of 60-110 beats/min results in minimal changes in cardiac output.[5] However, in situations where the myocardium has already been forced to increase its myocardial oxygen supply, heart rate changes may have a profound detrimental effect. As cardiac output is dependent upon heart rate and stroke volume, either tachycardia or bradycardia may result in reduction in stroke volume (SV) and cardiac output (CO). In addition, tachycardia exerts two potential detrimental effects upon cardiac performance. A reduction in ventricular filling is accompanied by an increase in myocardial oxygen

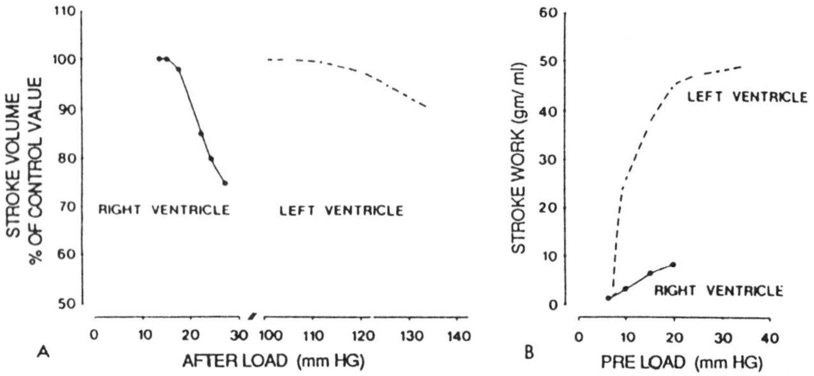

Figure 2. The effect of variations in preload and afterload on right and left ventricular function. (From McFadden ER, Braunwald E. Cor pulmonade and pulmonary thromboembolism. In: Braunwald E, ed. *Textbook of Cardiovascular Medicine*. Philadephia, PA: W.B. Saunders; 1980:1643-1680. With permission).

consumption. As a result, tachycardia, in patients with coronary artery disease has recently been associated with an increased incidence of perioperative ischemia.[6] On the other hand, bradycardia may result in an increased stroke volume per beat but overall cardiac output may be reduced.

Contractility, or inotropy, is defined as the capability of the cardiac muscle to shorten, i.e., develop force and velocity in response to a given stimulus. The intrinsic contractile performance (ejection fraction) is dependent upon preload and afterload and is usually measured in the pre- and postoperative periods via ventriculography via the following formula:

$$EF = \frac{EDV - ESV}{EDV}$$

EDV = end diastolic volume
ESV = end-systolic volume

nl = 70%

However, the intraoperative assessment of the inotropic state of the ventricle can be estimated by constructing a series of ventricular function curves (Fig. 3). By constructing these curves for individual patients, the impact of various pharmacological and hemo-

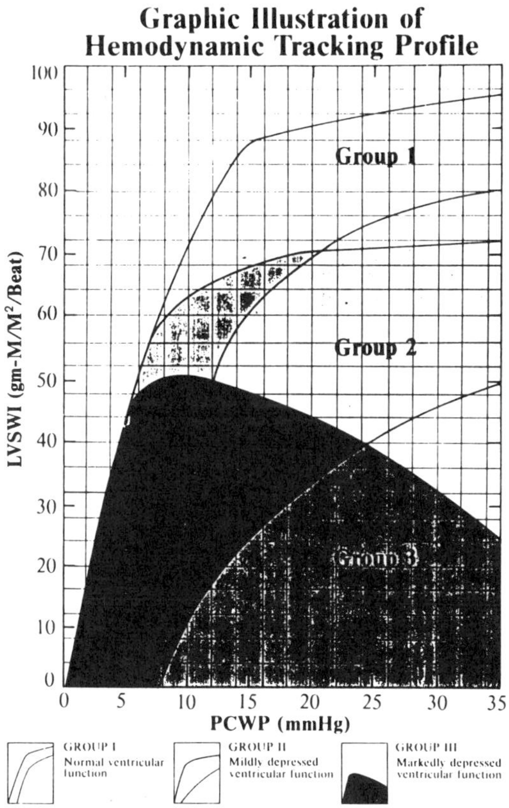

Figure 3. The pharmacological management of the patient with ventricular dysfunction is facilitated by constructing a series of ventricular function curves.

dynamic interventions are graphically displayed and may be compared to normal or baseline values.

Management Strategies

A successful management strategy for the treatment of perioperative myocardial dysfunction will involve the utilization of all the previous identified factors (i.e., preload, afterload, contractility, and heart rate).[7,8] The order and importance of various interventions will be influenced by the etiology of this decreased cardiac performance (i.e., whether cardiac failure is acute or chronic).

Preload Augmentation

The goal here is to increase intravascular volume while avoiding pulmonary edema or a reduction in coronary perfusion pressure. Depending upon the specific clinical setting, blood, blood components (packed red cells or whole blood) colloid solutions (albumin or hydroxyethyl starch) or crystalloid solution may all be utilized. Preload augmentation will be most effective in the treatment of acute ventricular dysfunction.

Afterload Reduction

Vasodilation of the patient with compromised myocardial contractility should allow for an increase in stroke volume and cardiac output with a minimal increase in myocardial work or oxygen consumption. In fact, the lower wall tensions permitted by the vasodilation may even decrease the oxygen expenditure in spite of an increase in cardiac output. This is the case is both acute and chronic ventricular dysfunction.

In the management of chronic failure vasodilators serve as one of the principal modalities to augument ventricular performance.[8,9] Although the nitrates do cause an increase in arterial compliance and promote left ventricular ejection, other dilators are much more efficacious. It has been long recognized that sodium nitroprusside is beneficial in the treatment of congestive failure.[10] There have been many studies that have examined the clinical effect and outcome of adding various arterial dilators to standard nitrate therapy.[11-13] The addition of hydralazine to nitrate therapy has been shown to improve the arterial dilator effect of nitrates alone.[14] It has also been demonstrated that the addition of hydralazine to nitrate therapy increases exercise tolerance, improves ejection fraction and prolongs survival over nitrates alone.[15] However, the choice of arterial vasodilator seems to be important.[16,17]

Unfortunately, the chronic use of nitrates in the treatment of congestive heart failure has its limitations. One characteristic of nitrate therapy that has long been recognized is the development of tolerance after prolonged exposure to the drug. Some investigators fear the beneficial effects of nitrate therapy may decrease over time. Indeed it is possible to demonstrate decreasing hemodynamic effectiveness of nitrate therapy with continued or repeated doses.[12,13] However, the lessening effect of the drugs on hemodynamic parameters are not well correlated with subjective clinical relief from symptoms. Despite the decreasing effects on preload reduction and arterial compliance, nitrates continue to deliver clinical relief from symptoms of congestive failure.[11,13]

In addition to nitrates and hydralazine, other vasodilators have been used in the treatment of congestive cardiac failure. The angiotensin converting enzyme (ACE) inhibitors captopril and enalapril have been evaluated for their efficacy in this clinical scenario.[18-22] In studies of patients with severe congestive failure (NYHA Class IV), currently treated with digoxin, diuretics and often other vasodilators, administration of enalapril was associated with increased survival over placebo.[21] This study was also able to demonstrate a subjective decrease in symptoms and an objective decrease in heart size among the enalapril treated patients. Similar beneficial effects of the administration of catopril to patients with severe failure have been reported.[17,18]

Angiotensin converting enzyme inhibitors have also been studied in less clinically severe patient populations. Here also their beneficial effects are demonstrable. Several studies have shown increased exercise tolerance and improved clinical status with the addition of ACE inhibitors to a digoxin and diuretic treatment regimen.[17,21] However, in patients with relatively minor symptoms of congestive failure (NYHA Class II), there has been little clinical difference between digoxin alone and ACE inhibitor alone in the improvement of exercise tolerance or increased ejection fraction.[21]

Inotropic Agents

An ideal inotropic agent must enhance the contractility of the failing ventricle. However, this augmentation in inotropic activity should be accomplished without any significant increase in heart rate, preload, afterload or myocardial oxygen consumption.[23] Clinically, sympathomimetic drugs are the pharmacologic agents that are capable of providing both inotropic and/or vasopressor activity (Fig. 4). Traditionally, catecholamines have served as the sympathomimetic agents of choice for augmenting cardiac output and/or altering (usually increasing) vascular tone.[24,25] Based upon their derivation, catecholamines are divided into synthetic or endogenous classes (Table I). All catecholamines (endogenous or synthetic) exert their inotropic and vascular effects by stimulating adrenergic-mediated receptors in the sympathetic nervous system.[26,27] As a result, catecholamines are known as adrenergic sympathomimetic agents. These adrenergic receptors are classified as α (1 and 2), β (1 and 2) and dopaminergic (Table II).[27] Catecholamines yield their hemodynamic effects by direct or indirect action

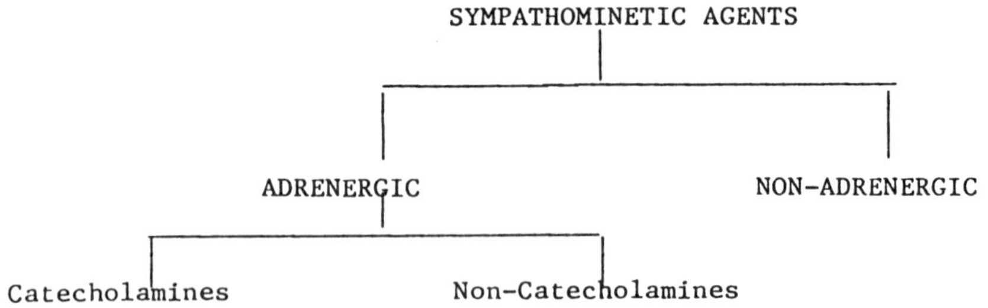

Figure 4. Classification of sympathomimetic agents based upon their mode of action.

Table I
Classification of Cathecholamines

CATHECHOLAMINES

ENDOGENOUS	*SYNTHETIC*
Epinephrine	Isoproterenol
Norepinephrine	Dobutamine
Dopamine	
Phenylephrine	

Table II
Site and Action of Adrenergic Receptors

Receptor	*Site*	*Action*
α_1	Postsynaptic-vascular smooth muscle	■ Vasoconstriction
α_2	Presynaptic (minimal postsynaptic)	■ Inhibits norepinephrine
β_1	Postsynaptic-myocardium	■ Increased inotropy ■ Increased chronotropy ■ Increased conduction velocity
β_2	Postsynaptic — vascular smooth muscle — bronchial smooth muscle —uterine smooth muscle	■ Decreased vascular tone ■ Increased bronchodilation ■ Uterine atony
DA_1	Postsynaptic-renal and mesenteric vasculature ? coronary	■ Vasodilatation
DA_2	Presynaptic	■ Inhibits norepinephrine release

on these adrenergic receptors (Table III). Indirect acting catecholamines produced their effects by stimulating the release of stored neurotransmitter from sympathetic nerve terminals while direct acting agents act directly at the adrenergic receptor site. Some

Table III
Receptor Stimulation of Catecholamines

	Receptors					
Agent	a_1	a_2	b_1	b_2	DA_1	DA_2
Epinephrine	+++++	+++	++++	++	o	o
Norepinephrine	+++++	++++	++	o	o	o
Dopamine	++→+++++	?	++++	++	+++	?
Isoproterenol	o	o	+++++	+++++	o	o
Dobutamine	o → +	?	++++	++	o	o
Phenylephrine	++++	?	±	o	o	o

(Reprinted with permission from: Durrett L, Lawson N. Autonomic nervous system physiology and pharmacology. In: Barash PG, Cullen BF, Stoelting RK, eds. *Clinical Anesthesia*. Philadelphia, PA: Lippincott; 1989:195.)

agents (dopamine and ephedrine) are capable of either direct or indirect stimulation depending upon the dose administrated.[28,29]

Regardless of their mode of action, (direct or indirect) all catecholamines exert the positive inotropic action by stimulation of the β_1 receptor. This results in the activation of the "second messenger" pathway that stimulates the release of cyclic adenosine monophosphate (cAMP).[30] By stimulating cAMP, calcium channel influx into the cell is increased and dp/dt (force of contractility) is augmented. However, in addition to providing positive inotropic support, these augmented cAMP concentrations may also result in chronotropic (increasing heart rate) and vasoactive effects. These vasoactive actions may result in either vascular constriction (α) or vascular dilatation (β_2) depending upon the specific agent chosen (Table IV).[31] In addition, the stimulation of β_1 receptors is also associated with the potential for dromotropic (increased conduction velocity) and dysrhythmic) activity.

The clinical effectiveness of any particular adrenergic agent will be influenced by the availability (i.e., density) and responsiveness (i.e., affinity) of the β-receptors. A syndrome of β-receptive "down regulation" has been previously described by Bristow et al.[32] In patients suffering from chronically elevated levels of plasma catecholamines (such as those in CHF or hypertension) a reduction in the number and the sensitivity of β-receptors has been reported.[33] Conversely, in patients who have been receiving chronic β-adrenergic antagonists therapy, a significant increase in the number of β-receptors has been shown. Although initially thought to develop only in situations of chronic elevations in plasma catecholamine levels, β-receptor down regulation has now been observed with short-term exposure to the β-agonists as well. A recent report by Marty et al. demonstrated a significant postoperative increase in β-receptor density and a decrease in receptor afinity for β agonists in patients undergoing noncardiac procedures who experienced intraoperative adrenergic activation.[34] Therefore, even in the setting of an acute activation of the adrenergic system, β-adrenergic responsiveness may be altered. In summary, to insure the maximal hemodynamic effectiveness of adrenergic agents the following factors must be taken into consideration: (1) the concentration of the receptor agonist; (2) the number and binding affinity of the adrenergic receptors and (3) the availability of calcium ions.[31]

Table IV
Dose-Related Hemodynamic Effects of Sympthomimetic Agents

Drug	*IV Push Adult*	*IV Infusion Rate*	*CO*	*Inotropy*	*HR*	*VR*	*TPR*	*RBF*
Phenylephrine (10 mg/250 mL)*	50–100 mcg	0.015–0.75 mg.kg.min	±↓	—	reflex ↓	↑↑↑	↑↑	—↓
Norepinephrine (4 mg/250 mL)*	NR	0.5–7 mcg/kg/min	—↓	↑	reflex ↓	↑	↑↑↑	↓↓↓
Epinephrine (1 mg/250 mL)*	0.3–.05 mL 1:1000	0.01–0.05 mcg/kg/min	↑↑	↑↑	↑	↑	↑	↑
		.05–.1 mcg/kg/min	↑—	↑↑	↑↑	↑	↑↑	↓—
		.10 mcg/kg/min	↑—↓	↑↑	↑↑	↑	↑↑↑	↓
Dopamine (200 mg/250 mL)*	NR	.05–2.0 mcg/kg/min	±↑	— —	— —	±↑	+↓	↑↑
		2–5 mcg/kg/min	↑	— —	— —	↑	—↓	↑
		5–10 mcg/kg/min	↑—↓	↑↑	↑↑↑	↑	↑↑	—↓
Dobutamine (250 mg/250 mL)*	NR	5–10 mcg/kg/min	↑↑	↑↑	↑↑	?	—	↑
Isoproterenol (4 mg/250 mL)*	.015 mcg/kg/min	.015 mcg/kg/min	↑—↓	↑↑↑	↑↑↑	↓	↓	—↑
Amrinone (250 mg/250 mL)*	NR	1–3 mg/kg (loading dose) 5–20 mcg/kg/min	↑	↑↑	±↑	±↓	↓↓	±↑

NR = not recommended; * suggested concentration for continuous infusion; CO = cardiac output; HR = heart rate; VR = venous resistance; TPR = total peripheral resistance; RBF = renal blood flow. Adapted and reprinted with permission from Durrett L, Lawson N. Autonomic nervous system physiology and pharmacology. In: Barash PG, Cullen BF, Stoelting RK, eds. *Clinical Anesthesia.* Philadelphia, PA: Lippincott; 1989: 201.

Adrenergic Agents

Phenylephrine

Phenylephrine is a pure arterial vasoconstrictor, its use results in an increase in arterial blood pressure. In addition, a transient venous constriction may also occur with a net effect of increasing pressure and flow (i.e., cardiac output).[35] However this effect of acute venoconstriction, may cause a decreased output in patients with underlying ventricular dysfunction (ischemia, CHF) by acutely increasing afterload.[36] Clinically, the starting dose for an infusion of phenylephrine is 0.15 μg/kg/min. However, the drug may also be administered in boluses of 50-150 mcg in situations where a rapid, but transient vasoconstriction is desired.[37] In clinical situations where peripheral vascular resistance is low such as septic shock, the arterial vasoconstriction seen with phenylephrine may result in a dramatic increase in perfusion pressure. In a setting of acute ventricular dysfunction where the principle abnormality is a decreased preload (i.e., idiopathic hypertropic subaortic stenosis spinal or epidural anesthetics), phenylephrine is the agent of choice for supporting and maintaining perfusion pressure.[35-37]

Norepinephrine

Norepinephrine is the naturally occurring neurotransmitter released at the sympathetic postganglionic fibers. Its hemodynamic effects are the result of stimulation of both α- and β-receptors, in a dose-related manner. The net effect is an increase in cardiac output and heart rate secondary to β-receptor stimulation.[38] However, at higher doses, the positive inotropic effect of the β-receptorg may be masked by the intense α-adrenergic stimulation.[39]

As a result of its intensive vasoconstriction properties the use of phenylephrine in the clinical setting is often met with a significant amount of concern. These concerns revolve around the fear that the associated vasoconstriction will increase the work of an already failing ventricle and that secondary organ ischemia may develop.

However, with appropriate physiologic monitoring, cardiac output can be maximized via the β effects of this agent, while the α-adrenergic mediated vasoconstrictive can be minimized.[31] Reflex bradycardia can occur, but is usually seen only in dosing exceeding 0.05-.010 mcg/kg/min. As with phenylephrine, norepinephrine is extremely useful in combination with β-agonist for the treatment of syndromes associated with low peripheral resistance, such as septic shock and anaphylaxis.[40,41] Norepinephrine has also been alone or in comination with phosphodiesterase (PDE-III) inhibitors to aid in the separation of patients from cardiopulmonary bypass.[42] However, in patients who have received an internal mammary artery (IMA) graft, animal data suggest that the use of norepinephrine may result in decreased IMA graft flow.[43] Opponents argue that since IMA flow is pressure dependent, simply by increasing perfusion pressure, therapy with norepinephrine may secondarily increase IMA graft flow.

Epinephrine

The cardiovascular effects of epinephrine results from the direct stimulation of both α- and β-receptors.[44] The predominant hemodynamic effect (i.e., α or β) will depend upon the dose of epinephrine administered. Epinephrine produces a mixed peripheral vascular effect with α stimulation occurring in the skin, muscle and kidney. In contrast, the β stimulation (β_2) actions predominant in the vascular muscle giving rise to vasodilation. As a result, at therapeutic doses of 0.01-0.05 mcg/kg/min the β_2 effects predominant resulting in an decrease in SVR. However, constriction may be maintained in the renal and cutaneous beds because of its α action at these sites. In addition, due to venoconstrictive properties, renal and splenic blood flow may be reduced.

Clinically, however, as a result of its potent β_1 stimulating actions, epinephrine is the most frequently employed agent to use in the separation of patients from cardiopulmonary bypass.[45-47] Perhaps one of the main reasons for its popularity is the wide range of effects (β, α, or mixed β/α) that can be observed with varying doses ranges. With doses in the range of 0.01 to 0.05 mcg/kg/min, the major hemodynamic responses will be one of positive inotropic support with minimal vaso- or venoconstrictive activity. Despite its high degree of chronotropic activity, associated ventricular dysrhythmias are infrequently observed when the dose is maintained at this level. However, if the infusion is increased to greater than 0.05 mcg/kg/min, dysrhythmias may be encountered.[48,49] Increasing the infusion rate to 0.1 mcg/kg/min results in a predominance of of α-adrenergic effects with minimal if any residual β activity. These α-adrenergic effects may also stimulate constriction of the pulmonary vasculature, therefore exacerbating preexisting pulmonary hypertension and/or right ventricular dysfunction.

Isoproterenol

Isoproterenol is a nonspecific β-adrenergic catecholamine. In addition to stimulating β_1 cardiac receptors, resulting in a tachycardia, isoproterenol also acts upon β_2 receptors resulting in pulmonic and systemic vasodilation.[50] As a result of its pulmonary effects, isoproterenol is frequently used as the inotropic of choice in patients with pulmonary hypertension who require positive inotropic therapy.[51] Also in patients with right ventricular failure, the pulmonary dilating effects of isoproterenol may prove beneficial by combining pulmonary vasodilation with inotropic support. The major clinical concerns surrounding the use of isoproterenol center around the potential for dysrhythmias that are frequently encountered due to its potent β_1 stimulating activity. In addition to tachycardia, a reduction in coronary diastolic perfusion pressure occurs with isoproterenol infusion (secondary to its β_2 effects). The combination of increased myocardial oxygen demand (secondary to tachycardia), and reduced oxygen supply (via decreased coronary perfusion pressure) has been associated with the extension of a previously ischemic area.[52] However, isoproterenol's ability to increase heart rate, may be advantageous in situations of heart block, particularly, those secondary to β blocker or calcium channel antagonist overdoses. The clinical dose range for administration of isoproterenol to obtain the positive inotropic and vasodilating effects occurs at 0.01-0.02 mcg/kg/min. However, for the treatment of pharmacologically induced heart block, or bradycardia, doses as high as 0.1 mcg/kg/min may be necessary.[31]

Dopamine

Dopamine is the natural precursor of norepinephrine. Its pharmacological properties are unique as it is the only catecholamine that is capable (in a dose related fashion) of simulating all types of adrenergic receptors (α, β, and dopaminergic).[53-56] At low doses, < 2 mcg/kg/min, dopamine selectively stimulates dopaminergic receptors resulting in an increase in renal perfusion and a diuresis.[57-59] With increasing doses of 2-5 mcg/kg/min, β_1 receptors stimulation occurs with secondary increases in heart rate, cardiac output, and stroke volume. At these doses, there is little if any effect on peripheral resistance. Unfortunately, dopamine (in β stimulation doses) is associated with a significant potential for tachycardia. Clinically this tachycardia often limits the usefulness of dopamine as a positive inotropic agent.[28,60-62] The effects of α-adrenergic receptor stimulation is seen at approximately 7 mcg/kg/min. At these higher doses, increased systemic arterial and venous pressures associated with higher left ventricular filling pressures become apparent.[63] In addition, decreased splenic and renal blood flow can occur at these higher dose levels. The effect of dopamine on coronary blood flow is also dose-dependent.[64,65] At < 5 mcg/kg/min, coronary blood flow is increased in response to increased myocardial oxygen work and dopaminergic mediated dilatation of the coronary arteries. These effects are reversed at doses > 7 mcg/kg/min when the α effects may lead to an increased coronary vascular resistance.

Dopamine's effect on dopaminergic receptors ($\leq$ 2 mcg/kg/min) may be used to stimulate renal perfusion.[28,57-59] Dopamine is frequently administered in the dopaminergic ranges, in combination with "stronger" β agonists such as epinephrine or dobutamine.[66,67] This combination has gained clinical popularity in that it promotes both increaed inotropy with an independent increase in renal perfusion. At higher doses, (5-10 mcg/kg/min) the venoconstrictive effects and positive inotropic effects may be useful to support cardiac output and maintain systemic perfusion pressure.[68] However, in septic shock, dopamine will be ineffective, at any dose, due to the inhibition of dopamine β hydroxylase by endotoxin.[69]

Dobutamine

Dobutamine is a synthetic, direct acting catecholamine that is related to both dopamine and isoproterenol. However, unlike isoproterenol, it has little effect on β_2 receptors and unlike dopamine it does not stimulate the release of norepinephrine or stimulate α receptors.[70-72] Dobutamine increases cardiac output, stroke volume, and at higher doses (> 10 mg/kg) heart rate.[73] Of note, dysrhythmias have been reported in patients with a history of atrial fibrillation or other tachydysrhythmias even at these lower doses (5-10 mcg/kg/min). Changes in cardiac output are mainly the result of positive inotropic product support with minimal if any β_2 vasodilatory effects.[72,74] Any fall in vascular resistance or filling pressures results from an increased cardiac output not from the direct stimulation of β_2 receptors. Dobutamine does possesses some, although weak, α-arterial vasoconstrictive effects that are usually balanced by its weak β_2 effects. Clinically, tachyphylaxis has been reported with prolonged dobutamine infusions.[75] In the treatment of medical patients, dobutamine has been shown to be most effective in patients suffering from acute or chronic congestive heart failure based upon an ischemic etiology.[71,72,74,76] Gilespe and colleagues[71] administered dobutamine to 16 patients with the diagnosis of acute myocardial infarction. In this population they found that the drug improves ventricular performance without any further increase in myocardial injury (unlike isoproterenol).

In the cardiac surgical arena, dobutamine may be used during the weaning of patients from cardiopulmonary bypass.[77,78] As dobutamine is principally a β_1 antagonist, its efficacy in this patient population is the result of an increase in inotropy. However, if vasodilation either at the systemic or pulmonary beds is desired, the addition of vasodilators may be required. Butterworth et al.[73] designed a study to evaluate the hemodynamics occurring following dobutamine and epinephrine infusions in patients following coronary artery bypass surgery. Their study addresses the questions of tachycardia and increases in cardiac performance (as assessed by stroke volume) observed with epinephrine and dobutamine infusion in patients who developed left ventricular dysfunction following cardiac surgery. In this study, the authors evaluated the hemodynamic effects of dobutamine at doses of 2.5 and 5.0 mcg/

kg/min and epinephrine at 10 and 30 ng/kg/min in the treatment of postbypass left ventricular dysfunction. Their results demonstrated that both drugs (dobutamine and epinephrine) significantly increased heart rate, stroke volume and cardiac index. However, dobutamine at 5 mcg/kg/min caused a significantly greater increase in heart rate than did epinephrine at 30 ng/kg/min. Of note, this increase in heart rate seen with a higher dose of dobutamine, was accompanied by smaller increases in cardiac output and stroke volume than were observed with a 30 ng/kg/min dose of epinephrine.

Nonadrenergic Agents

All of the agents described within this class exert their vasoactive and positive inotropic actions via nonadrenergic mechanisms (Table V). In the treatment of acute perioperative ventricular dysfunction, calcium, and the phosphodiesterase inhibitors are the most frequently used nonadrenergic agents. As a result, the discussion will focus on the hemodynamic effects of these agents.

Calcium chloride is often used to treat decreases in myocardial contractility of relatively short duration resulting from conditions that can be reversed by the admnistration of calcium salts.[80] These include (1) rapid transfusion of large quantities of citrate preserved blood products in patients with poor ventricular function (2) myocardial depression immediately after or during separation from cardiopulmonary bypass and (3) transient cardiac depression from a channel entry blocker.[81]

Intravenous administration of calcium results in increases in contractility (↑ dp/dt), stroke volume and decreases in left ventric-

Table V
Nonadrenergic Sympathomimetic Agents

Calcium
Glucagon
Digitalis
Phosphodiesterase-III Inhibitors
Xanthines

ular end diastolic pressure and heart rate. However, these effects are only significant if hypocalcemia is present. In situations of nomocalcemia only minimal changes in hemodynamic parameters are observed. Any changes that occur in systemic vascular resistance, will depend upon the calcium level prior to $CaCl_2$ therapy. In conditions of nomocalcemia, SVR will increase significantly while little or no change in SVR is seen in the presence of hypocalcemia.[81]

Phosphodiesterase Inhibitors

There are a variety of phosphodiesterase inhibitors (PDE-III inhibitors) in various stages of development (Table VI). All of these agents have a similar mode of action as they are noncatecholamine and nonadrenergic. Therefore, they do not rely upon β-receptor stimulation for their positive inotropic activity. Although the precise mechanism of action is yet to be elucidated, the proposed theory of action involves the inhibition of type III phosphodiesterase inhibitors found predominantly in cardiac muscle.[82,83] This inhibition of phosphodiesterase results in a secondary increase in cAMP that leads to an increase in calcium channel entry into the cell (↑ dp/dt). In addition to providing positive inotropic support these agents also produce systemic and pulmonary vasodilatation.[64,85,86] As a result of this combination of hemodynamic effects, i.e., positive inotropic support and vasodilatation, the term inodilators has been coined to describe this new class of agents. For the purpose of classification, the phosphodiesterase inhibitor agents are divided into groups based upon their biochemical properties. They are either byperidines; amrinone, and milrinone, or

Table VI
Phosphodiesterase Inhibitors

Amrinone
Milrinone
Persatine
Aminophylline
Enoximone
Piroximone

immidazoles; enoximone, and piroximone. As amrinone is the only PDE-III inhibitor currently available for clinical use, the following discussion will focus upon its applications.

Amrinone

As a biperidine PDE-III inhibitor, amrinone is yellow in color. In addition to its ability to augment contractile performance by increasing cAMP, amrinone produces systemic and pulmonary vasodilatation which appear to be mediated via a direct effect on vascular smooth muscle.[87-89] Following the administration of amrinone, the hemodynamics that occur are the result of its combined positive inotrope and vasodilator properties. Amrinone produces an increase in cardiac output and a decrease in systemic vascular resistance (SVR), pulmonary vascular resistance (PVR), pulmonary capillary wedge pressure (PCWP), and right atrial pressure (RAP) (Table VII).[86] Of clinical note, the hemodynamic effects are accomplished without any significant increase in either heart rate or myocardial oxygen consumption (MVO_2). This decrease (or lack of change) in MVO_2 may be the result of either improved relaxation of the cardiac muscle, improved vasodilatation or, some combination of both. However, any changes that are seen in systemic arterial pressure occur indirectly from an increased cardiac output. In addition, amirnone appears to improve renal blood flow, although indirectly, via increased cardiac output, as it does not stimulate dopaminergic receptors.[88]

Amrinone's effectiveness is not altered by previous β blockade therapy or reduced in patients who may experience β-receptor down regulation. When used in comination with β-agonists, PDE-III inhibitors have been shown to result in an additive effect in the improvement of myocardial performance.[90-93] Gage et al.[91] were the first to demonstrate that the combination of PDE-III inhibitors and β-agonists (in this case dobutamine) resulted in an additive effect on overall myocardial performance. Subsequent reports have demonstrated the beneficial therapeutic effects of amrinone in combination with other sympathomimetic agents such as norepinephrine and dopamine.[90-93] This is important clinically, as the PDE-III inhibitors may be used to attenuate the vasoconstrictive

Table VII

Hemodynamic Effects of Amrinone: Congestive Heart Failure due to Coronary Artery Disease

Period	*Cardiac Index (L/min)*	*Mean PCWP (mm Hg)*	*Mean PAP (mm Hg)*	*LVSWI (g.m/m²)*	*O_2 (mL/L)*	*MVO_2 (mL/min)*
Before	1.3 ± 0.4	31 ± 5	44 ± 8	10.6 ± 3.0	129 ± 19	27 ± 14
After	2.2 ± 0.7	26 ± 4	37 ± 4	19.2 ± 6.3	109 ± 17	19 ± 9
P	<.001	<0.01	<0.0005	<0.0025	<0.005	<0.01

PCWP = Pulmonary capillary wedge pressure; PAP = Pulmonary artery pressure; LVSWI = Left ventricular stroke work index; O_2 = Oyxgen concentration-difference between systemic arterial and coronary sinus blood concentration; MVO_2 = Myocardial oxygen consumption.

effects of the catecholamines, while the combination of agents (i.e., catecholamines and PDE-III) results in an increased cardiac performance.

The clinical use profile of the phosphodiesterase inhibitors extends over a wide variety of medical, as well as surgical settings. As initially reported in the medical literature, amrinone is especially used for the treatment of patients with acute heart failure.[87,88] Amrinone has also been used effectively to manage noncardiac surgical patients who develop perioperative congestive heart failure or who experience cardiogenic shock.[85] In addition, in the surgical arena during noncardiac surgery, amrinone has been used to manage ventricular dysfunction following aortic cross clamping during vascular surgery and right ventricular function secondary to pulmonary hypertension.[94-96]

In the area of cardiac surgery, amrinone has been used in all three phases of patient care: preoperatively, intraoperatively, and postoperatively in the intensive care unit.[90,93] Preoperatively, amrinone has been used to effectively stabilize patients following failed angioplasty. Amrinone may be used to increase cardiac output in patients requiring inotropic support during the prepump period, particularly in those who have a history of arrhythmias. Amrinone has also been used effectively as a primary agent either alone or in combination with β-agonist therapy to wean patients successfully from CPB.[92,93] Postoperatively, amrinone may be useful either alone or in combination with catecholamine therapy to manage patients in the cardiothoracic intensive care unit, especially those who present with low cardiac and high filling pressures.[97] One of the most recent clinical indications of the phosphodiesterase inhibitors has been focused on the ability of these agents to augment right ventricular performance particularly in those patients with concomitant pulmonary hypertension.[94-96] In this setting, amrinone's beneficial effects result predominantly from afterload reduction.

Another potential clinical advantage of the PDE-III inhibitor amrinone is its ability to improve or augment diastolic dysfunction.[98] Finally, amrinone has been shown effective in treatment in patients with right sided failure who are awaiting cardiac transplantation.[95,96]

The appropriate dosing of amrinone has been the focus of much confusion and debate. Initial work performed by Benotti et al.[86] recommended a loading dose of 0.75 mg/kg followed by continuous infusion of 5-10 mcg/kg/min. Using this protocol the mean elimination half-life in patients with congestive heart failure was approximately 5.8 hours. However, for the management of acute ventricular dysfunction, present recommendations now suggest a loading dose of 1–2 mg/kg followed by continuous infusion of 10-20 mcg/kg/min.[97] Goen et al.[98] were the first to report on the efficacy of amrinone therapy in cardiac surgical patients suffering from low cardiac output syndrome in the postoperative period. In their study, the authors administered 2 mg/kg of amrinone as loading dose following by a continuous infusion of 20 mcg/kg/min. This regimen resulted in a significant increase in cardiac output and a reduction in pulmonary capillary wedge pressure (PCWP). More recent data by Levy et al.[99] suggest that if amrinone is used during the weaning from cardiopulmonary bypass (CPB), that at least 1.5 mg/kg must be administered into the CPB venous reservoir with a simultaneous infusion of 10 mg/kg/min. These authors further suggest that if therapy after CPB is desired, a loading dose of 1.5-2 mg/kg followed by a continuous infusion of 10 mcg/kg/min will result in the maximum therapeutic effect. Data from this study also reveal an elimination half-life following cardiopulmonary bypass of approximately 3.5 ± 2 hours. However, as with all pharmacologic agents, the most effective dose regimen for amrinone will vary according to a particular patient's clinical situation.

With regard to potential side effects of the PDE-III inhibitors, none carry an incidence greater than 3%. The two complications that appear to be most clinically significant, are those of hypotension and potential thrombocytopenia. With appropriate monitoring and maintenance of adequate filling volume, hypotension should not be a major clinical problem. In addition, by extending the time of administration of the loading dose to 10-20 minutes the potential for hypertension during the loading dose administration is further reduced. Dose-related thrombocytopenia, which was initially reported as a complication following oral phosphodiesterase therapy, occurred as a result of an accelerated peripheral loss of platelets.[100] Thrombocytopenia, however was mild and reversible in all cases, and there were no episodes of clinical bleeding associated with this thrombocytopenia. Recently, the acute administration of intravenous amrinone on platelet number and function was evaluated in patients following cardiopulmonary bypass.[101] Patients received amrinone as a loading dose of 1 to 3 mg/kg followed by a continuous infusion of 10-20 mcg/kg/min. However, none of these patients received more than 25 mg/kg/day of amrinone within a 24-hour period. The acute administration of intravenous amrinone (< 25 mg/kg in a 24-hour period) did not produce any abnormalities of either platelet function or platelet number in patients receiving the drug following CPB.[101]

Milrinone

This is a second-generation phosphodiesterase III inhibitor with a similar hemodynamic profile to amrinone.[101] This agent combines both positive inotropic and vasodilating activities. However, its positive inotropic action is approximately 12-15 times that of amrinone. In addition, recent data suggest that milrinone may improve myocardial relaxation and augment coronary perfusion.[102-104] Drexler et al.[105,106] also reported an increase in splenic and skeletal blood flow. However, milrinone is not yet clinically available.

Enoximone

Enoximone's cardiac and vascular profile are similar to other phosphodiesterase fraction III inhibitors.[107] Choraria evaluated the efficacy of enoximone in a double blind cross over comparison with placebo in patients with CHF.[108] Symptom limited exercise capacity and ejection fraction at rest improved with enoximone. Heart rate and blood pressure remained unchanged. Enoximone's role in the management of acute ventricular dysfunction is presently under investigation.

Agents That May be Used to Decrease Heart Rate

Both calcium and β blocking agents exert their cardiac effects by reducing the net amount of calcium influx through the slow calcium channels of cardiac cell membranes, resulting in impaired cardiac conduction and a reduction in ventricular contractility. β-Adrenergic blockers reduce the number of calcium channels in the active configuration for calcium influx, while the calcium channel blockers interfere directly with the calcium channel.

Calcium Channel Blockers

Presently available calcium channel blockers include nifedipine, verapamil, and diltiazem (Table VIII). All of these agents are effective in either acutely or chronically lowering arterial blood pressure, as a result of a reduction in systemic vascular resistance.[109-111] Nifedipine is the most potent dilator of these three. Unfortunately, nifedipine is extremely light sensitive, and therefore, there is no presently available intravenous form of the drug. Also, its profound vasodilator effects result in a significant reflex tachycardic response.[112] However, nifedipine has little if any antiarrhythmic action. Verapamil is a less potent vasodilator, with conduction interfering effects at usual clinical doses. In addition, it possesses the most potent negative inotropic properties of the calcium channel blockers and therefore must be used cautiously in patients with impaired ventricular performance. Diltiazem is relatively sparing of ventricular function and it shares similar conduction effects with verapamil, i.e., slowing of AV node conduc-

Table VIII
Hemodynamics and Pharmodynamic Properties of the Calcium Blocking Agents

	Calcium Channel Blockers		
	Verapamil	*Nifedipine*	*Diltiazem*
Blood Pressure	↓↓	↓↓↓	↓↓
Contractility	↓↓	↑↓	↓
AV Conduction	↑↑↑	o	↓↓
SVR	↓↓	↓↓↓	↓
TVR	↓↓	↓↓↓	↓↓↓
T½ (hr)	2–7	4–6	4–6

tion.[113] All of the calcium channel blockers are highly protein bound with elimination half-lifes ranging from 2-7 hours.

β-Adrenergic Blockers

β Blocking agents work via blockade of β-adrenergic receptors (Table IX).[114] Blockade of β_1 receptors reduces resting and exercise-induced rises in heart rate, decreases the rate of spontaneous depolarization of ectopic pacemakers, and prolongs atrioventricular conduction.[115] Cardiac effects result in a decrease in cardiac output and blood pressure with a potential increase in ventricular volume and end diastolic pressure. These myocardial depressant effects are not caused by direct depression of the myocardium, but occur rather as a result of the inhibition of intrinsic sympathetic activity.[116] As a result, these agents should be used with caution in patients with a history of congestive heart failure that may be compensated for by an increased level of sympathetic activity (i.e., tachycardia). The decrease in heart rate, ventricular systolic wall tissue and contractility occurring with β blockade therapy reduces myocardial oxygen consumption. Although coronary blood flow is reduced, a favorable oxygen supply/demand ratio is maintained due to a greater decrease in myocardial oxygen consumption. This may be particularly advantageous in the perioperative management of patients with coronary artery disease. Several recent studies have documented the ability of β blockade to decrease or prevent perioperative ischemia in this patient population.

Table IX
A Comparison of the Cardioselectivity, Potents and Half-Lives of Selected β Blockers

	Parenteral β Blockers		
	Cardioselectivity	*Potency*	*T½ (min)*
Propranolol	o	1	360
Esmolol	+	0.03	9
Labetalol	o	0.3	300
Metoprolol	+	1	240

Historically, one of the greatest problems surrounding the use of perioperative β blockade has been the lack of β_1-specific agents (Table IX). That is, until recently all of the available β-adrenergic blockers resulted in nonselective blockade, i.e., blockade of both β_1 and β_2 receptors. This was particularly predominant in patients with lung disease as blockade of the β_2 receptor frequently leads to bronchospasm or CHF. The development of newer β_1 selective blocking agents has all but erased these concerns. Presently available selective, β_1 antagonists include metoprolol and esmolol (Breviblock® [Dupont Pharmaceuticals Inc., Manoti, Puerto Rico]).[117,118] Esmolol has an additional advantage, a short half-life. Previously available β blockers had half-lives of 4-6 hours. Esmolol was developed to meet the demand for a cardioselective (i.e., greater β than β_2 blocking potency in clinical doses) agent with a short half-life. As a result of biochemical modifications, esmolol undergoes rapid hydrolysis (by red blood cell esterase) resulting in a half-life of 7-9 minutes. Clinical studies have documented the efficacy of esmolol to control the ventricular rate of both supraventricular tachycardia and atrial fibrillation. Additional uses include the control of perioperative hypertension and as a modality to reduce the incidence of perioperative tachycardia.[119]

Mixed α and β-Adrenergic Blocking Agents: Labetalol

Labetalol is a mixed α and β antagonist resulting in peripheral vasodilation (via α blockade). As the drug also posseses β blocking properties this vasodilation occurs without reflux tachycardia.[120,121] The ratio of β to α blocking potency has been estimated as being in a ratio of 7:1 (IV) or 4:1 (po). Unfortunately however, the β blocking properties are nonspecific, much like those of propranolol. Therefore, caution should be exercised with the use of labetolol in patients with a history of bronchospastic disease, congestive heart failure or impaired intracardiac conduction. Of note, the half-life of labetolol is approximately 240 minutes and may be of concern if hypotension develops.

Management of Right Ventricular Failure

Management of the patient with right ventricular (RV) failure remains controversial. Hemodynamics of RV failure include: (1)

increased right atrial and right ventricular end diastolic pressures, (2) normal left atrial and left ventricular end diastolic pressures, (3) decreased cardiac output. Treatment strategies have emphasized: (1) volume loading, (2) vasodilators, (3) inotropic support, (4) vasoconstrictors, and (5) mechanical assist devices, and (6) maintenance of normal AV conduction. The appropriate sequences of the therapeutic intervention depend in a large part on the status of the pulmonary vascular resistance, i.e., the RV afterload and the contractile state of the right ventricle (Fig. 5).

Volume expansion is the foundation of treatment in situations of RV failure when the pulmonary vascular resistance and RV contractility are normal. This increased volume, in the normal highly compliant RV, will create maximal RV myocardial fiber stretch and maintain cardiac output. The dilation of the RV is the major compensatory mechanism for augmenting RV contractility. However, the restraining influence of the pericardium limits this treatment with volume expansion to a ventricular filling pressure of approximately 12 mm Hg.[122]

Right ventricular volume overload has been shown to distort the intraventricular septum, leading to a reduction in both LV volume and septal contractility.[122-124] Any further increase in RV volume overload may exacerbate the already decreased LV compliance. In view of these facts, use of volume loading therapy for patients with acute RV infarction should be questioned. Inotropic support may be preferable for these patients, as it maintains com-

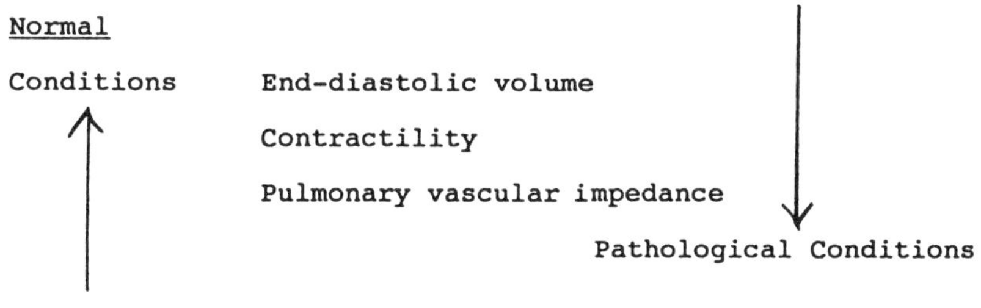

Figure 5. Factors affecting right ventricular performance. Under conditions of normal RV contractility perfusion is governed by preload, contractility and pulmonary vascular impedance (PVR). However, in pathological states (i.e., pulmonary hypertension), afterload becomes the most important factor governing RV performance.

pliance of both ventricles.[125] The effects of volume loading, dobutamine, and nitroprusside were compared in patients with acute RV infarction.[126] By itself, volume loading did not improve output, despite a rise in cardiac filling pressures. However, following appropriate volume loading, dobutamine administration improved cardiac output and RVEF significantly more than did nitroprusside.

Laver[124] demonstrated the ability of vasoconstrictive therapy to maintain RV perfusion pressure while treating RV dysfunction. Right ventricular dysfunction was produced in a canine model with myocardial ischemia by progressive occlusion of the main pulmonary artery. This was accompanied by a pronounced rise in right ventricular end diastolic pressure. The infusion of phenylephrine produced a dramatic increase in aortic diastolic pressure, thereby improving right ventricular perfusion.

When increased RV afterload is the principal cause of RV dysfunction, agents that result in pulmonary vasodilatation are the principal modalities of therapy. All of the following agents will produce a decrease in pulmonary vascular resistance: nitroglycerin, nitroprusside, theophylline, dobutamine, amrinone, aminophyline, prostacylin and prostaglandins (PGE_1). When choosing a pulmonary vasodilating agent, the best agent will be one that exerts the greatest effect of the pulmonary vasculature and the least effect upon the systemic vasculature. Clinically, nitroglycerin and nitroprusside are both excellent pulmonary vasodilators. However, nitroprusside generally results in a greater decrease in perfusion pressure for a given change in vascular resistance than does nitroglycerin.

New modalities of pharmacologic therapy that have been advocated for use in the treatment of RV failure secondary to pulmonary hypertension are the prostaglandins most notably PGE_1, and the phosphodiesterase inhibitor, amrinone.[94,127] D'ambra et al.[127] have reported their results in the infusion of prostaglandin E_1 to dilate the pulmonary vasculature and improve RV function in patients undergoing mitral valve replacement. Unfortunately, PGE_1 is not a selective pulmonary vasodilator and frequently system hypotension is a complication with this therapeutic technique. In the D'ambra study, to circumvent this problem, doses of PGE_1 were administered via a right atrial line while concomitant left atrial infusions of norepinephrine were administered to maintain systemic perfusion pressures in these patients. A more recent study evaluated the ability of PGE_1 to be a selective pulmonary vasodilator.[128]

Recently, the fraction III phosphodiesterase inhibitors, for example amrinone, have been successfully utilized to reduce pulmonary vascular resistance and augment right ventricular function in patients with mitral valve disease and concomitant pulmonary hypertension. Hess et al.[94] reported on the pulmonary vasodilator effects of amrinone in this patient population. When amrinone was administered as a bolus of 1.5 mg/kg, followed by continuous infusion of 10 mcg/kg/min, cardiac index increased by 30%, mean PAP decreased by 10%, and PVR decreased by 40%. Similarly, because of its ability to significantly decrease PVR, amrinone has been effective in stabilizing patients with a right sided myocardial dysfunction awaiting cardiac transplantation.

When a depression of contractility is the principal modality affecting RV performance then agents that augment contractility are vital to restoring normal RV function. Numerous clinical situations have been associated with a direct reduction in RV contractility. These include: ischemia, high levels of positive pressure ventilation (PEEP > 20 cm of water), cardiopulmonary bypass (either from air or direct trauma to the RV), and protamine administration.[129-131] All of the previously described sympathomimetic agents such as: dopamine, dobutamine, epinephrine, and isoproterenol may be used to increase RV contractility in these situations. However, the RV dysfunction that may be observed following protomine administration is best explained as an anaphylatoid type reaction mediated via complement activation. As a result, epinephrine would be the pharmacological agent of choice for reversing the associated hemodynamic derangements.

However, if RV dsyfunction is precipitated by a combination of reduced contractility and increased afterload (↑ PVR) agents that possess both positive inotropic and pulmonary vasodilating properities should be administered. In this situation, isoproterenal, epinephrine, or amrinone all are capable of producing the desired effects. If however, contractility is depressed secondary to a low right coronary artery perfusion pressure (i.e., ischemia, CBP, then agents such as norepinephrine will result in an increased perfusion pressure.[124] Caution must be excerised here to ensure that pulmonary vascular resistance is not elevated.

The value of maintaining normal atrioventricular conduction and contraction is essential to maintaining normal RV function. The loss of the sinoatrial activity contributes to a decrease in RV efficiency in much the same way that loss of the atrial decreases left ventricular efficiency.

In addition to pharmacological agents, the use of mechanical assist devices (right atrial to pulmonary artery pumps) has also been suggested for the treatment of refractory right ventricular dysfunction. This device is initially used to treat postpericardiotomy right ventricular failure. However, this device is only useful in patients with depressed RV performance with normal pulmonary vascular resistance. A promising alternative is the right atrial to pulmonary artery bypass pump and using a biomedicus that is a standard roller, centrifical pump. In patients whose right ventricular dysfunction is principally a matter of pulmonary hypertension, Miller[132] has successfully utilized the pulmonary artery balloon counterpulsation (PABC) device to wean a patient with RV dysfunction from cardiopulmonary bypass. This device has been effective in RV failure to principally to pulmonary hypertension or acute RV infarction with pulmonary hypertension. It must be emphasized that both of these devices are temporizing measures and may be used in that regard or as a bridge to cardiac transplantation (Fig. 6).

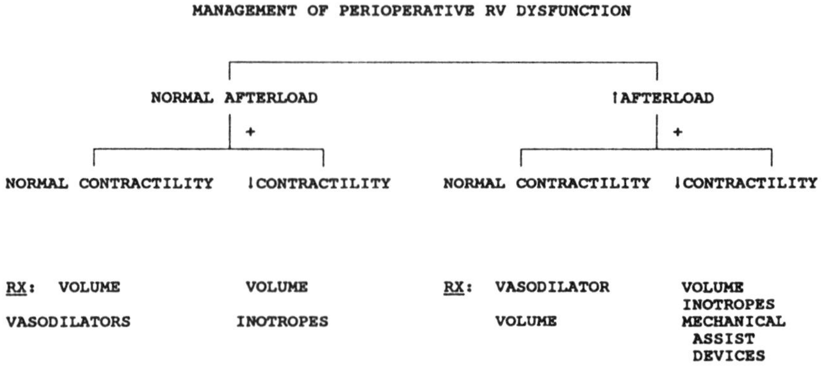

Figure 6.

End stage right ventricular failure secondary to irreversible pulmonary vascular disease is presently treated using combined heart/lung transplantation. This operation was first successfully performed in Stamford in March of 1981 and is presently performed at multiple centers throughout the country. This procedure is associated with an approximately 65% 1-year survival rate and has an accompanying perioperative mortality rate of 30%.

Summary

The successful management of perioperative ventricular dysfunction is a complex process involving the identification, diagnosis, and treatment of the underlying pathophysiologic processess. With increasing sophisicated methods for the monitoring of intraoperative cardiac performance combined with newer approaches to pharmacological therapy a significant positive impact on patient care should be accomplished.

REFERENCES

1. Guyton AC. Cardiac output, venous return and their regulation. In: Guyton AC, ed. *Textbook of Medical Physiology.* Philadelphia, PA: WB Saunders; 1981:274-288.
2. Sarnoff SJ. Myocardial contractility as described by ventricular function curves. *Physiol Rev* 35:107-122, 1955.
3. Shibutani K, Del Guerico LRM. Preoperative hemodynamic assessment of the high-risk patient. *Semin Anesth* 11:221-240, 1983.
4. Little RC, Little WC. Cardiac preload, afterload, and heart failure. *Arch Intern Med* 142:819-822, 1982.
5. Berne RM, Levy MN. Control of the heart. In: Berne RM, Levy MN, eds. *Cardiovascular Physiology.* St. Louis, MO: CV Mosby; 1977:155-190.
6. Slogoff S, Keats PS. Does perioperative myocardial ischemia lead to postoperative myocardial infarction? *Anesthesiology* 62:107-114, 1985.
7. Rahmintoola SH. The pharmacologic treatment of chronic congestive heart failure. *Circulation* 80:693-699, 1989.
8. Cohn JN. Current therapy of the failing heart. *Circulation* 78:1099-1107, 1988.

9. Leier CV, Huss P, Magorien RD, et al. Improved exercise capacity and differing arterial and venous tolerance during chronic isosorbide dinitrate therapy for congestive heart failure. *Circulation* 67:817-822, 1983.
10. Guiha NH, Cohn JN, Mikulic E, et al. Treatment of refractory heart failure with infusion of nitroprusside. *N Engl J Med* 291:587-592, 1974.
11. Franciosa JA, Blank RC, Cohn JN. Nitrate effects on cardiac output and left ventricular outflow resistance in chronic congestive heart failure. *Am J Med* 64:207-213, 1978.
12. Franciosa JA, Goldsmith SR, Cohn JN. Contrasting immediate and long-term effects of isosorbide dinitrate therapy on exercise capacity in congestive heart failure. *Am J Med* 69:559-566, 1980.
13. Franciosa JA, Mikulic E, Cohn JN, et al. Hemodynamic effect of orally administered isosorbide dinitrate in patients with congestive heart failure. *Circulation* 50:1020-1024, 1974.
14. Pierpont GL, Cohn JN, Franciosa JA. Combined oral hydralazinenitrate therapy in left ventricular failure. Hemodynamic equivalency to sodium nitroprusside. *Chest* 73:8-13, 1978.
15. Cohn JA, Rector TS. Prognosis of congestive heart failure and predictors of mortality. *Am J Cardiol* 62:25A-30A, 1988.
16. Cohn JA, Archibald DG, Ziesche S, et al. Effect of vasodilator therapy on mortality in chronic congestive heart failure. Results of a Veterans Administration Cooperative Study (V-HeFT). *N Engl J Med* 314:1547-1552, 1986.
17. The Captopril Multicenter Research Group I: A cooperative multicenter study of captopril in congestive heart failure: Hemodynamic effects and long-term response. *Am Heart J* 110:439-447, 1985.
18. Massie BM, Kramer BL, Topic N. Long-term captopril therapy for chronic congestive heart failure. *Am J Cardiol* 53:1316-1320, 1984.
19. Captropril Multicenter Research Group. A placebo-controlled trial of captropril in refractory chronic congestive heart failure. *J Am Coll Cardiol* 3:755-763, 1983.
20. Creager MA, Massie BM, Faxon DP, et al. Acute and long- term effects of enalapril on the cardiovascular response to exercise and exercise tolerance in patients with congestive heart failure. *J Am Coll Cardiol* 6:163-170, 1985.
21. The Captopril-Digoxin Multicenter Research Group. Comparative effects of therapy with captopril and digoxin in patients with mild to moderate heart failure. *J Am Med Assoc* 259:539- 544, 1988.
22. Beaune J. Comparison of enalapril versus digoxin for congestive heart failure. *Am J Cardiol* 63:22D-25D, 1989.
23. Evans DB, Weishaar RE, Kaplan H. Strategy for the discovery and development of a positive inotropic agent. *Pharmocol Ther* 16:303-330, 1982.
24. Chernow B, Rainey TG, Lake CR. Catecholamines in critical care medicine. In: Ziegler MG, Lake CR, ed. *Frontiers of Clinical Neuroscience. Volume 2, Norepinephrine.* Baltimore, MD: Williams and Wilkins; 1983:368-383.

25. Schmid PG, Eckstein JW, Abboud FM. Comparison of the effects of several sympathomimetic amines on resistance capacitance vessels in the forearm of man. *Circulation* 34: 209-210, 1966.
26. Motulsky JH, Insel PA: Adrenergic receptors in man. *N Engl J Med* 302:18-29, 1982.
27. Ariens EJ, Simonis AM. Physiological and pharmacological aspects of adrenergic receptor classification. *Biochem Pharmacol* 32:1539-1545, 1983.
28. Goldberg LI. Dopamine—clinical uses of an endogenous catecholamine. *N Engl J Med* 291:707, 1974.
29. Ramanthan S, Grant GJ. Vasopressor therapy for hypotension due to epidural anesthesia for cesarean section. *Acta Anaesthesiol Scand* 32:1-7, 1988.
30. Levitzki A. From epinephrine to cyclic Amp. *Science* 241:800-806, 1988.
31. Lawson N. The use of inotropes and vasopressors. *ASA Refresher Course in Anesthesiology* 18:195-223, 1990.
32. Bristow MR, Ginsberg R, Minobe W, et al. Decreased catecholamine sensibility and β-adrenergic receptor density in failing human hearts. *N Engl J Med* 307: 205-211, 1982.
33. Fowler Mm, Laser JA, Hopkins GL, et al. Assessment of the β-adrenergic receptor pathway down-regulation and subsensitivity to agonist response. *Circulation* 74:1290, 1986.
34. Marty J, Nimier M, Rocchiccioli C, et al. β-Adrenergic receptor function is acutely altered in surgical patients. *Anesth Analg* 71:1-8, 1990.
35. Kollgen H, Drexler H. Use of inotropes in the critical care setting. *Crit Care Med* 18(1):556-560, 1990.
36. Zimmerman BG, Abboud FM, Eckstein JW. Comparison of the effects of sympathomimetic amines upon venous and total vascular resistance in the foreleg of the dog. *J Pharmacol Exp Ther* 139:290-295, 1963.
37. Schwinn DA, Reves JG. Time course and hemodynamic effects of α_1 adrenergic bolus administration in anesthetized patients with myocardial disease. *Anesth Analg* 68(5):571-578, 1989.
38. Allwood MJ, Cobbold AF, Ginsburg J. Peripheral vascular effects of noradrenaline, isopropylnoradrenaline and dopamine. *Br Med Bull* 19:132, 1963.
39. Butterworth JF, Piccione W, Berrizibetia LD, et al. Augmentation of venous return by adrenergic agonists during spinal anesthesia. *Anesth Analg* 65:612-616, 1988.
40. Desjars P, Pinaud M, Potel G, et al. A reappraisal of norepinephrine therapy in human septic shock. *Crit Care Med* 15:134-137, 1987.
41. Meadows D, Edwards JD, Wilkins RG, et al. Reversal of intractable septic shock with norepinephrine therapy. *Crit Care Med* 16:663-666, 1988.
42. Robinson RJS, Tchervenkov C. Treatment of low cardiac output after aortocoronary artery bypass surgery using a combination of norepinephrine and amrinone. *J Cardiothorac Anesth* 3:229-233, 1987.

43. Jeff GK, Arcido J, Dorsey M, et al. Vasoactive drug effects on blood flow in internal mammary artery and saphenous vein grafts. *J Thorac Cardiovasc Surg* 94(1):2-11, 1987.
44. Stratton JR, Pfeifer MA, Ritchie JL, et al. Hemodynamic effects of epinephrine: concentration-effect study in humans. *J Appl Physiol* 58(4):1199-206, 1985.
45. Balderman SC, Aldridge J. Pharmacologic support of the myocardium following aortocoronary bypass surgery: a comparative study. *J Clin Pharmacol* 26:175, 1986.
46. Rude RE. Pharmacologic support in cardiogenic shock. *Adv Shock Res* 10:35, 1983.
47. Steen PA, Tinker JH, Pluth JR, et al. Efficacy of dopamine, dobutamine, and epinephrine during emergency from cardiopulmonary bypass in man. *Circulation* 57:378, 1978.
48. Maze M, Smith CM. Identification of receptor mechanism mediating epinephrine-induced arrhythmias during halothane anesthesia in the dog. *Anesthesiology* 59:322, 1983.
49. Kapur PA, Flacke WE. Epinephrine-induced arrhythmias and cardiovascular function after verapamil during halothane anesthesia in the dog. *Anesthesiology* 55:218, 1981.
50. Goldstein DS, Zimlichman R, Stull R, et al. Plasma catecholamine and hemodynamic responses during isoproterenol infusions in humans. *Pharmacol Ther* 40:233, 1986.
51. Furman WR, Summer WR, Kennedy TP, et al. Comparison of the effects of dobutamine, dopamine, and isoproterenol on hypoxic pulmonary vasoconstriction in the pig. *Crit Care Med* 10:371, 1982.
52. Schmidt DH, Blau FM, Hendrix LJ, et al. Myocardial perfusion after aortocoronary bypass surgery: Measurements at rest and after administration of isoproterenol. *Circulation* 71:767, 1985.
53. Clark RB, Brunner JA. Dopamine for the treatment of spinal hypotension during cesarean section. *Anesthesiology* 53:514-517, 1980.
54. Leier CV, Heban PT, Huss P, et al. Comparative systemic and regional hemodynamic effects of dopamine and dobutamine in patients with cardiomyopathic heart failure. *Circulation* 58:466-475, 1978.
55. Vincent J, Reuse C, Kahn RJ. Effects on right ventricular function of a change from dopamine to dobutamine in critically ill patients. *Crit Care Med* 16:659-662, 1988.
56. Loeb HS, Ostrenga JP, Gaul W, et al. Beneficial effects of dopamine combined with intravenous nitroglycerin on hemodynamics in patients with severe left ventricular failure. *Circulation* 68:813, 1983.
57. Schaer GL, Fink MP, Parrillo JE. Norepinephrine alone vs norepinephrine plus low-dose dopamine: Enhanced renal blood flow with combination pressor therapy. *Crit Care Med* 14:492- 496, 1985.
58. Beregovich J, Bianchi C, Rubler S, et al. Dose-related hemodynamic and renal effects of dopamine in congestive heart failure. *Am Heart J* 87:550, 1974.

59. Yeh BK, McNay JL, Goldberg LI. Attenuation of dopamine renal and mesenteric vasodilation by haloperidol: evidence for a specific dopamine receptor. *J Pharmacol Exp Ther* 168:303, 1969.
60. Leier CV, Heban PT, Huss P, et al. Comparative systemic and regional hemodynamic effects of dopamine and dobutamine in patients with cardiomyopathic heart failure. *Circulation* 58:466, 1978.
61. Goldberg LI. Cardiovascular and renal actions of dopamine: potential clinical applications. *Pharmacol Rev* 24:1, 1972.
62. Goldberg LI, Rajfer SI. Dopamine receptors: applications in clinical cardiology. *Circulation* 72:245, 1985.
63. Lucchesi BR. Inotropic agents and drugs to support the failing heart. In: Anonaccio M, ed. *Cardiovascular Pharmacology*. New York, NY: Raven Press; 1977:337-375.
64. Toda N, Goldberg LI. Effects of dopamine on isolated canine coronary arteries. *Cardiovasc Res* 9:384, 1975.
65. Brooks HL, Stein PD, Matson JL, et al. Dopamine-induced alterations in coronary hemodynamics in dogs. *Circ Res* 24:699, 1969.
66. Goldberg LI, Hsieh Y, Resnekov L. Newer catecholamines for treatment of heart failure and shock: an update on dopamine and a first look at dobutamine. *Prog Cardiovasc Dis* 19:327, 1977.
67. Maekawa K, Liang C-S, Hood WB. Comparison of dobutamine and dopamine in acute myocardial infarction: effects of systemic hemodynamics, plasma catecholamines, blood flows, and infarct size. *Circulation* 67:750, 1983.
68. Stephenson LW, Blackstone EH, Kouchoukos NT. Dopamine vs epinephrine in patients following cardiac surgery: randomized study. *Surg Forum* 27:272, 1976.
69. Harari A, Martin E, Bouvier AM, et al. Decreased dopamine-β-hydroxylase activity in septic shock. *Anesthesiology* 51:S155, 1979.
70. Ruffolo RR, Yaden EL. Vascular effects of the stereoisomers of dobutamine. *J Pharmacol Exp Ther* 224:46-51,1982.
71. Gillespie TA, Ambos HD, Sobel BE, et al. Effects of dobutamine in patients with acute myocardial infarction. *Am J Cardiol* 39:588, 1977.
72. Lipman J, Plit M. A guide to the rational use of dopamine, dobutamine, and isoprenaline in patients who need inotropic support. *S Afr Med J* 65:506, 1984.
73. Butterworth J, Prielipp R, Zaloga G, et al. Is dobutamine less chronotropic than epinephrine after coronary bypass surgery? *Anesthesiology* A61, 1990, V73, 1003A.
74. Amin DK, Shah PK, Shellock FG, et al. Comparative hemodynamic effects of intravenous dobutamine and MDL 17,043, a new cardioactive drug, in severe congestive heart failure. *Am Heart J* 109:91-98, 1985.
75. Unverferth DV, Blanford M, Kates RE, et al. Tolerance to dobutamine after a 72-hour continuous infusion. *Am J Med* 69:262, 1980.
76. El Allaf D, Cremers S, D'Orio D, et al. Combined hemodynamic effects of low doses of dopamine and dobutamine in patients with acute

infarction and cardiac failure. *Arch Int Physiol Biochem* 92:S49-S59, 1984.
77. Uretsky BF, Lawless CE, Verbalis JG, et al. Combined therapy with dobutamine and amrinone in severe heart failure. *Chest* 92:657-662, 1987.
78. Makabali C, Weill MH, Henning RJ. Dobutamine and other sympathomimetic drugs for the treatment of low output cardiac failure. *Semin Anesth* 1:63-69, 1982.
79. d'Hollander A, Primo G, Hennart D, et al. Compared efficacy of dobutamine and dopamine in association with calcium chloride on termination of cardiopulmonary bypass. *J Thorac Cardiovasc Surg* 83:264, 1982.
80. Bull J, Band DM. Calcium and cardiac arrest. *Anesthesiology* 35:1006, 1980.
81. Shapira N, Scharf HV, White RD, et al. Hemodynamic effects of calcium chloride injection following cardiopulmonary bypass: response to bolus injection and continuous infusion. *Ann Thorac Surg* 37:133-140, 1984.
82. Gain KR, Appleman MM. Distribution and regulation of the phosphodiesterases of muscle tissues. In: George WJ, Ignarro LJ, eds. *Advances in Cyclic Nucleotide Research*. New York, NY: Raven Press: 1978:221-231.
83. Weishaar RE, Burrows SD, Kobylarz DC, et al. Multiple molecular forms of cyclic nucleotide phosphodiesterase in cardiac and smooth muscle and in platelets. Isolation, characterization, and effects of various reference phosphodiesterase inhibitors and cardiotonic agents. *Biochem Pharmacol* 35:787-800, 1986.
84. Alousi AA, Johnson DC. Pharmacology of the bipyridines: amrinone and milrinone. *Circulation* 73:III-10, 1986.
85. Konstam MA, Cohen SR, Weiland DS et al. Relative contribution of inotropic and vasodilator effects to amrinone-induced hemodynamic improvement in congestive heart failure. *Am J Cardiol* 57:242, 1986.
86. Benotti JR, Grossman W, Braunwald E, et al. Hemodynamic assessment of amrinone. *N Engl J Med* 299:1371-1377, 1987.
87. Benotti JR, Grossman W, Braunwald E, et al. Effects of amrinone on myocardial energy metabolism and hemodynamics in patients with severe congestive heart failure due to coronary artery disease. *Circulation* 62:28-36, 1980.
88. Colucci WS, Wright RF, Braunwald E. New positive inotropic agents in the treatment of congestive heart failure: mechanisms of action and recent clinical developments. *N Engl J Med* 314:349-358, 1986.
89. Likoff MJ, Weber KT, Andrews V, et al. Amrinone: a promising new cardiotonic agent in the treatment of chronic cardiac failure. *Herz* 8:199, 1983.
90. Olsen KH, Kluger J, Fieldman A. Combination high-dose amrinone and dopamine in the management of moribund cardiogenic shock after open heart surgery. *Chest* 94:503-506, 1988.

91. Gage J, Rutman H, Lucido D, et al. Additive effects of dobutamine and amrinone on myocardial contractility and ventricular performance in patients with severe heart failure. *Circulation* 74:367-373, 1986.
92. Robinson RS, Tchervenkov C. Treatment of low cardiac output after aortocoronary bypass surgery using a combination of norepinephrine and amrinone. *J Cardiol Anesth* 1:229-233, 1987.
93. Nakatuska M, Mobleg R. The combined use of noradrenalin, amrinone and nitroglycerine in the management of severe low cardiac output after coronary artery surgery. *Anaesth Intensive Care* 16:458-487, 1988.
94. Hess W, Arnold B, Veit S. The haemodynamic effects of amrinone in patients with mitral stenosis and pulmonary hypertension. *Eur Heart J* 7:800, 1986.
95. Deeb GM, Bolling SF, Guynn TP, et al. Amrinone versus conventional therapy in pulmonary hypertensive patients awaiting cardiac transplantation. *Ann Thorac Surg* (in press).
96. Bolling SF, Deeb GM, Crowley OC, et al. Prolonged amrinone therapy prior to orthotopic cardiac transplantation in patients with pulmonary hypertension. *Transplant Proc* 20:753-756, 1989.
97. Levy JH, Bailey JM, Rogers G, et al. Amrinone: is the recommended dose appropriate? (abstract) Society of Cardiovascular Anesthesiologists, 1990.
98. Goenen M, Pedemonte O, Baele P, et al. Amrinone in the management of low cardiac output after open heart surgery. *Am J Cardiol* 56:33B-38B, 1985.
99. Smith VE, Katz AM. Inotropic and lusitropic abnormalities as the basis for heart failure. *Heart Failure* 3(2):55-56, 1987.
100. Ansell J, Tiarks C, McCue J, et al. Amrinone induced thrombocytopenia. *Arch Intern Med* 144:949-952, 1984.
101. Hines R, Brasch PB. Amrinone associated thrombocytopenia: does it occur with short term adminstration? *Anesthesiology* 67(Suppl 3A):A599, 1987.
102. Alousi AA, Stankus GP, Stuart JC, et al. Characterization of the cardiotonic effects of milrinone, a new and potent cardiac bipyridine, on isolated tissues from several animal species. *J Cardiovasc Pharmacol* 5:804, 1983.
103. LeJemtel TH, Maskin CS, Mancini D, et al. Systemic and regional hemodynamic effects of captopril and milrinone administered alone and concomitantly in patients with heart failure. *Circulation* 72:364, 1985.
104. Monrad ES, Baim DS, Smith HS, et al. Effects of milrinone on coronary hemodynamics and myocardial energetics in patients with congestive heart failure. *Circulation* 71:972, 1985.
105. Drexler H, Faude F, Winterer H, et al. Central and regional vascular effects of milrinone in experimental heart failure: comparison to captopril and dobutamine. *Z Kardiol* 76:507, 1987.

106. Drexler H, Faude F, Hoing BS, et al. Blood flow redistribution within skeletal muscle during exercise in the presence of chronic heart failure: effect of milrinone. *Circulation* 76:1344, 1987.
107. Leier VC, Meiler SEL, Matthews S, et al. A preliminary report of the effects of orally administered enoximone on regional hemodynamics in congestive heart failure. *Am J Cardiol* 60:27C, 1987.
108. Choraria SK, Taylor D, Pilcher J. Double-blind crossover comparison of enoximone and placebo in patients with congestive heart failure. *Circulation* 76:1307, 1987.
109. Kapur PA. Calcium channel blockers. In: Stoelting RK, Barash PG, Gallagher TJ. eds. *Advances in Anesthesia*. Chicago, IL: Year Book Medical Publishers; 1985:167-206.
110. Kapur PA, Matarazzo DA, Fung DM, et al. The cardiovascular and adrenergic actions of verapamil or diltiazem in combination with propranolol during halothane anesthesia. *Anesthesiology* 66:122-129, 1987.
111. Merin RG: Calcium channel blocking drugs and anesthetics: is the drug interaction beneficial or detrimental? *Anesthesiology* 66:111-113, 1987.
112. Slogoff S, Keats AS. Does chronic treatment with calcium entry blocking drugs reduce perioperative myocardial ischemia? *Anesthesiology* 68:676-680, 1988.
113. Tosaki A, Szekeres L, Hearse DJ. Diltiazem and the reduction of reperfusion-induced arrhythmias in the rat: protection is secondary to modification of ischemia injury and heart rate. *J Molec Cell Cardiol* 19:441-451, 1987.
114. Menkhaus PG, Reves JG, Kissin I, et al. Cardiovascular effects of esmolol in anesthetized humans. *Anesth Analg* 64:327-334, 1985.
115. Bexton RS, Milne JR, Cory-Pearce R, et al. Effect of β blockade on exercise response after cardiac transplantation. *Br Heart J* 49:584, 1983.
116. Wallace AC, Schaal SF, Sugimoto G, et al. Electrophysiological effects of β-adrenergic blockade in cardiac denervation. *Bull NY Acad Med* 43:1119, 1967.
117. Reilly CS, Wood M, Koshakji RP, et al. Ultra-short-acting β-blockade: a comparison with conventional β-blockade. *Clin Pharmacol Ther* 38:579-585, 1985.
118. Gray RJ, Bateman TM, Czer LSC, et al. Use of esmolol in hypertension after cardiac surgery. *Am J Cardiol* 56:49F-56F, 1985.
119. Reves JG, Flezzani P. Perioperative use of esmolol. *Am J Cardiol* 56:57F-62F, 1985.
120. Gagnon RM, Morissett M, Priesant S, et al. Hemodynamic and coronary effects of intravenous labetalol in coronary artery disease. *Am J Cardiol* 49:1267, 1982.
121. Weidmann P, DeChiatel R, Ziegler WH, et al. α- and β-Adrenergic blockade with orally administered labetalol in hypertension. *Am J Cardiol* 41:570, 1978.

122. Taylor RR, Covell JW, Sonnenblick EH, et al. Dependence of ventricular distensibility effect on filling of the opposite ventricle. *Am J Physiol* 218:711, 1967.
123. Laver MB. Myocardial ischemia: dilemma between information available and information demand. *Br Heart J* 50:222-230, 1983.
124. Laver MB, Strauss WH, Robost GM. Herbert Shubin Memorial Lectures. Right and left ventricular geometry: adjustments during acute respiratory failure. *Crit Care Med* 7:509-516, 1975.
125. Ghignone M, Girling L, Prewitt R. Volume expansion versus norepinephrine in treatment of a low cardiac output complicating an acute increase in right ventricular aferload in dogs. *Anesthesiology* 69:132-135, 1984.
126. Dell'Italia L, Starling M, Blomhardt R, et al. Comparative effects of volume loading dobutamine and nitroprusside in patients with predominant RV infarction. *Circulation* 72:1327-1335, 1985.
127. D'Ambra M, La Raia P, Phellen D, et al. Prostaglandin El—a new therapy for refractory right heart failure and pulmonary hypertension after mitral valve replacement. *J Thorac Cardiovasc Surg* 89:567-572, 1985.
128. McLean R, Prielipp R, Rosenthal M, et al. Vasodilator therapy in microembolus procaine pulmonary hypertension. *Anesth Analg* 71:35-41, 1990.
129. Lowenstein E, Johnson W, Lappas D, et al. Catastrophic pulmonary vasoconstriction associated with the reversal of heparin. *Anesthesiology* 59:470-473, 1983.
130. Jardin F, Farcot JC, Boisanti C, et al. Influence of positive end expiratory pressure on left ventricular performance. *N Engl J Med* 304:387-392, 1981.
131. Biondi JW, Hines RL, Matthay RA, et al. Comparative right ventricular function during assist control, intermittent mandators and spontaneous ventilation. *Anesth Analg* 65:518, 1986.
132. Miller DC, Moreno-Cabral RT, Stinson EB, et al. Pulmonary artery balloon counterpulsation for acute right ventricular infarction. *J Thorac Cardiovasc Surg* 80:760-763, 1980.

Chapter 16

Vasodilator Therapy During Cardiopulmonary Bypass

George N. Vretakis, MD,
Phillip Fyman, MD,
and Charles M. Fermon, MD

Hypothermic cardiopulmonary bypass causes significant physiologic alterations, among them changes in the systemic vascular resistance (SVR). These alterations are not a reflection of inadequate anesthesia but rather a consequence of the actions of the bypass. To minimize the adverse effects, vasodilators are often used. Proper use of these drugs requires an understanding of both bypass-induced changes and drug actions.

Components of the Systemic Vascular Resistance and Bypass Effects

Arteriolar tone is a primary determinant of SVR and is regulated by the neuroendocrine and renin-angiotensin systems. During

From Casthely PA, Bregman D, (eds): *Cardiopulmonary Bypass: Physiology, Related Complications, and Pharmacology.* Mount Kisco, NY, Futura Publishing Company, Inc., © 1991.

cardiopulmonary bypass, nonvascular components such as temperature, packed red blood cell volume, red blood cell rheology, plasma viscosity, cardiac output, pump flow rate,[1-3] and the type of pump flow (pulsatile vs. nonpulsatile)[4] also influence the SVR.

At the initiation of cardiopulmonary bypass, hemodilution acutely decreases the plasma viscosity by lowering the hematocrit and the fibrinogen concentration.[2,3,5,6] The lowered viscosity results in a drop in the SVR, which may lower the perfusion pressure to the major organs. As cardiopulmonary bypass continues, the SVR rises primarily because of vasoconstriction.

The sympathoadrenal and renin-angiotensin systems are key elements in this increase in arteriolar tone.[7-11] The circulating catecholamine concentration increases during cardiopulmonary bypass. In fact, a substantial rise in catechol levels occurs as cardiopulmonary bypass is instituted,[12] which may be secondary to an inability of the lungs to extract circulating epinephrine and norepinephrine from the blood as a result of their exclusion from the circulation. Another contributing factor may be the myocardial hypoxia and acidosis that develop as the heart is bypassed. This triggers a cardiac reflex[12] involving the sympathetic efferent limb, which causes the adrenomedullary release of epinephrine and regional sympathetic discharge of norepinephrine during the period that the aorta is cross clamped.[13] Because the circulating concentration of epinephrine exceeds that of norepinephrine by a ratio of four to one, the adrenomedullary system bears the predominant responsibility for this increase in the vascular resistance.[12] A third explanation is that hypothermia cools the fibers that send vagal afferent impulses to the cardiovascular centers of the medulla, effectively blocking input from the arterial and cardiac baroreceptors.[14] Therefore, the mean arterial pressure (MAP) rises steadily.

The renin-angiotensin system also influences the peripheral vascular resistance. During cardiopulmonary bypass, circulating levels of angiotensin II increase[1,15,16] when the granular cells of the renal juxtaglomerular apparatus secrete renin in response to the decreases in blood volume, renal perfusion, serum sodium concentration, or delivery of sodium chloride to the macula densa.[4,17,18] This renin promotes the conversion of angiotensinogen to angiotensin I. In the lungs, angiotensin I is converted into the potent vasoconstrictor angiotensin II, which then causes an increase in MAP not only by increasing the SVR, but also by stimulating aldosterone secretion. Aldosterone promotes sodium resorption by the distal renal tubules and collecting ducts. Water passively follows the reabsorbed sodium and expands the intravascular volume, leading to an increased MAP.

The sympathetic nervous system can also activate the renin-angiotensin-aldosterone system. Epinephrine and norepinephrine, in concentrations found in the plasma during cardiopulmary bypass, increase the renal vascular resistance, which decreases renal blood flow. In response to this decrease in perfusion,[19] the juxtaglomerular apparatus secretes renin. As noted, this ultimately results in raising the serum angiotensin II levels.[15] In this way, an increase in sympathetic outflow leads to an increase in angiotensin II. Moreover, local vasoconstriction in the superficial cortex induces the kidney to retain sodium[8] resulting in intravascular volume expansion and increased MAP.

The renin-angiotensin system nevertheless appears to have an effect on the SVR independent of the neuroendocrine axis, as captopril, an angiotensin-converting enzyme inhibitor, significantly decreases the MAP.[16] During cardiopulmonary bypass, the MAP varies directly with the SVR assuming the pump flow is constant. With specific blocking of the renin-angiotensin system, the SVR falls independent of any effect on the sympathetic nervous system.

The type of pump flow also affects the total SVR. For example, nonpulsatile cardiopulmonary bypass produces a greater increase in the peripheral vascular resistance than does pulsatile bypass.[9] Also, nonpulsatile flow causes an increase in angiotensin II,[9] epinephrine, norepinephrine, and renin levels, whereas pulsatile flow diminishes renin stimulation.[4]

During hypothermic cardiopulmonary bypass, other factors also raise the SVR. Hypothermia, for example, raises the vascular resistance by promoting both vasoconstriction and an increase in the plasma viscosity.[20] Serotonin, circulating freely in the plasma after being released from platelets that are destroyed during passage through the bypass pump, increases the SVR solely by inducing vasoconstriction.[21] Elevated levels of arginine vasopressin, which also occur during cardiopulmonary bypass, likewise promote vasoconstriction.[22]

On the other hand, the red blood cell concentration primarily determines the viscosity. Increased rouleaux formation directly raises the viscosity.[3] Moreover, any elevation of the plasma fibrinogen concentration enables the red blood cells to aggregate more easily and magnifies rouleaux formation.[3,5] To a lesser extent, elevated plasma protein concentrations, decreased erythrocyte flexibility, and narrowed blood vessel lumens increase the viscosity of blood.[5]

The plasma cortisol concentration increases after the initial phase of cardiopulmonary bypass.[12,23] At the inception of bypass, cortisol concentrations decrease secondary to hemodilution. As bypass continues, however, the adrenal cortex secretes greater amounts of cortisol into the plasma.[23] Marked rises in the circulating plasma levels of antidiuretic hormone also occur in response to the stress of bypass.[23]

In view of this heightened stress response, some clinicians believe that the hemodynamic changes outlined above are secondary to an inadequate depth of anesthesia. However, several studies[24-26] suggest that no plasma concentration of narcotic will block the increases in cortisol, epinephrine, norepinephrine, or vasopressin levels during cardiopulmonary bypass. Not only does the SVR increase progressively during bypass, but the potential for marked elevations in MAP exists. Also, there appears to be a heightened response to phenylephrine, and probably vasopressors in general, during hypothermic cardiopubnonary bypass.[20] This results from an increased sensitivity of the peripheral vasculature to vasoconstrictors, irrespective of the amount of anesthetic administered to the patient.

Except for using a rapidly acting angiotensin-converting enzyme inhibitor to block the renin-angiotensin system, the only options for treating hypertension during cardiopulmonary bypass are to decrease the pump flow or to counteract the increasing peripheral vascular resistance with vasodilators. Because there is a limit to how much one can reduce the pump flow, and because lowering the flow rate of the pump can raise SVR by increasing the plasma viscosity, vasodilators are frequently used. The ensuing reduction of the SVR permits higher pump flows and potentially better perfusion of vital organs during hypothermic cardiopulmonary bypass.[26,27] There are numerous drugs to choose from. Although they may all be classified as "vasodilators," they differ with regard to mechanism and site of action, systemic effects, toxicity, and other features. In order to obtain the maximum benefit from these drugs, it is important to appreciate the differences.

Sodium Nitroprusside

In 1929, Johnson first documented the usefulness of sodium nitroprusside (SNP) in the treatment of hypertension in humans.[28] In spite of its known efficacy, however, its use was limited because of the fear of cyanide (CN) toxicity. A renewed interest in SNP developed in the 1920s when various studies demonstrated its ability to improve cardiac function in patients with left ventricular failure,[29,30] and the US Food and Drug Administration (FDA) approved SNP for clinical use as an antihypertensive in 1974. Because of its potential for the treatment of cardiac dysfunction and its capacity to control blood pressure precisely, it was enthusiastically received and has been extensively used.

Action

Sodium nitroprusside is remarkably specific for the relaxation of vascular smooth muscle,[31] resulting in vasodilatation of both arteries and veins. However, its exact mechanism of action is not known. Needleman et al.[32] have obtained data from studies of aortic strips that support the hypothesis that SNP, along with other vasodilators, acts on the outer membrane via sulfhydryl (SH) receptors. Because of its rapid (almost immediate) onset and short duration (2-3 minutes) of action, it is likely that SNP itself and not a metabolite is responsible for vasodilatation.

Toxicity

The potential for toxicity with SNP is apparent when one considers its chemical structure, ($Na_2[Fe(CN)_5(NO)]^2H_20$) (Fig. 1), which contains five CN groups. Through an unknown mechanism, the molecule is rapidly broken down in the blood, and CN is released. This is converted to thiocyanate by a mitochondrial enzyme system, rhodanese, which facilitates the transfer of CN to sulfur. Thiocyanate is ultimately excreted in the urine.

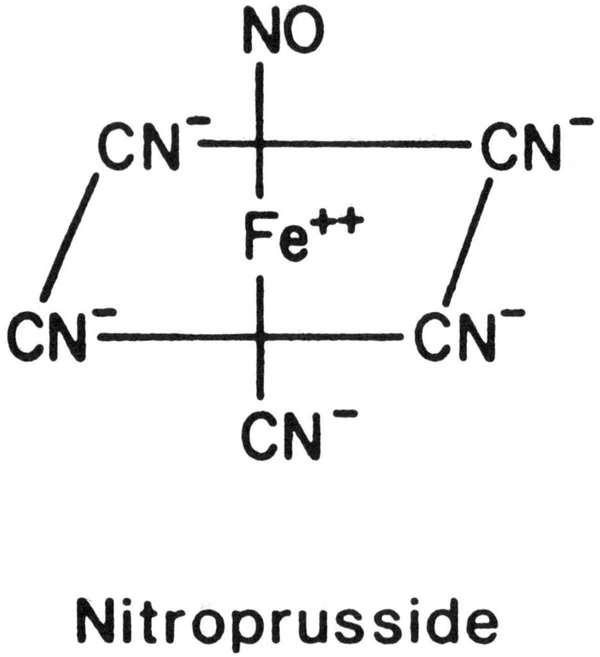

Figure 1.

In order to prevent CN toxicity, a sulfur donor and functioning rhodanese system therefore are needed. Certain pathologic sites exist in which CN and thiocyanate metabolism are abnormal, and use of SNP is therefore contraindicated. These include Leber's optic atrophy, tobacco amblyopia, severe liver disease, hypothyroidism, malnutrition, vitamin B_{12} deficiency, and severe renal disease.

In attempting to prevent or treat CN toxicity, the goal is to prevent CN binding with cytochrome C and to remove CN from the blood. Several different approaches are possible. Infusion of thiolsulfate, which serves as a sulfur donor, is effective as the sulfur binds with CN to form thiocyanate. Methemoglobin can be formed with the administration of sodium nitrite. The compound cyanomethemoglobin results, freeing more cytochrome C and permitting more aerobic respiration. Cottrell et al.[33] demonstrated that an infusion of hydroxocobalamin decreases erythrocyte CN levels and tissue hypoxia during SNP administration when the hydroxocobalamin combines with the CN.

Diagnosing CN toxicity may be difficult. Metabolic acidosis is usually the earliest sign, and, if this condition is unexplained, SNP should be discontinued. Cyanide and thiocyanate levels are frequently difficult to measure and the results may be misleading, precluding their use as a diagnostic tool.

Various maximum doses of SNP have been recommended, ranging from 1 mg to a total of 3.5 mg. Rarely does toxicity result with an infusion rate of 3 mcg/kg per minute or less.

Nitroglycerin

Nitroglycerin (NTG) was first synthesized in 1846 by Sobrero, but it was not until 1897 that William Murrel established its usefulness in the treatment of angina pectoris. The drug is effective when applied to the skin or mucous membranes or administered intravenously. For this reason, it is available in various forms: tablets, ointment, aerosol, and injectable solution. The intravenous has been commercially available since 1981.

Action

After IV administration of NTG, there is a rapid distribution and metabolism of the drug. Its half-life is short, as indicated by the rapid return of the hemodynamic alterations almost to normal. This occurred within 9 minutes in one study[34] and within 6 minutes in another.[29]

The exact mechanism by which NTG works at the cellular level is unclear. It has been postulated that the drug interacts with a specific receptor in the vascular wall.[32] The effect is then mediated via a pathway common to all vasodilators, which is activated by an SH receptor. Although venodilatation is the predominant effect, arteriolar dilatation also can occur, especially with higher doses.[35,36] This is in contrast to the effect of SNP, which affects the venous and arteriolar beds equally[37]

Toxicity

The liver is the prinicpal site of NTG degradation.[38] This reaction is dependent on the enzyme organic nitrate reductase, and only partial denitration occurs. Because of the liver's large capacity to metabolize NTG, metabolism is in the one-pass category. What effect liver disease has on NTG metabolism is unknown. Partial denitration can produce methemoglobin, but the clinical significance of this has not been determined, and methemoglobinemia must be rare.

Hypotension is the most common adverse effect of NTG and is dose-related. When the drug is discontinued, the effect is rapidly reversed. No other toxicities of NTG are known. Acute withdrawal symptoms have been noted in munition workers after long-term NTG exposure but this effect has not been reported after stopping of nitrates in patients with classic angina pectoris.[39]

Calcium Entry Blockers

Calcium entry blockers (CEBs) that can cause vasodilatation have been used in the treatment of Prinzmetal's angina,[40,41] classic angina,[42,43] hypertension,[44] and dysrhythmias.[45,46]

In view of the key role that calcium ion plays in the electromechanical activity in many cardiovascular functions, it is not surprising that alteration of calcium fluxes by CEBs can modify many of these activities. Although these agents are grouped in one broad category and all decrease the levels of intracellular calcium, their mechanisms of action may be different. For example, it is postulated that diltiazem acts by stimulating calcium extrusion, whereas verapamil works by inhibiting calcium influx. Possibly because of the different mechanisms of action, the various CEBs have different potencies in affecting coronary vascular tone, electrical activity, and myocardial contractility. Because of this difference in selectivity, one agent may be preferable to another in particular circumstances.

Phentolamine

Regitine

Phentolamine was introduced into clinical practice as an antihypertensive agent. Its action is mediated through α-adrenergic blockade. Although some investigators felt that phentolamine also had some intrinsic β-agonist activity,[47] it now appears that increases in inotropy and heart rate are reflexively induced.[48] The beneficial effects of phentolamine-induced afterload reduction in patients with congestive heart failure have been demonstrated. In patients with left ventricular failure secondary to ischemic heart disease, 5 mg was administered as a bolus intravenously, and an infusion of 1-2 mg/min was started until the MAP was decreased to 95-105 mmHg. Systemic vascular resistance and left ventricular end diastolic pressure were decreased significantly, whereas cardiac output increased significantly, and the heart rate remained unchanged. The drug's ability to improve low cardiac output states associated with high SVR was subsequently confirmed. Forearm vascular resistance and venous tone were also measured to determine the site of drug action. It was found that phentolamine predominantly affects the systemic arterial vessels, NTG predominantly affects venous vessels, and SNP's action is balanced between arterial and venous vessels.

Sodium nitroprusside and NTG have largely replaced phentolamine in clinical situations requiring vasodilators, mainly because of their easier titratability and higher potency.

Trimethaphan

Arfonad

Action

Trimethaphan, a vasodilator, was introduced into clinical practice in 1953. Indications for administration include treatment of hypertension, induced hypotension, and severe vasoconstriction. The drug's effects are mediated through direct vasodilatation and ganglionic blockade.[49] Coronary and renal blood flows are decreased to a greater extent by trimethalphan-induced hypotension than by SNP-induced hypotension. Bradycardia secondary to inhibition of cardiac sympathetic fibers can be beneficial through its improvement of myocardial oxygen balance. This contrasts with reflex tachycardia that can be produced by most of the other vasodilators.

Toxicity

There are a number of undesirable side effects associated with trimethaphan infusion. These effects are secondary to ganglionic blockade and include bladder and intestinal atony, xerostomia, and anhidrosis. Cycloplegia can also occur, which may hinder the postoperative evaluation of the patient undergoing neurosurgery or open heart surgery.

Tachyphylaxis is a common problem, and none of the many counteractants has been successful. These techniques include use of intermittent bolus doses of trimethaphan during infusion, increasing the rate or concentration of the infusion, and phenoxybenzamine, guanethidine, and halothane administration.

Because of the drawbacks associated with trimethaphan usage, other vasodilators are more commonly used.

Hydralazine

Hydralazine is a direct-acting vascular smooth-muscle relaxant that has a predominant effect on arterial beds and no direct action on the heart. The vasodilatory effects are not uniform, being more pronounced in the coronary, cerebral, renal, and splanchnic circulations.

Although its most frequent indication is control of hypertension, hydralazine has been used perioperatively as a vasodilator. Hydralazine 2.5-5 mg was administered intravenously to cardiac surgical patients with a low cardiac index, an elevated SVR, and high pulmonary capillary wedge pressure. After administration of hydralazine, there was a significant increase in cardiac index with a significant decrease in SVR and essentially no change in blood pressure or PCWP.

The peak hemodynamic effects of hydralazine may not occur for 60 minutes. Intraoperatively or in the immediate postoperative period, a faster response is frequently desired, and for this reason, other vasodilators that have a faster onset of action and are easier to titrate usually are administered.

Miscellaneous Agents

Potent Inhalation Agents

Isoflurane,[51] enflurane, and halothane[52] are inhalation anesthetics that cause vasodilation through their relaxant effect on smooth muscle and their depression of the central nervous system, inhibiting sympathetic activity and decreasing vascular tone. However, their potencies differ in this respect, isoflurane producing the most profound vasodilatation, enflurane being intermediate, and halothane resulting in the least decrease in vascular resistance. This effect is dose-related, and may be affected by the duration of anesthesia in the case of halothane. That is, vasodilatation increases with the duration of halothane administration, whereas the vasodilatation produced by isoflurane is unrelated to duration of anesthesia.

Although all the potent inhalation agents produce coronary artery vasodilation, isoflurane has a greater effect than halothane[53] or enflurane.[54] Their effects on myocardial perfusion are likewise not uniform. Whereas isoflurane increases myocardial perfusion, equipotent doses of halothane decrease it.[55] Isoflurane may result in a coronary steal phenomenon in patients with atherosclerotic heart disease.[56-58] In studies of patients with stable coronary artery disease who were undergoing major vascular procedures, coronary perfusion pressure was decreased during isoflurane adminstration with coronary blood flow being unchanged, indicating a reduction in coronary vascular resistance. However, in one study 10 out of 21 patients developed ECG and metabolic alterations consistent with ischemia. Patients who did not develop ECG changes did not experience any metabolic changes indicative of ischemia, i.e., a decrease in lactate extraction. The investigators concluded that isoflurane may cause a redistribution of myocardial blood flow, resulting in regional ischemia in patients with coronary artery disease. However, the decrease in coronary perfusion pressure could not be ruled out as the cause of these alterations.

These findings were supported in a canine model of chronic coronary occlusion. Regional myocardial perfusion was assessed by 9-μm radioactive microspheres, and regional contraction was measured with piezoelectric crystal sets. During isoflurane administration, there was a decrease in coronary vascular resistance, with total coronary flow remaining the same. However, there was a redistribution of flow from the collateral dependent zone to the normal zone. In addition, contractility decreased in the collateral zone and increased in the normally perfused area. This study provides further evidence that isoflurane may cause intracoronary steal in patients with critical coronary artery stenosis.

The potent inhalation agents have been administered as vasodilators during cardiopulmonary bypass via a vaporizer interposed in the oxygen line. However, all of these agents can cause significant myocardial depression.[59-62] With the availability of vasodilators that have no direct effect on myocardial contractility, the use of potent inhalation agents has become less frequent during and after cardiopulmonary bypass, a time when contractility may already be impaired by various metabolic abnormalities, such as ischemic arrest during aortic cross-clamping, hypothermia, trauma from manual manipulation, and cardioplegia solution.

Chlorpromazine

Chlorpromazine is a major tranquilizer with α blocking action. It has been used during cardiopulmonary bypass as a vasodilator to permit higher pump flows when vasoconstriction limits this. The hemodynamic effects of chlorpromazine-induced vasodilatation have been investigated in cardiac surgical patients in the early postoperative period.[26] The cardiac index increased 26% with a decrease in SVR of 31%. However, there was an increase heart rate of 20%, which could increase in myocardial oxygen consumption, offsetting the beneficial effects. Because of this and the production of sedation, which may not be desired, and the lesser control over hemodynamics than is possible with SNP or NTG, chlorpromazine is less frequently used than in the past for its vasodilating effect.

Droperidol

Droperidol possesses α blocking activity and has been used to treat increases in SVR during cardiopulmonary bypass. One study[63] used dosages of 0.15 mg/kg to 0.30 mg/kg, which resulted in transient decreases in the blood pressure secondary to α-adrenergic blockade[64] that were not dose-dependent. The magnitude of the blood pressure decline was greatest when the preinjection level of the peripheral vascular resistance was the highest. Therefore, droperidol exerted its greatest effects during nonpulsatile cardiopulmonary bypass. Moreover, injection via the bypass oxygenator, an intra-arterial injection, resulted in a quicker and a more prolonged decrease in MAP, than intravenously administered droperidol. Such injections via the oxygenator blunted peripheral vasoconstriction attributable to epinephrine and norepinephrine for a period of about 10 minutes.[65]

In addition to this transitory effect on the arteriolar resistance vessels, there was an increase in venous capacitance secondary to venous dilatation. This effect, although not as rapid as that on the arterioles, lasted longer[63] and theoretically could have proved detrimental during bypass if significant reduction in the blood return to the bypass pump occurred.

Conclusion

Hypothermic cardiopulmonary bypass induces a number of changes, among them hypertension. This undesirable effect is often counteracted with vasodilators. Sodium nitroprusside and nitroglycerin are among the most popular drugs for this application because of the precision with which their effects can be controlled. Their use, like that of other vasodilators, requires a clear understanding both of the specific effects one wishes to achieve and of the peculiarities of each drug.

REFERENCES

1. Thacker U, Geary V, Chalmers P, et al. Low systemic vascular resistance during cardiac surgery: case reports, brief review, and management with angiotensin II. *J Cardiothorac Anesth* 4:360-363, 1990.
2. Putman EA, Manners JM. Vascular resistance during cardiopulmonary bypass. *Anaesthesia* 38:635-643, 1983.
3. Putnam TC, Kevy SV, Replogle RL. Factors influencing the viscosity of blood. *Surg Gynecol Obstet* 124:547-552, 1967.
4. Landymore W, Murphy DA, Kinley CE, et al. Does pulsatile flow influence the incidence of postoperative hypertension. *Ann Thorac Surg* 28: 261-266, 1979.
5. Editorial: haemorheology, blood flow and venous thrombosis *Lancet* 2:113-114, 1975.
6. Gordon RJ, Ravin M, Rawitshcher RE, et al. Changes in arterial pressure, viscosity, and resistance during cardiopulmonary bypass. *J Thorac Cardiovasc Surg* 69:552-561, 1974.
7. Hayase S, Shimizu T, Nakajima M. Role of sympathoadrenal and renin-angiotensin system in hemodynamic state after coronary artery bypass grafting. *Nagoya J Med Sci* 49:1-15, 1987.
8. Diedericks BJS, Roelofse JA, Shipton EA, et al. The renin-angiotensin-aldosterone system during and after cardiopulmonary bypass. *S Afr Med J* 64:946-949, 1983.
9. Taylor KM, Bain WH, Morton JJ. The role of angiotensin II in the development of peripheral vasoconstriction during open heart surgery. *Am Heart J* 100:935-936, 1980.
10. Taylor KM, Casals JG, Mitra SM, et al. Hemodynamic effects of angiotensin-converting enzyme inhibition after cardiopulmonary bypass in dogs. *Cardiovasc Res* 40:199-205, 1980.
11. Gray RJ. Post-cardiac surgical hypertension. *J Cardiothorac Anesth* 5:678-682, 1988.
12. Brown AM. Coronary pressor reflexes. *Am J Cardiol* 44:849, 1979.
13. Reves JG, Karp RB, Buttner EE, et al. Neuronal and adrenomedullary catecholamine release in response to cardiopulmonary bypass in man. *Circulation* 66:49-55, 1982.
14. Donald DE, Shepherd JT. Cardiac receptors: normal and disturbed function. *Am J Cardiol* 44:873, 1979.
15. Taylor KM, Morton IJ, Brown JJ, et al. Hypertension and the renin-angiotensin systems following open heart surgery. *J Thorac Cardiovas Surg* 74:840-845, 1977.
16. Taylor KM, Brannan JJ, Bain WH, et al. Vasoconstriction during cardiopulmonary bypass. *Cardiovasc Res* 13:269-273, 1979.
17. Covino BG, Beavers WR. Hind limb blood flow during immersion hypothermia. *J Appl Physiol* 10:146-150, 1957.
18. Prough DS, Foreman AS. Anesthesia and the renal system. In: Barash PG, Cullen BF, Stoelting RK, eds. *Clinical Anesthesia*. Philadelphia, PA: JB Lippincott; 1989:1081.

19. Jacobson WE, Hammarsten JF, Heller BI. The effects of adrenaline upon renal function and electrolyte excretion. *J Clin Invest* 30:1503, 1959.
20. Baraka A. Altered response to vasopressors before and during cardiopulmonary bypass. *Anesthesiology* 70:1024-1025, 1989.
21. James TN, Hageman GR, Urthaler F. Anatomic and physiologic considerations of a cardiogenic hypertensive chemoreflex. *Am J Cardiol* 44:852, 1979.
22. Feddersen K, Aurell K, Deun J, et al. Effects of cardiopulmonary bypass on prostacyclin, plasma catecholamines, angiotensin II, and arginine-vasopressin. *Acta Anaesthesiol Scand* 29:224-230, 1985.
23. Oka Y, Wakayama S, Oyama T, et al. Cortisol and antidiuretic hormone responses to stress in cardiac surgical patients. *Can Anaesth Soc J* 28:334-338, 1981.
24. Flezzani P, Croughwell ND, McIntyre RW, et al. Isoflurane decreases the cortisol response to cardiopulmonary bypass. *Anesth Analg* 65:117-122, 1986.
25. Sebel PS, Bovill JG, Schellekens APM, et al. Hormonal responses to high-dose fentanyl anesthesia. *Br J Anaesth* 53:941-948, 1981.
26. Stinson EB, Holloway EL, Derby GC, et al. Control of myocardial performance early after open-heart operations by vasodilator treatment. *J Thorac Cardiovasc Surg* 73:523-529, 1977.
27. Kaplan JA, Jones EL. Vasodilator therapy during coronary artery surgery: comparison of nitroglycerin and nitroprusside. *J Thorac Cardiovasc Surg* 77:301-309, 1979.
28. Johnson CC. The factors and toxicity of sodium nitroprusside. *Arch Int Pharmacodyn Ther* 35:480-416, 1929.
29. Franciosa J, Guiha N, Lima C, et al. Improved left ventricular function during nitropusside infusion in acute myocardial infarction. *Lancet* 1:650, 1972.
30. Guiha N, Cohn J, Mikulic E, et al. Treatment of refractory heart failure with infusion of nitroprusside. *N Engl J Med* 291:587, 1974.
31. Page I, Corcoran AC, Dustan HP, et al. Cardiovascular actions of sodium nitroprusside and hypertenisve patients. *Circulation* 11:188, 1955.
32. Needleman P, Jakschik B, Johnson E. Sulfhydryl requirement for relaxation of vascular smooth muscle. *J Pharmacol Exper Ther* 187:324, 1973.
33. Cottrell JE, Casthely PA, Brodie J, et al. Prevention of nitroprusside-induced cyanide toxicity with hydroxycobalamin. *N Engl J Med* 298:809, 1978.
34. Fahmy N. Nitroglycerin as a hypotensive drug during general anesthesia. *Anesthesiology* 49:17, 1978.
35. Petrovich L, Smith G, Quinones M, et al. Hemodynamic effects of nitroglycerin vs. pure preload reduction masked dilatory effect. *Circulation* 58:223, 1978.
36. Kates RH. Antianginal drug therapy. In: Kaplan J, ed. *Cardiac Anesthesia*. 1979:451-465.

37. Miller RR, Vismara CV, Williams DO, et al. Mechanisms of ventricular unloading in heart failure. *Circulation* 52:76, 1975.
38. Needleman P, Dlehm D, Harkey A, et al. The metabolic pathway in the degradation of glyceryl nitrate. *J Pharmacol Exper Ther* 179:347, 1971.
39. Hill NS, Antman EM, Green LH, et al. Intravenous nitroglycerin. *Chest* 79:69, 1981.
40. Muller JF, Gunther SJ. Nifedipine therapy for Prinzmetal's angina. *Circulation* 57:137-139, 1978.
41. Endo M, Kanada I, Hosoda S, et al. Prinzmetal's variant form of angina pectoris. *Circulation* 52:33-37, 1975.
42. Freedman B, Dunn RF, Richmond DR, et al. Coronary artery spasm: treatment with verapamil. *Circulation* 60:11-249, 1979.
43. Sandler G, Clayton GA, Thornicroft SG. Clinical evaluation of verapamil in angina pectoris. *Br Med J* 3:244-247, 1968.
44. Aoki K, Kondo S, Mochizuki A, et al. Antihypertensive effect of cardiovascular Ca_2-antagonist in hypertensive patients in the absence and presence of β-adrenergic blockade. *Am Heart J* 96:218-226, 1978.
45. Singh BN, Collett JT, Chew CYC. New perspectives in the pharmacologic therapy of cardiac arrhythmias. *Prog Cardiovasc Dis* 22:243, 1980.
46. Waxman HL, Myerburg RJ, Apple R, et al. Verapamil for control of ventricular rate in paroxysmal supraventricular tachycardia and atrial fibrillation or flutter. *Ann Intern Med* 94:1-6, 1981.
47. Singh JB, Hood WB, Abelmannn WH. β Adrenergic mediated inotropic and chronotropic actions of phentolamine. *Am J Cardiol* 26:660, 1970.
48. Magid PA, Sharma B. Phentolamine for vasodilator treatment of severe heart failure. *Lancet* 719:23, 1971.
49. Wang HH, Liu LM, Kate RL. A comparison of the cardiovascular effects of sodium nitroprusside and trimethaphan. *Anesthesiology* 46:40-48, 1977.
50. Sladen RN, Rosenthal MD. Specific afterload reduction with parenteral hydralazine following cardiac surgery. *J Thorac Cardiovasc Surg* 78:125-202, 1979.
51. Stevens WC, Cromwell TH, Halsey MJ, et al. The cardiovascular effects of a new inhalation anesthetic, forane, in human volunteers at constant arterial carbon dioxide tension. *Anesthesiology* 35:8-16, 1970.
52. Calverley RK, Smith NT, Prys-Roberts C, et al. Cardiovascular effects of enflurane anesthesia during controlled ventilation in man. *Anesth Analg* 57:619-628, 1976.
53. Reiz S, Balfors E, Gustavsson B, et al. Effects of halothane on coronary hemodynamics and myocardial metabolism in patients with ischemic heart disease and heart failure. *Acta Anaesthesiol Scand* 26:113, 1982.
54. Rydvall A, Haggmark S, Nyhman H, et al. Effects of enflurane on coronary hemodynamics in patients with ischemic heart disease. *Acta Anaesthesiol Scand* 28:690-695, 1984.
55. Gelman S, Fowler K, Smith L. Regional blood flow during isoflurane and halothane anesthesia. *Anesth Analg* 63:557-565, 1984.

56. Reiz S, Balfors E, Sorenson M, et al. Isoflurane—a powerful vasodilator in patients with coronary artery disease. *Anesthesiology* 59:91-97, 1983.
57. Reiz S, Ostman M. Regional coronary hemodynamics during isoflurane-nitrous oxide anesthesia in patients with ischemic heart disease. *Anesth Analg* 64:570-576, 1985.
58. Buffington CW, Romson JL, Duttlinger NL., Does isoflurane cause coronary steal? *Anesthesiology* 63:A9, 1985.
59. Morrow DH, Morrow AG. The effects of halothane on myocardial contractile force and vascular resistance. *Anesthesiology* 22:537-541, 1961.
60. Brown BR, Cront JR. A comparative study of the effects of five general anesthetics on myocardial contractility. *Anesthesiology* 34:236-245, 1971.
61. Sonntag H, Donath M, Hillebrand W, et al. Left ventricular ventricular function in conscious man during halothane anesthesia. *Anesthesiology* 48:320-324, 1978.
62. Kemmotsu O, Hashimoto Y, Shimosato S. Inotropic effects of isolated cat papillary muscles from normal and failing hearts. *Anesthesiology* 39:470-477, 1973.
63. Videcoq M, Desmonts JM, Marty J, et al. Effects of droperidol on peripheral vasculature: use of cardiopulmonary bypass as a study model. *Acta Anaesthesiol Scand* 31:370-374, 1987.
64. Muldoon SM, Janssens WJ, Verbeuren TJ, et al. α-Adrenergic blocking properties of droperidol on isolated blood vessels of the dog. *Br J Anaesth* 49:211-215, 1977.
65. Whitwan JG, Russell WJ. The acute cardiovascular changes and adrenergic blockade by droperidol in man. *Br J Anaesth* 43:581-590, 1971.

Chapter 17

Thoracic Aortic Aneurysm Repair: Hemodynamic Changes and Complications

Youngick Lee, MD
and Ayad Jihayel, MD

Aortic Aneurysms

While aortic aneurysms may arise from many causes including infections, congenital problem such as Marfan's Syndrome, disruption of a graft suture line, dilation of the graft itself in association with pregnancy and secondary to trauma, by far the most common cause is atherosclerosis. Aortic dissections may result in compression of the true lumen of the aorta, occlusion of major tributaries of the aorta, and/or death from rupture of the aorta or accompanying sequelae. Mortality rates associated with acute aortic dissection range from 74% to 89%.[1] Two basic systems are in wide use to classify aortic dissections. (Table I).

Thoracic aortic dissection occurs two to three times more frequently in males than females. Approximately 57% of dissections

From Casthely PA, Bregman D, (eds): *Cardiopulmonary Bypass: Physiology, Related Complications, and Pharmacology.* Mount Kisco, NY, Futura Publishing Company, Inc., © 1991.

Table I
Classification of Thoracic Aortic Dissections

DeBakey Classification	
Type I:	Originates in the ascending aorta and involves aortic arch and beyond.
Type II:	Limited to the ascending aorta.
Type III:	Originates beyond the left subclavian artery and extends distally for various distances.
Daily Classification	
Type A:	Dissection where there is any involvement of the ascending aorta.
Type B:	Dissection begins distal to the left subclavian artery.

begin in the proximal ascending aorta, 10% begin just proximal to the innominate artery, 28% start just distal to the left subclavian artery, 3% occur in the descending aorta, and 2% start distal to the renal arteries.[1] Type A dissections are associated with approximately a twofold mortality rate during the first 2 weeks when compared to type B dissections. Type A dissections tend to occur in younger patients. Patients with type B dissections are more likely to be hypertensive on admission and have a greater incidence of associated arteriosclerosis. Aortic regurgitation is present in approximately 50% of type A dissections compared to 10% in type B.[2] Patients may present with back and shoulder pain, hematuria or oliguria, Horner's syndrome, hoarseness, pulsating neck masses, suprasternal ecchymoses, heart block, dyspnea, murmur, or neck vein distension. Serum chemistries and urinalysis are usually nonspecific. On chest X-ray, one may see a widening of the mediastinum, separation of the aortic intima calcification from the outer edge of the aorta, and/or blurring or obliteration of the aortic knob. Computed tomography is one of the most reliable noninvasive techniques available. The definitive method of diagnosis is contrast aortography. Patients with type A dissections are usually surgical candidates unless the patient is exhibiting evolving neurologic symptoms associated with their dissection.

Cross Clamping of Descending Thoracic Aorta: Pathophysiologic Consequences

Blood flow interruption of the thoracic aorta can generate sudden increase in afterload secondary to the aortic occlusion,[3,4] resulting in proximal hypertension, left ventricular strain by elevated end diastolic pressure, pulmonary congestion, and increase in cerebrospinal fluid (CSF) pressure.[4,5] Experimental studies by Alexis Carrel[6] and data by Hug and Carlson[4,7] have conclusively shown that a temporary diversion of the aortic blood flow may prevent those untoward events during thoracic aortic occlusion. Nitroprusside or nitroglycerin are commonly used to decrease systemic vascular resistance (SVR), pulmonary capillary wedge pressure (PCWP), and counteract the increase in arterial pressure and small doses of propranolol, esmolol, labetalol, or verapamil are effective in controlling heart rate. Nitroprusside and the anesthetic agent isoflurane both decrease SVR, however, both have been reported to produce intracardic "steals" in some patients and may promote myocardial ischemia while many researchers have challenged the steal effect of isoflurane.[8-10] Some authors prefer the use of nitroglycerin, thorazine, an α blocker, or other agents to counteract the hypertension associated with aortic cross clamping. The unstable hemodynamics associated with unclamping has a variety of etiologies including: (1) reactive hyperemia, (2) a decrease in peripheral vasomotor tone, (3) redistribution of blood from the upper to the lower body, and (4) the systemic effects of the acidosis and metabolites from the lower extremities. The decrease in cardiac performance secondary to the acidosis is usually transient and rarely requires administration of bicarbonate. Slow unclamping with an adequate or moderately elevated preload will diminish the severity of declamping hypotension. The transient use of vasopressors such as phenylephrine may be necessary in some cases. A cell saver can prove to be useful in retrieving shed blood and returning it to the patient, decreasing the number of transfused units. A large amount of blood transfusion and crystalloid infusion may result in a dilutional coagulopathy requiring administration of platelets and fresh frozen plasma.

In addition, distal organ ischemia involving kidneys and spinal cord is also an important sequelae of thoracic aortic interruption. Renal tolerance to reduced blood flow below 45 to 50 mL per minute is markedly diminished during cross clamping, resulting in reduction of urine output. The urine output, however, improves to the level of 74% to 83% of the baseline value around 60 minutes following the release of the cross clamp.[4]

When the thoracic aorta is cross clamped beyond the origin of the left subclavian artery, diminished blood supply to the spinal cord may result in paraplegia or paraparesis,[11] in which the incidence of paraplegia increases with the duration of aortic cross clamping (Fig. 1).[12] Proposed factors include: (1) proximal hypertension with associated increased cerebral fluid pressure (resulting in either compression of nutrient arteries or alteration of the pressure gradient between the CSF and the abdominal aorta below the clamp, (2) intraoperative hypotension, (3) prolonged clamping with distal ischemia, and (4) disruption of vital intercostal arteries.[13] The spinal cord ischemia may also be increased by a concomitant increase in intracranial and intraspinal pressure. The two posterior spinal arteries arise from the posterior inferior cerebellar arteries, but are not the major contributors to the cord. The single

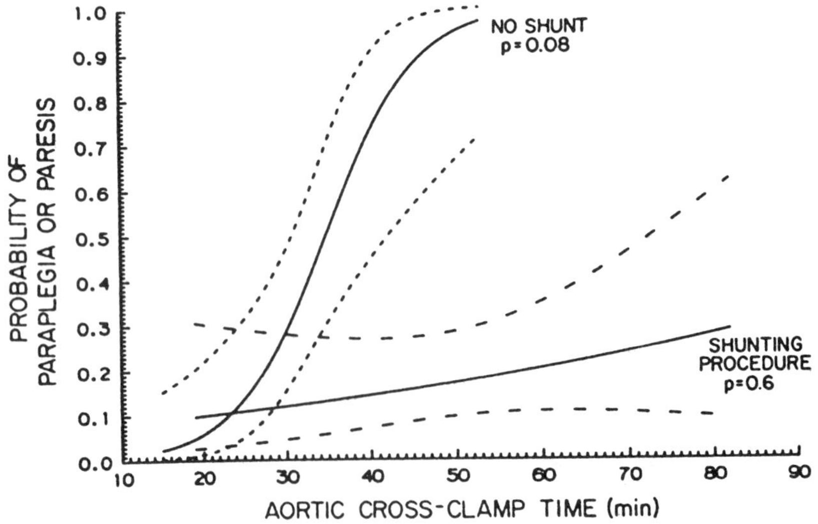

Figure 1. Nomogram of the logistic equations (Table V) relating the probability of evidence for spinal cord injury (paraplegia or paresis to aortic cross clamp time (minutes) for patients in whom no shunting procedure was used and for those in whom it was used. The dashed lines are the 70% confidence limits. (Reprinted with permission from Katz NM, et al. Incremental risk factors for spinal cord injury following operation for acute traumatic aortic transection. *J Thorac Cardiovasc Surg* 81:669-674, 1981.)

anterior spinal artery is formed by the union of branches or each vertebral artery and receives spinal branches from the vertebral, deep cervical, ascending cervical, posterior intercostal, lumbar, and lateral sacral arteries. Spinal cord perfusion pressure (SPPP) can be defined as spinal artery pressure (MAP) minus cerebral spinal fluid pressure (CSFP) [SCPP = MAP - CSFP]. A driving pressure of greater than 30 mm Hg is usually necessary for adequate cord perfusion. It is interesting to note that the anatomic variation of the blood supply to the spinal cord also determines the tolerance of the individual to the cross clamping.[12] Therefore, ligation of a particularly large radicular artery, the artery of Adamkiewicz, can produce paraplegia or paraparesis.[13] This artery arises between T-9 and T-12 (the level of thoracic vertebrae) in 60%, between T-5 and T-8 in 15%, and from L-1 or lower in about 25% of the population. Accordingly, the cross clamp of the aorta immediately distal to the left subclavian artery for 45–60 minutes can potentially induce permanent spinal cord damage in 90% of patients. The cross clamp at the level of the diaphragm for 45–60 minutes may subject 25% of the population to the development of paraplegia or paraparesis. Furthermore, the length of the excluded segment is also inversely related to the increased incidence of paraplegia. For example, in patients with coarctation of the aorta with multiple complete collateral circulation, the aorta can probably be cross clamped indefinitely without spinal cord injury. However, most patients we operate on for thoracic aneurysm have aorta with little or no intercostal arterial flow since degenerative changes of atherosclerosis contribute to the thrombotic occlusion involving the origin of the intercostal arteries.

Barbiturates may provide a protective effect in focal ischemia with little protection in global ischemia. The latter point has been challenged by a recent report where approximately 40 mg/kg of thiopental was used during normothermic cardiopulmonary bypass.[14] The potential CNS protective effects of this dose of thiopental must be weighed against the potentially delirious effects on the cardiovascular system. Nimodipine, a calcium channel blocker, has been shown to decrease the severity of neurologic deficits in primates when given after a period of ischemia.[15] Gelmers et al.[16] reported that nimodipine therapy initiated within 24 hours of the onset of symptoms of an acute ischemic stroke significantly improved neurologic outcome and significantly decreased mortality.

Isoflurane has been shown to produce an isoelectric EEG at two times the minimum alveolar concentration (2MAC) and appears to have an effect on $CMRO_2$ similar to that of barbiturates.[17] Nehls et al.[18] reported that in baboons isoflurane in concentrations sufficient to maintain burst suppression was not protective against temporary occlusion of the middle cerebral artery; in comparison, four of six thiopental treated animals were normal. Modest increases in serum glucose at the time of an ischemic event has been shown to worsen neurologic outcome in the primate.[19] Other agents less well studied and with less convincing evidence for protection include iron chelators such as deferoxamine, superoxide dismutase, benzodiazepines, etomidate, naloxone, lidoflazine, flunarizine, and acetazolamide. Magnesium therapy has been reported to lower the incidence of dysrrhythmias and hypertension. Magnesium can be replaced emergently at a rate of 2 gm in 10 mL D5W over 10 minutes. In addition to hypothermia, Vacanti and Ames, and Kass et al. have reported that Mg^{++} may be protective against central nervous system ischemia.[20-22] Grum has reported that isoflurane may be associated with a decrease in spinal cord perfusion pressure, while intrathecal papaverine may produce an increase in blood flow to the spinal cord.[23] Drainage of CSF or avoiding increase of CSFP may help prevent spinal cord damage during aortic cross clamping.[24-26]

Rationale for Distal Perfusion

The etiology of spinal cord injury during the cross clamp of the thoracic aorta is multifactorial. Thus, attempts to support the distal circulation may only reduce, but not eliminate, the risk of paraplegia or paraparesis. In spite of the experiences of Robert, Crawford, and Najafi,[3,5,27] advocates of bypass or shunts to support the distal circulation have reported a decreased incidence of paraplegia. The distal circulation support also reduces the afterload on the heart, and preserves distal organ perfusion especially in patients with preexisting renal dysfunction.[7] Aortic occlusion could incite the development of acute left heart failure with mitral insufficiency, elevated left atrial pressure, and congestion and hemorrhage of the lung.[4] Therefore, the overall objectives of distal perfusion include: (a) lowering the metabolic demand of the ischemic spinal cord during the period of aortic cross clamping, (b) prevention of proximal hypertension, and (c) any increase in CSF pressure by maximizing the collateral blood flow. The techniques to achieve these goals, which will be discussed, are cumbersome when compared with currently popular techniques called "clamp and sew." However, they eliminate several contributing factors of paraplegia following resection of descending or abdominal aorta. However, the efficacy of the individual technique to be described below, remains to be proven by further prospective clinical studies.

Methods of Minimizing Paraplegia and Paraparesis

Perfusion of the Distal Aorta

Perfusion of the distal aorta by any one of several methods to be described, prevents spinal cord ischemia and paraplegia. Distal aortic perfusion, however, prevents paraplegia only when the excluded segment of the aorta by a pair of clamps does not contain the origin of radicular arteries, critical for the spinal cord. The mean distal perfusion pressure should be at least 60 mm Hg to prevent paraplegia according to the studies by Laschinger and his colleagues.[28]

Whole Body Hypothermia

Experimental studies by Hufnagel[29] and Beattie,[30] confirmed by Pontius and colleagues,[31] demonstrated that hypothermia clearly prolonged the safe ischemic time for the spinal cord. These studies indicate that the spinal cord can regain its normal function following a 60-minute ischemia at a whole body temperature of 30°C. However, cooling the whole body to 30°C requires formal surface cooling, which is time consuming, especially in large patients.

Regional Hypothermia

Animal experiments performed by Coles and his colleagues[31] have shown that perfusion cooling of the excluded aorta with sanguinous hypothermic solution of 5°C over a 3-minute period substantially protected the spinal cord against irreversible injury during a 30-minute aortic occlusion. In recent years, substantial progress has been made in treating aneurysms located in the ascending or descending aorta with perfusion techniques using profound hypothermia with or without circulatory arrest.[32]

Reattachment of the Intercostal and Lumbar Arteries

Success of this method depends on the preservation of spinal cord integrity during the period before the intercostal or lumbar arteries are reattached. Recommendation of the modified technique of resection, namely to leave posterior wall of the aorta that contain the origins of intercostal arteries, has been proposed by some,[31] but not by all.

Pharmacological Agents

No single pharmacological agent has been proven effective in preventing paraplegia. However, prolonging a tolerable time period before the onset of spinal cord infarction has been achieved by various pharmacological agents. The most commonly used are: steroids, thiopental, calcium channel blockers, and free radical scavengers.[33-36]

Cerebrospinal Fluid Drainage

It is well recognized that the CSF pressure increases during aortic cross clamping which, in turn, further diminishes the spinal cord perfusion pressure in which the circulation is already compromised.[24,38] The spinal cord perfusion pressure can be obtained by subtracting the CSF pressure from the spinal artery pressure. This increased CSF pressure is merely a reflex response to the proximal hypertension occurring in aortic cross clamp. Cerebrospinal fluid drainage alone is of limited value in preventing ischemic injury of the spinal cord. Recently, a beneficial effect on the spinal cord ischemia was shown when maneuvers of the CSF drainage was combined with the intrathecal infusion of papaverine hydrochloride that dilates the spinal artery. This procedure increases the perfusion pressure by lowering the CSF pressure.[36] Although these maneuvers did not prevent paraplegia completely during simple aortic cross clamping, it is a promising palliative adjunct.

Monitoring the Spinal Cord Ischemia with Somatosensory Evoked Potentials (SEP)

This technique has been popularized by Laschinger and colleagues.[28] Essentially, this technique recognizes the cord ischemia by detecting decreased somatosensory potential of the lower extremities, and therefore allows one to provide more blood to the distal portion from the site of cross clamp. The baseline somatosensory evoked potential (SEP) can be routinely obtained prior to the aortic cross clamp as well as during the period of cross clamping. The measurements can also be obtained serially during the entire period of the aortic cross clamp. The pressure of radial and femoral arteries are monitored simultaneously by using a heparinized Gott shunt or femora-femoral bypass to ensure the distal perfusion and the maintenance of SEP during the aortic cross clamp. The loss of SEP following the aortic cross clamp indicates the involvement of critical intercostal arteries in the excluded aortic segment (Figs. 2 and 3). At times, direct perfusion of critical intercostals may be important to prevent neurologic injuries. Lesions located at unfavorable sites such as aortoiliac disease, extensive thoracoabdominal aneurysm, and distal aortic dissection, preclude the use of this technique because an adequate distal perfusion is very difficult when treating such lesions. In these cases, SEP monitoring may not be helpful and the incidence of paraplegia may vary according to the time elapsed before the intercostals are reimplanted blindly.

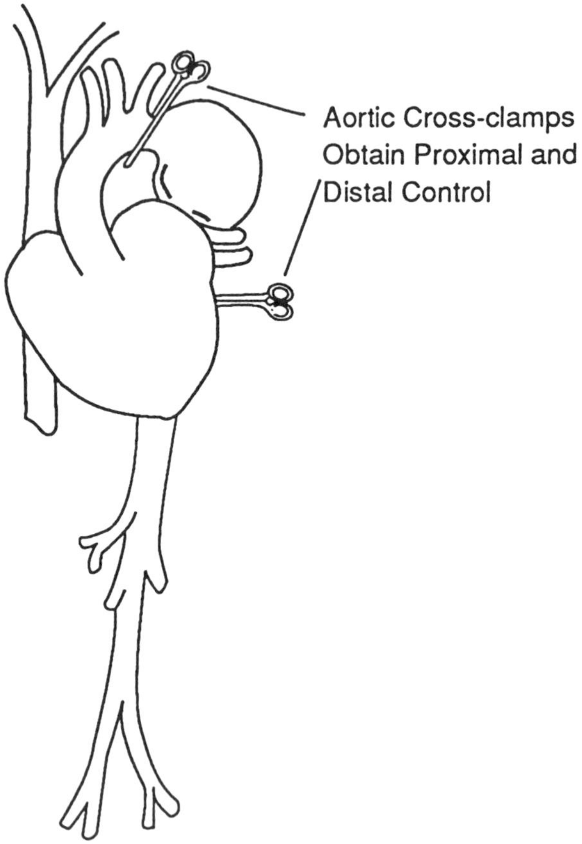

Figure 2. Aortic cross clamping without shunt or bypass.

Renal Complications

Infrarenal aortic cross clamping is associated with a 30% decrease in renal blood flow and a 75% increase in renal vascular resistance.[38] Cross clamping the aorta at the thoracic level will result in an 85% to 94% reduction in renal blood flow. The incidence of renal failure following elective repair of AAA is approximately 5% compared to 18%–20% following emergency procedures. Stenosis of the renal arteries or multiple renal arteries may

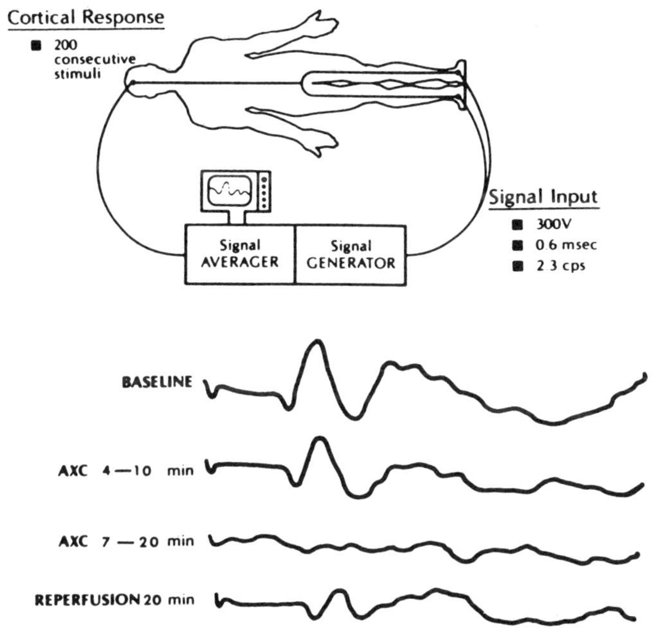

Figure 3. (Top) Schematic representation of clinical technique of SEP monitoring. (Bottom) Type I SEP response: Loss of SEP because of spinal cord ischemia after proximal aortic cross clamping (AXC) without distal aortic perfusion. (Reproduced with permission from Cunningham JN Jr, Laschinger JC, Spencer HC. Monitoring of somatosensory evoked potentials during surgical procedures on the thoracoabdominal aorta. *J Thorac Cardiovasc Surg* 94:275-285, 1987.

be present in up to 20% of patients with AAA. Most authors recommend maintaining an adequate urine production (½–1 mL/kg/hour) and augmentation of cortical blood flow by administering 25 g of mannitol approximately 30 minutes prior to aortic cross clamping.[39] Warm ischemic time to the spinal cord and kidneys is approximately 30 minutes. Some authors recommend retrograde perfusion of the kidneys via a femoral artery shunt. Renal hemodynamic deterioration seen with aortic cross clamping may persist for at least an hour after unclamping. This may be secondary to stimulation of the renin-angiotensin system during aortic cross clamping. The use of renin or calcium antagonists may attenuate the intensity of these effects or their duration. Woolley et al.[40] reported that verapamil injected into the renal artery of sheep prior to renal ischemia was somewhat protective. Low-dose dopamine (3 μg/kg/min) may be warranted to increase renal blood flow.

Methods of Distal Perfusion

The purpose of perfusing the descending thoracic and abdominal aorta is to lower the metabolic demand of the ischemic spinal cord and to prevent the proximal hypertension during the period of aortic cross clamping. The paraplegia is quite rare after cardiopulmonary bypass because the blood flow in thoracic or abdominal aorta below the distal clamp, although reduced, is sufficient enough to supply the spinal cord to prevent paraplegia, provided that the excluded segment lacks the intercostal arteries critical to the spinal cord blood flow. A flow of 1 L/min/m^2 of body surface at normothermia appears adequate to prevent paraplegia. There are several methods that provide such a level of blood flow.

Passive Bypass

Passive bypass can be accomplished by a conduit of either silastic or a heparin-coated Gott shunt[41] without using any pumping device. This technique does not require heparin unless silastic tubing is used.

Aorto-aortic shunt

To perfuse the descending and abdominal aorta, the Gott shunt can be used (Fig. 4). The Gott shunt tubing is 7 or 9 mm in diameter and 90 cm in length (9 mm size is often preferred). Because the Gott shunt is heparin-coated, anticoagulation is not necessary. A ¼-inch silastic tubing, a component of cardiopulmonary bypass, is a cheaper alternative. However, it requires one-half the usual dose of heparin (1.5 mg/kg). The cannulae are inserted into the aorta

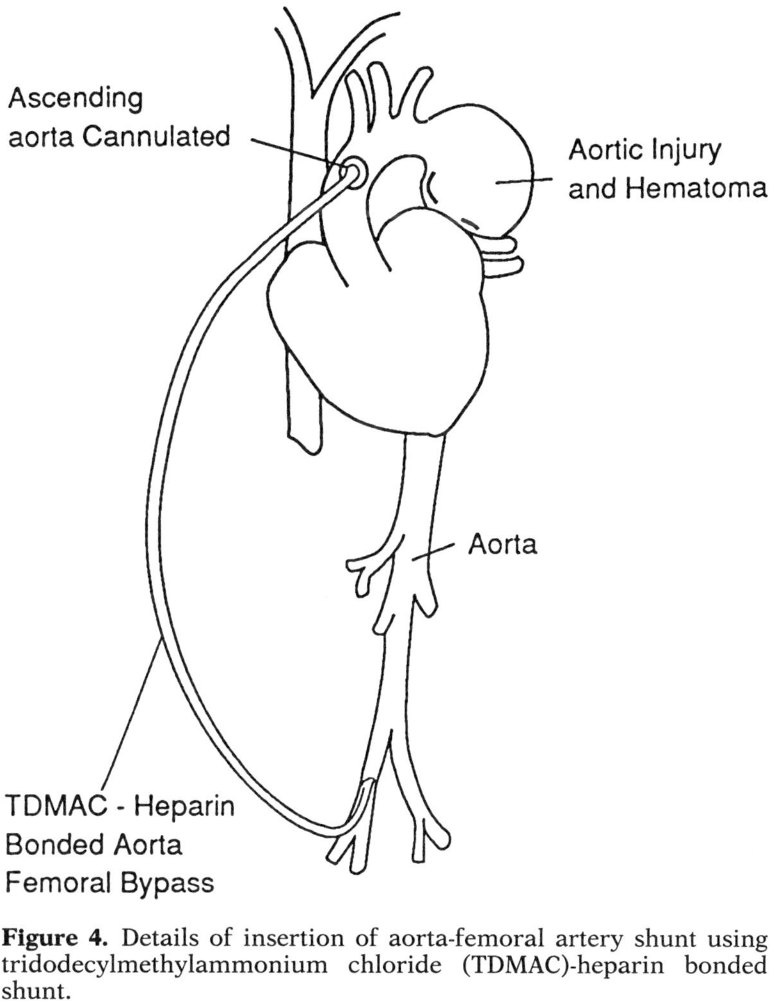

Figure 4. Details of insertion of aorta-femoral artery shunt using tridodecylmethylammonium chloride (TDMAC)-heparin bonded shunt.

(proximal and distal) through purse strings sutures. The proximal end of the shunt can be placed in the transverse arch, subclavian artery, or the ascending aorta, and the distal end in the femoral artery (Fig. 4). During aortic cross clamping the arterial pressure is simultaneously monoclonal via two cannulae inverted in the right radial artery (proximal) and the femoral artery (distal). A Swan-Ganz thermodilution catheter is inserted to monitor cardiac output, right and left heart pressures.

Left ventricular-femoral or iliac artery shunt

In 1965, English[42] placed a shunt into the left ventricular apex achieving direct left ventriculofemoral bypass in a patient who had anomalous subclavian arteries. Since then, many investigators[43-47] have demonstrated that a bypass can be achieved by direct ventriculoaortic, ventriculofemoral, or iliac artery diversion with heparin-bonded shunts as an alternative to the cannulation of the left subclavian artery or ascending aorta. This procedure is achieved by a standard left thoracotomy in which the shunt passes through the anterior end of the incision and does not obstruct exposure of the transverse arch and descending aorta. In patients who have associated abdominal and head injuries, the use of the heparinized shunt bypass without anticoagulation, may be lifesaving. Following aortic cross clamping, the blood from the left ventricle to the iliac artery averages about 33% of the left ventricular output. Some reversal of the flow during diastole can be observed occasionally that amounted to about 10% of the forward flow through the shunt.[47] Such reversal flow does not have serious adverse effects on cardiac output.

These studies have also shown that there was an adequate blood flow to the visceral arterial bed, adequate urine output and no histological evidence of renal ischemia for prolonged period during cross clamping. Because the mean pressure in the peripheral arterial bed is higher than those of the left ventricle, a reversal of flow from iliac or femoral artery to the left ventricle occurs if the shunt is opened before the cross clamping of aorta.

In conclusion, the ventriculoaortic, the ventriculoiliac, or the femoral artery bypass with heparin-bonded shunt is a safe and reliable technique for left heart decompression that can maintain satisfactory renal and intestinal blood flow. Potential complications include bleeding from the cannulation site, arrhythmia during manipulation of the heart, and air embolism.

Active Pump Bypass

This technique requires heparinization and pump oxygenator or reservoir.

Femora-femoral bypass

This method, popular among surgeons, requires full heparinization and partial cardiopulmonary bypass. After isolation of both the femoral artery and vein in the groin, the arterial cannula is inserted, secured, and then attached to the pump oxygenator. A long venous cannula, 28 to 30 F in diameter is introduced into the femoral vein, and advanced up to the inferior vena cava in order to produce an adequate venous drainage. To assure a satisfactory position, the tip of the cannula should be at least 3–4 cm above the sacral promontory. The perfusate temperature is kept at 35°C and the flow of 1.0–1.5 L/min/$m^2$of body surface is maintained. During the perfusion, anesthesiologists can monitor the cardiovascular system with an appropriate medication to maintain the pulmonary artery diastolic pressure at around 15 mm Hg and the arterial pressure of the upper body to slightly higher than normal. When the perfusion is finished, heparin reversal is accomplished with slow administration of protamine. Occasionally we have encountered some difficulty in cannulating the femoral vein.

Left atriofemoral bypass

In this procedure, a disposable bubble oxygenator is used only for the purpose as a reservoir. This method is technically more difficult. Nevertheless, it is useful in situations when the use of a Gott shunt is not appropriate. The left atrium is approached by opening the pericardium in front of the phrenic nerve through left thoracotomy and cannulated with a 7–8 mm cannula. The return cannula is inserted into the external iliac artery. The flow is maintained about 1.5 L/min/m^2 body surface and left atrial pressure around 5–8 mm Hg.

Left atrial femoral bypass with centrifugal pump without reservoir

The left atrium is cannulated in the usual fashion through a left thoracotomy, then the left common femoral or the external

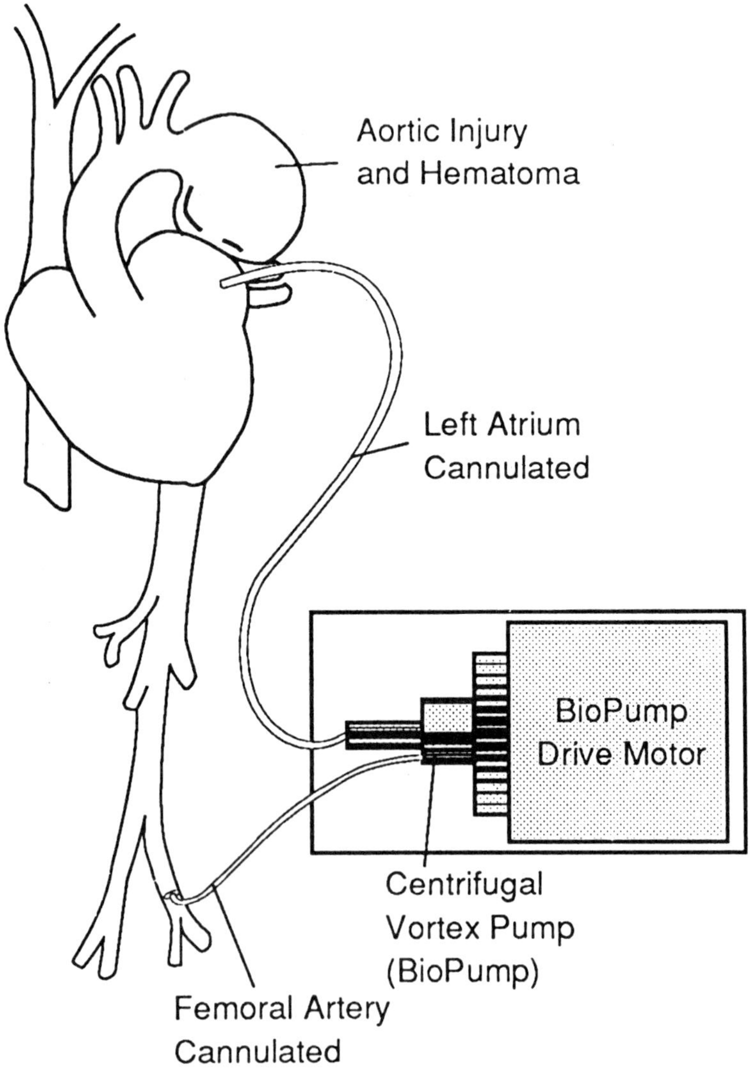

Figure 5. Details of insertion of left atrial-femoral artery bypass without heparin.

iliac artery and the cannulae are connected to a BioMedicus Centrifugal Pump (Fig. 5). No systemic heparin is used. However, when heparin is used, a minimal amount to maintain an activated clotting time in the range of 150–200 seconds appears sufficient. The limited amount of heparin is the main advantage when used in patients with multiple injuries.[48,49] The flow through these pumps can be set initially at 1 L/min/m^2, then the flow is adjusted accordingly to prevent stasis within the pump, and to reduce the afterload. The mean pressure of the upper body should be maintained between 50–75 mm Hg and the distal perfusion should provide at 60 mm Hg or above. The centrifugal BioMedicus pump has several advantages over the roller pump. Low-density micro-air bubbles will remain in the center of the vortex within the pump head, making air embolism a very rare complication. This pump is also less traumatic to blood elements.[50] Minimal doses of heparin (150 μ/kg) are administered to maintain the activated clotting time around 150–200 seconds when the pump is used without a membrane or reservoir in the circuit. Direct arterial bypass can also be accomplished with the BioMedicus pump without cannulating the heart. This technique has replaced many of the other methods used to bypass the thoracic to abdominal aorta during aortic aneurysm repair. One disadvantage with the BioMedicus pump is its somewhat inflexibility to volume change. Ergin[51] modified the BioMedicus pump technique in which a cannulation of the left ventricular apex and the left femoral artery was performed using a 20F cannula, that was connected to the centrifugal pump. Heparin, 1 mg/kg, was given, and the flow was maintained at 1.5 to 2.2 L/min/m^2. The temperature of the perfusate was kept cool at 33°C to 34.5°C. The pressures of the pulmonary, radial, and femoral arteries were also monitored. Cross clamp and bypass time were 60 $\pm$ 28 and 61 $\pm$ 33 minutes, respectively. Among 22 patients operated on for descending thoracic aneurysm, one patient was reoperated for bleeding and one patient developed chylothorax. Most importantly, only one patient developed paralysis and there was no mortality. Thus, this method appears to be an ideal perfusion technique in minimizing spinal cord injury.

REFERENCES

1. Ergin MA, Galla JD, Lansman S, et al. Acute dissections of the aorta. Current surgical treatment. *Surg Clin N Am* 65:721-741, 1985.

2. Diehl JT, Cali RF, Hertzer NR, et al. Complications of abdominal aortic reconstruction: an analysis of perioperative risk factors in 557 patients. *Ann Surg* 197:49-56, 1983.
3. Robert AJ, Nova JD, Hughes WA, et al. Cardiac and renal responses to cross-clamping of the descending thoracic aorta. *J Thorac Cardiovasc Surg* 86:732-741, 1983.
4. Hug HR, Taber RE. Bypass flow requirements during thoracic aneurysmectomy with particular attention to the prevention of left heart failure. *J Thorac Cardiovasc Surg* 57:203-213, 1969.
5. Crawford ES, Walker HS, Saleh SM, et al. Graft replacement of aneurysm in descending thoracic aorta: results without bypass or shunting. *Surgery* 89:73-85, 1981.
6. Carrel A. On the experimental surgery of the thoracic aorta and the heart. *Ann Surg* 52:83-95, 1910.
7. Carlson DE, Karp RB, Kouchoukos NT. Surgical treatment of aneurysms of the descending thoracic aorta: an analysis of 85 patients. *Ann Thorac Surg* 35:58-69, 1983.
8. Gilbert M, Roberts SL, Mori M, et al. Comparative coronary vascular reactivity and hemodynamics during halothane and isoflurane anesthesia in swine. *Anesthesiology* 68:243-253, 1988.
9. Moffitt EA, Barker RA, Glenn JJ, et al. Myocardial metabolism and hemodynamic responses with isoflurane anesthesia for coronary artery surgery. *Anesth Analg* 65:53-61, 1986.
10. Goldstein RE. Coronary vascular response to vasodilator drugs. *Prog Cardiovasc Dis* 24:419-436, 1982.
11. Adams HD, Van Geertruyden HH. Neurologic complications of aortic surgery. *Ann Surg* 144:574, 1956.
12. Katz NM, Blackstone EEH, Kirklin JW, et al. Incremental risk factors for spinal cord injury following operation for acute traumatic aortic transection. *J Thorac Cardiovasc Surg* 81:669-674, 1981.
13. Wadouh F, Lindemann EM, Arndt CF, et al. The arteria radicularis magna anterior as a decisive factor influencing spinal cord damage during aortic occlusion. *J Thorac Cardiovasc Surg* 88:1-10, 1984.
14. Nussmeir NA, Arlund C, Slogoff S. Neuropsychiatric complications after cardiopulmonary bypass: cerebral protection by a barbiturate. *Anesthesiology* 64:165-170, 1986.
15. Steen PA, Gisvold SE, Milde JH, et al. Nimodipine improves outcome when given after complete cerebral ischemia in primates. *Anesthesiology* 62:406-414, 1985.
16. Gelmers HJ, Gorter K, de Weerdt CJ, et al. A controlled trial of nimodipine in acute ischemic stroke. *N Engl J Med* 318:203-207, 1988.
17. Newberg LA, Milde JH, Michenfelder JD. The cerebral metabolic effects of isoflurane at and above concentrations that suppress cortical electrical activity. *Anesthesiology* 66:453-464, 1987.
18. Nehls DG, Todd MM, Spetzler RF, et al. A comparison of the cerebral protective effects of isoflurane and barbiturates during temporary focal ischemia in primates. *Anesthesiology* 66:453-464, 1987.

19. Lanier WL, Stangland KJ, Scheithauer BW, et al. The effects of dextrose infusion and head position on neurological outcome after complete cerebral ischemia in primates: examination of a model. *Anesthesiology* 66:39-48, 1987.
20. Gambling DR, Birmingham CL, Jenkins LC. Magnesium and the anaesthetist. *Can J Anaesth* 35:644-654, 1988.
21. Vacanti FX, Ames A III. Mild hypothermia and Mg^{++} protect against irreversible damage during CNS ischemia. *Stroke* 15:695-698, 1984.
22. Kass IS, Cottrell JE, Chambers G. Magnesium and cobalt, not nimodipine protect neurons against anoxic damage in the hippocampal slice. *Anesthesiology* 69:710, 1988.
23. Grum DF, Svensson LG, Blum J. Intrathecal papaverine for thoracic aortic aneurysm resection: a preliminary report. *Anesthesiology* 69:A894, 1988.
24. Myamoto K, Ken A, Wada T, et al. A new and simple method of preventing spinal cord damage following temporary occlusion of the thoracic aorta by draining the cerebrospinal fluid. *J Thorac Cardiovasc Surg* 1:188-197, 1960.
25. Laschinger JC, Owen J, Rosenbloom NT, et al. Detrimental effects of sodium nitroprusside on spinal cord motor tract perfusion during thoracic aortic cross-clamping. *Surg Forum* 38:195-196, 1987.
26. Marini CP, Grubbs PE, Toporoff B, et al. Effect of sodium nitroprusside on spinal cord perfusion and paraplegia during aortic cross-clamping. *Ann Thorac Surg* 47:379-383, 1989.
27. Najafi H, Javid H, Hunter J, et al. Descending aortic aneurysmectomy without adjuncts to avoid ischemia. *Ann Thorac Surg* 30:326-335, 1980.
28. Laschinger JC, Cunningham JN Jr, Ctainella FP, et al. Detection and prevention of intraoperative spinal cord ischemia after cross-clamping of the thoracic aorta: use of somatosensory evoked potential. *Surgery* 92:1109-1117, 1982.
29. Hufnagel CA, Gross RE. Coarctation of the aorta: experimental studies regarding its connection. *New Engl J Med* 223:283, 1945.
30. Coles JG, Wilson GJ, Sima AF, et al. Intraoperative management of thoracic aortic aneurysm. *J Thorac Cardiovasc Surg* 35:292-299, 1983.
31. Poutius RG, Brockman HL, Hardy EG, et al. The use of hypothermia in the prevention of paraplegia following temporary aortic occlusion: experimental observations. *Surgery* 36:33, 1954.
32. Sweeney MS, Cooley DA, Reul GJ, et al. Hypothermic circulatory arrest for cardiovascular lesions: technical considerations and results. *Ann Thorac Surg* 40:498, 1985.
33. Wakabayashi A, Connolly JE. Prevention of paraplegia associated with resection of extensive thoracic aneurysms. *Arch Surg* 111:1186, 1971.
34. Laschinger JC, Cunningham JN Jr, Cooper MM, et al. Prevention of ischemic spinal cord injury following aortic cross-clamping: use of corticosteroids. *Ann Thorac Surg* 38:500-507, 1984.
35. Wadouh F, Arndt CF, Opperman E, et al. The mechanism of spinal cord injury after simple and double aortic cross-clamping. *J Thorac Cardiovasc Surg* 92:121-127, 1986.

36. Svenson LG, Von Ritter CM, Groeneveld HT, et al. Cross-clamping of the thoracic aorta: influence of aortic shunts, papaverine, calcium channel blocker, allopurinol and superoxide dismutase on spinal cord blood flow and paraplegia. *Ann Surg* 204:38-47, 1986.
37. Casthely PA, Dluzneski J, Jones R, et al. Comparison of superoxyde dismutase, thiopental and nimodipine for maintenance of somatosensory evoked responses during aortic cross clamping and declamping in dogs. *Cardiothoracic Soc J* 2:792-797, 1988.
38. Gamulin Z, Forster A, Morel D, et al. Effects of infrarenal aortic cross-clamping on renal hemodynamics in humans. *Anesthesiology* 61:394-399, 1984.
39. Casthely PA, Fyman PN, Abrams LM, et al. Anesthesia for aortic arch aneuruysm repair: experience with 17 patients. *Can Anaesth Soc J* 32:73-78, 1985.
40. Woolley JL, Barker GR, Jacobson WK, et al. Effect of the calcium entry blocker verapamil on renal ischemia. *Crit Care Med* 16:48-51, 1988.
41. Gott VL. Heparinized shunts for thoracic vascular operation. *Ann Thorac Surg* 14:219, 1972.
42. English TAH. Direct left ventriculofemoral bypass during resection of the aorta with anomalous subclavian arteries. *Thorax* 20:36, 1965.
43. Jamieson CW, Goodwin DP, Storrs JA, et al. Emergency bypass of the thoracic aorta: experimental evaluation of a simple method. *Br J Surg* 57:661, 1970.
44. Hayden WG, Hirshorn S, Blank RH. Left ventriculoaortic shunt: a laboratory investigation. *Am Surg* 40:345, 1974.
45. Murray GF, Young WG Jr. Thoracic aneurysmectomy utilizing direct left ventriculofemoral shunt (TDMAC-heparin) bypass. *Ann Thorac Surg* 21:26-29, 1976.
46. Ketharanathan V, McConchie IM, Westlake GW. Left ventricle-femoral artery shunt in the management of acute traumatic rupture of the descending thoracic aorta. *J Thorac Cardiovasc Surg* 88:1, 1984.
47. Frantz PT, Murray GF, Shallal JA, et al. Clinical and experimental evaluation of left ventriculoiliac shunt bypass during repair of lesions of the descending thoracic aorta. *Ann Thorac Surg* 31:551-557, 1981.
48. Dixon CM, Magovern GJ. Evaluation of the bio pump for long-term cardiac support without heparinization. *J Extracorporeal Tech* 14:331, 1982.
49. Olivier HF Jr, Maher TD, Liebler GA, et al. Use of the BioMedicus Centrifugal pump in traumatic tears of the thoracic aorta. *Ann Thorac Surg* 38:586-591, 1984.
50. Lynch MF, Peterson D, Baker V. Centrifugal blood pumping for open heart surgery. *Minn Med* 61:536, 1978.
51. Ergin MA, Griepp R. Personal communication, 1990.

Chapter 18

Anesthetic Management of Cardiac Transplantation

James Harding, MD,
Ellise Delphin, MD,
and Douglas Jackson, MD

Cardiac transplantation has become an accepted therapy for patients with end stage heart disease over the last decade. A dramatic increase in the number of heart transplants has occurred since 1980, with approximately 2,500 operations performed yearly around the world.[1] Moreover, the number of centers performing cardiac transplants has risen from 114 in 1986 to 202 in 1989.[1] Survival after this procedure has also improved; most centers report 1 year survival rates of at least 80% and 5-year survival rates of 60%–70%.[2]

Clearly, all physicians will have an ever-expanding role in the care of these patients as the number of procedures continues to rise and as the survival of transplant patients continues to improve. The cardiac surgeon, cardiologist, and cardiac anesthesiologist are intimately involved in the perioperative management of these patients and it is essential that they be familiar with the many aspects

From Casthely PA, Bregman D, (eds): *Cardiopulmonary Bypass: Physiology, Related Complications, and Pharmacology.* Mount Kisco, NY, Futura Publishing Company, Inc., © 1991.

of their care. This knowledge must include a familiarity with the medical evaluation of a potential recipient and patient selection criteria, an understanding of the anesthetic management intraoperatively and in the postoperative period, as well as a familiarity with the long term complications of transplantation that may be encountered in a cardiac transplant recipient presenting for noncardiac surgery.

The history of heart transplantation began in 1905 when Carrel and Guthrie performed the first heterotopic heart transplant in dogs.[3] Their work showed that transplantation and reliable vascular anastomoses were possible. Over the next 60 years, research conducted by a number of investigators yielded answers to difficulties in surgical technique and myocardial preservation.

The modern era of cardiac transplantation began on December 3, 1967 when Christiaan N. Barnard performed the first successful human heart transplant at Groote Schuur Hospital in Capetown, South Africa. Although his work reawakened a great deal of interest in this field, initial enthusiasm quickly waned due to the disappointing survival of the early recipients. However, at a small number of centers, notably Stanford, continued research in this area during the 1970s yielded the advances in operative technique and immunosuppression that have made heart transplantation standard therapy today.[4]

What Factors are Involved in the Assessment and Selection of a Potential Recipient?

Since transplantation is frequently performed emergently with little time for preoperative assessment, familiarity with the general medical evaluation of potential recipients and the criteria used for their selection are necessary.

It has been reported that the incidence of congestive heart failure in the United States is increasing.[5] Moreover, given the potential 30% to 50% mortality within 1 year of diagnosis shown by recent studies, cardiac transplantation is clearly becoming a therapeutic option for a growing number of patients in this country.[6] In fact, it has been estimated that up to 15,000 transplants could be performed in this country each year.[7] However, the availability of donors is limited; therefore, potential recipients must be subjected to a selection process.

As a result of the large number of patients with "stable" heart failure as well as a typical waiting period of 6 to 9 months before transplantation, attempts have been made to identify those patients with the most limited survival.[8] Unfortunately, there are no reliable indicators of disease progression of congestive heart failure for an individual patient. For instance, Figulla et al. reported that 52% of their patients had stabilization or spontaneous improvement in ventricular function.[9] On the other hand, Massie et al. suggest that 30% to 50% of deaths in patients with heart failure occur suddenly.[6] Despite the apparent complexity of this disease process, recent studies have shown several variables to correlate with survival.

The factors that have been predictive of the most limited survival include abnormal hemodynamics, especially elevated cardiac filling pressures and depressed cardiac output, low ejection fraction, presence of left ventricular hypertrophy, worsening symptoms and exercise tolerance, frequent arrhythmias, activation of the sympathetic nervous system, and a depressed serum sodium.[5,6] For example, Keogh et al. reported a 6-month survival of only 17% in patients with an ejection fraction of less than 10%. Moreover, no patient in their study with an ejection fraction of greater than 20% died within 6 months.[10] In the selection process for a recipient, the above variables are examined in conjunction with the clinical history in order to identify those patients that should receive a high priority for transplantation and whose probable survival is less than 6 months to a year.

Potential recipients are further examined for contraindications that have evolved from clinical experience. Frequently quoted contraindications to transplantation are listed below:[5,7,11]

1. Pulmonary hypertension—Early experience at Stanford revealed that an elevated pulmonary vascular resistance (PVR) was associated with a poor outcome.[12] Although no one value has been selected as a strict guideline, it is generally felt that a PVR of less than 6 Wood units is preferable.[7,13] If the PVR is high, an attempt to determine the reversibility of the elevation with a vasodilator such as nitroprusside is undertaken. A fixed elevation is felt to preclude transplantation although alternatives such as the use of a large donor heart or an

auxillary heterotopic transplant may be considered to prevent right heart failure postoperatively.

2. Pulmonary infarction—Recent pulmonary infarction has been associated with an increased incidence of pulmonary abscess formation after immunosuppression is instituted.[11] Moreover, any undefined pulmonary process should be investigated prior to surgery.
3. Renal or hepatic failure—Cyclosporine-induced nephrotoxicity can be expected to affect virtually all patients to some degree in the postoperative period.[14] Hepatic toxicity is less frequent, but may occur. Therefore, irreversible renal and hepatic failure are strong contraindications to transplantation.
4. Severe hypertension—Virtually all patients receiving cyclosporine will develop significant postoperative hypertension even if none existed beforehand.[15] Severe preoperative hypertension therefore is undesirable.
5. Chronic obstructive pulmonary disease and chronic bronchitis—Pulmonary infections are a leading cause of morbidity and mortality in the transplant recipient. Chronic obstructive pulmonary disease (COPD) and chronic bronchitis are felt to contribute to prolonged weaning from mechanical ventilation in addition to a higher rate of pulmonary infection in the postoperative period.
6. Active infection—Infectious complications are the leading cause of mortality in the immunosuppressed transplant recipient.[1] Therefore, all infectious processes should be resolved prior to transplantation.
7. Vascular disease—Given the side effects of prednisone and cyclosporine, it is likely that cerebrovascular and peripheral vascular disease will progress in the postoperative period. Symptomatic vascular disease is felt to be a strict contraindication, whereas asymptomatic disease is only a relative contraindication.
8. Age—Before the advent of cyclosporine, patients greater than 50 years of age were not considered for transplantation. Now, however, more and more patients greater than age 50 are being transplanted with survival rates at 1 and 5 years comparable to those of younger patients as recently reported by the Registry of the International Society of Heart Transplantation.[16]
9. Diabetes Mellitus—At one time a strict contraindication, diabetes has become a relative one as cyclosporine has allowed

smaller steroid doses to be used in immunosuppressive regimens. Several studies have recently reported similar post-transplant survival in diabetic and nondiabetic patients.[17,18]

10. Cachexia—A state of severe malnutrition has been associated with a higher postoperative mortality.[11]
11. Noncompliance and substance abuse—Cooper et al.[19] have reported that noncompliant behavior is predictive of poorer outcome. Substance abuse and other psychosocial disorders are difficult issues; however, it is generally felt that patients without these problems are better equipped to handle the rigors of transplantation.
12. Malignancy—In general, malignancy and any other illness with a poor prognosis tend to preclude transplantation due to the risk of immunosuppression and the shortage of transplant donors.
13. Peptic ulcer disease—Perioperative stress, infection, and high-dose steroid use may exacerbate underlying peptic ulcer disease (PUD) and result in gastrointestinal bleeding or bowel perforation.
14. Obesity—Complications such as prolonged mechanical ventilation, wound dehiscence, and infection that are frequently seen in obese patients result in a higher perioperative morbidity in this group.
15. Other illnesses—Finally, any illness that may interfere with perioperative management or prolong the recovery phase may be considered a contraindication to transplantation.

Table I summarizes the strict and relative contraindications to transplantation. If a patient without these contraindications is referred for transplantation, a further assessment of their medical status is initiated as outlined in Table II.

Of note, a cardiac catheterization is generally performed in all patients to obtain an endomyocardial biopsy and to define the cardiac anatomy in order to rule out any reversible conditions that could be treated medically or by other cardiac surgery. As noted above, a determination of the pulmonary vascular resistance (PVR) is made, as an elevated PVR has been associated with a poorer surgical outcome.[12] At our institution, a determination of the PVR is made approximately every 6 months.

Critically ill patients with hemodynamic instability are a group that deserves special attention. Decisions whether or not to transplant these patients are frequently difficult. These patients are increasingly encountered as our ability to support them with inotro-

Table I
Strict and Relative Contraindications to Transplantation[5,7,11]

Strict
- Pulmonary hypertension
- Recent pulmonary infarction
- Irreversible renal or hepatic failure
- Symptomatic vascular disease
- Severe hypertension
- Cachexia
- Noncompliant behavior or substance abuse
- COPD and chronic bronchitis
- Ongoing infection
- Malignancy or other illness with poor prognosis

Relative
- Diabetes mellitus
- Peptic ulcer disease
- Extreme age
- Asymptomatic vascular disease
- Diverticulitis
- Obesity

Table II
Medical Evaluation of Potential Recipient[8,20]

1. Initial consultation by cardiologist.
2. Baseline laboratory data including full chemistry panel and hematologic profile, ECG, CXR, and urinalysis.
3. Serologic and culture data including tests for CMV, HSV, HIV, EBV, hepatitis B, varicella, toxoplasma, tuberculosis, and stool ova & parasites.
4. Determination of ABO blood type.
5. Panel reactive antibody screen for hyperacute rejection
6. Pulmonary evaluation with spirometry as well as nuclear scanning or pulmonary angiography as indicated.
7. Cardiac evaluation with echocardiography, nuclear imaging, and exercise testing as indicated.
8. Full cardiac catheterization.
9. Social, dental, and neuropsychiatric evaluations.

pic drugs and mechanical assist devices improves. Moreover, they often have the highest transplant priority.

The use of mechanical assist devices as a bridge to transplantation in the critically ill patient is a recent and exciting field. As of December 31, 1988, the Combined Registry for the Clinical Use of Mechanical Ventricular Assist Pumps and the Total Artificial Heart reported that 219 patients had received such support as a bridge to transplantation. Of those, 73% were eventually transplanted, and 62 percent of the recipients were discharged from the hospital.[21] Assist devices currently in use are of two basic designs: pulsatile flow is provided by pumps that displace blood from a chamber, whereas continuous flow is provided by pumps that propel blood with high-speed rotors. The spectrum of the devices includes the intra-aortic balloon pump commonly in use, the uni- or biventricular assist devices, and finally, the total artificial heart. Despite current limitations imposed by problems such as infection, limb ischemia, bleeding, and thromboembolism, the anesthesiologist may encounter this technology more frequently in the future.[22]

When a potential recipient is selected according to the guidelines outlined above, the transplantation may proceed when a suitable donor is found. A donor should preferably be less than 40 years of age, free of cardiac disease or systemic infection, and compatible in terms of body size, blood type, and cytomegalovirus (CMV) status. Donor selection and management has been reviewed recently by Frist and Fanning.[23]

What are Important Aspects of Intraoperative Anesthetic Care During Transplantation?

At our institution, the first contact between patient and anesthesiologist occurs on the day of surgery. Often the patient has been alerted to report to the hospital within hours of the proposed surgery. Other patients—usually those with more advanced cardiac failure—are already inpatients.

Initial assessment is directed at obtaining a brief history concerning the extent of symptoms of heart failure. It is particularly important to identify the subset of patients who have underlying coronary artery disease. In addition, the most recent cardiac catheterization results must be checked to determine pulmonary pressures and ejection fraction. Arterial blood gases are the simplest way to evaluate pulmonary function in the setting of a failing heart.

We routinely discuss the outlines of the anesthetic plan with our patients and familiarize them with the need for postoperative ventilation. Although these patients are among the best informed surgical patients, we never forget the extreme stress placed on these patients when the time for surgery is approaching.

We place two large bore peripheral intravenous lines and a radial arterial line in all patients. We also routinely place pulmonary artery (PA) catheters in all patients. Although there is some debate concerning the need for PA lines before bypass,[24] we feel that the enhanced ability to maintain ideal preload outweighs the risk of infection. In addition, if the patient has elevated pulmonary pressures, we attempt to keep these pressures as low as possible with an infusion of nitroglycerine, nitroprusside, and/or dobutamine prior to cardiopulmonary bypass (CPB). If the timing of the arrival of the donor heart requires an urgent start to surgery, we will place the PA line as soon as is practical following induction.

Our choice of anesthetic technique reflects the underlying pathology. These patients are all suffering from heart failure. It is important to keep in mind certain aspects of the pathophysiology of this disease. A defect in myocardial contraction results in three primary compensatory mechanisms to maintain cardiac output:[25] (1) augmentation of blood volume leading to increased preload and improved cardiac output by virtue of the Frank-Starling mechanism, (2) increased sympathetic stimulation resulting in improved inotropy, and (3) myocardial hypertrophy. Of course, when these mechanisms are overwhelmed by the extent of myocardial disease, clinical heart failure becomes evident. Unfortunately, the anesthesiologist's options for manipulating these variables intraoperatively are limited.

The patient in heart failure maintains cardiac output by increasing end diastolic volume. The Frank-Starling curve of the failing heart, however, is typically flattened and cardiac reserve is generally not available for improving output by adjusting preload.[26] Thus, unless a patient presents with intravascular volume depletion secondary to diuretic therapy, it is unlikely that fluid administration will improve cardiac output in a patient with marginal hemodynamics. The patient may, in fact, be able to increase his cardiac output only through the mechanism of increased heart rate.[27] At the same time, failure to maintain adequate preload can result in a precipitous drop in cardiac output and must be avoided. An important caveat is that patients with dilated cardiomyopathies often have a rightward shift of their left ventricular passive volume-pressure curves.[28] This can lead to an underestimation of end diastolic volume when using LVEDP as a gauge of preload.

The impaired contractility that results in the flattened shape of the Frank-Starling curve also limits the response of the myocardium to inotropic agents. The dramatic leftward shift of the Frank-Starling curve seen in the normal heart with the administration of inotropic agents is not attainable with the failing heart.[25] Adding to this problem is the abnormal response of the failing heart to endogenous and exogenous catecholamines. In heart failure, there is a persistent increase in levels of circulating catecholamines that results in the down-regulation of β receptors.[29] The patient thus has an abnormally depressed response to stress.[30] In addition, the response to exogenous inotropic agents, almost all of which are mediated by β receptor stimulation, is decreased. Therefore, the anesthesiologist must anticipate an impaired response to the addition of inotropic agents, and any inotropic agents the patient is receiving must be continued until CPB.

These pathophysiological considerations have led us to adopt a technique of high-dose narcotic anesthesia for our transplant patients. We seek to avoid agents that will depress contractility, heart rate, or that will increase afterload. We typically administer either fentanyl (50–100 μg/kg) or sufentanil (15–20 μg/kg) along with a paralyzing dose of vecuronium (0.2 mg/kg). Pancuronium or atropine is used to maintain heart rate if bradycardia develops after narcotic administration. Small doses of diazepam are typically added, however, because of the hypotension seen when adding benzodiazepines to high dose narcotics,[31] this is done slowly and cautiously. If cardiac output is marginal and preload manipulation does not produce adequate hemodynamics, an inotrope is promptly added. We prefer dobutamine because it increases inotropy without increasing afterload.[32]

A brief comment should be made concerning those patients with a full stomach. It is not infrequent that a patient arrives in the operating room having recently eaten. While we recognize that there may be a small increase in the risk of aspiration,[24] we do not adopt a full rapid sequence procedure. Rather, we proceed with a slow narcotic induction with administration of succinylcholine as the patient loses consciousness. Cricoid pressure with positive pressure ventilation by mask is maintained as additional narcotic is administered. The endotracheal tube is placed only when the hemodynamic response to intubation is felt to be adequately blunted.

Following the institution of cardiopulmonary bypass, the heart is arrested and cooled, and attention is then directed to assuring that adequate levels of anesthesia and muscle relaxation are maintained. After completion of the surgical anastamoses and rewarming of the transplanted heart, efforts are now directed at restoring electrical activity to the heart. Prior to the release of the cross clamp, lidocaine (1.5 mg/kg) is administered, and the heart is defibrillated as needed. The goal of therapy is to achieve a sinus rhythm at a rate of 110–120 beats/min. This requires the administration, in virtually every case, of isoproterenol (.05–.15 μg/kg/min). Because of the impaired automaticity of the heart, only rarely is the isoproterenol ever totally discontinued during the first 72 hours. If turned off because of excessive heart rate, it is always left attached to the patients central line. We also routinely begin an infusion of dopamine (3–5 μg/kg/min) to augment cardiac contractility.

In addition to the usual criteria for separation from bypass, three key considerations must be kept in mind. First, although the donor heart should ultimately have near-normal cardiac function,[33] it has just undergone a period of up to 5 hours of global ischemia intraoperatively. Depressed response to preload and inotropic agents is to be expected.[34] Because these ventricles have a leftward shift of their compliance curves, higher than normal filling pressures will be needed to maintain adequate end diastolic volume. The transplanted heart is also abnormal in its response to stress. Normal patients initially increase cardiac output by increasing heart rate, while only later raising end diastolic volume and stroke volume through a Frank-Starling mechanism.[35] Pope et al.[36] have shown that the denervated heart, on the other hand, relies primarily on a Frank-Starling mechanism to maintain cardiac output, with changes in heart rate occurring later as serum catecholamines rise.[36] This again stresses the need to maintain adequate cardiac filling post-CPB.

A second important consideration is that the transplanted heart is denervated. Although β receptors of the transplanted heart will respond to circulating catecholamines and exogenously administered agents, the heart is free of any direct autonomic influence and lacks the ability to alter its performance through autonomic reflex pathways.[37] This has an important effect on the selection of agents for use post-CPB. In general, only drugs that have some direct effect upon myocardial receptors are useful. Epinephrine, isoproterenol, and propranolol produce clinical effects similar to those seen in normal hearts.[38] Norepinephrine, however, raises heart rate through a direct β effect on the donor sinus node, an effect that is suppressed in the normal heart by a baroreceptor response to rising blood pressure.[39] Dopamine and ephedrine exert their effects directly as well through indirect catecholamine release; they have both been shown to produce essentially normal drug responses in the transplanted heart.[40] Although there is some concern about and evidence for a denervation hypersensitivity to cathecholamines in the transplanted heart, the clinical significance of this is unclear.[35,39]

Drugs that solely act through an indirect autonomic mechanism would be expected to have no effect on the denervated heart. Therefore, drugs such as atropine, pancuronium, and the anticholinesterases will have no effect on heart rate.[41] Drugs that possess both direct and autonomic modes of action will exert only their direct effect. Thus, digoxin has no effect on heart rate, but may maintain its positive inotropic effect.[35] In addition, quinidine and disopyramide produce a paradoxical slowing of the heart rate in the transplanted heart resulting from their direct effects as well the absence of their vagolytic effects.[35] Verapamil does appear to directly decrease sinus rate and AV node conduction in the denervated heart; nifedepine, on the other hand, appears to have little effect on heart rate, as its usual acceleration of heart rate is primarily autonomically mediated.[35,39,42]

The third important consideration upon separating from bypass is the danger of right heart failure. In our experience, this is the most common cause of failure to separate from the pump. Right heart failure appears to be secondary to increased pulmonary pressures. Whether these increased pressures reflect preexisting disease or a response to bypass is unclear.[43] What is certain is that the signs of right heart failure, e.g., increasing CVP, decreased CO, and hypotension, must be treated aggressively. We initially treat this condition with pulmonary vasodilators and inotropes; we prefer a combination of dobutamine and nitroglycerine.[44] If this combination is unsuccessful, or if systemic hypotension is a limiting factor, we administer nitroglycerine directly into the pulmonary artery while giving norepinephrine through a left atrial line. We also administer prostaglandin E_1 (30–150 ng/kg/min) when further therapy is needed.[43]

What are Important Aspects of the Operative Technique for Orthotopic Transplantation?

After all monitoring lines are placed, and the patient is anesthetized as described in the previous section, a median sternotomy is performed and preparation is made for the institution of cardiopulmonary bypass (CPB). If there is a markedly enlarged heart, tenuous hemodynamic status, or history of previous cardiac surgery, a femoral artery and vein should be noted or isolated preoperatively so that femoral-femoral bypass can be initiated promptly in the event of hemodynamic deterioration or bleeding after sternotomy. Once the chest is open, the aortic and venous cannulae are placed in the usual fashion for CPB. However, in order to preserve a large cuff of atrial tissue for anastomosis to the donor heart, the venous cannulae are placed directly into the caval vessels or into the posterior right atrium near the orifice of the vena cava. Only when the donor heart is in the vicinity of the recipient hospital is total CPB initiated and systematic cooling to 28–30 °C begun. In order to limit the ischemic time of the donor heart to under 4 hours and to minimize the duration of CPB, cardiectomy begins prior to the arrival of the donor heart in the operating room.

After the aorta has been cross clamped and the native heart further decompressed by a left ventricular vent, excision of the native heart takes place, leaving behind large cuffs of right and left posterior atrial tissue with the interatrial septum and pulmonary venous system intact (as shown in Figure 1). Long cuffs of aorta and pulmonary artery are also preserved.[45] The use of a left atrial cuff was first described by Goldberg *et al.* in 1988, and the creation of a right atrial cuff was reported by Cass and Brock in 1959.[3,4] These techniques greatly simplified the pulmonary venous and caval anastomoses. Finally, prior to the implantation of the donor

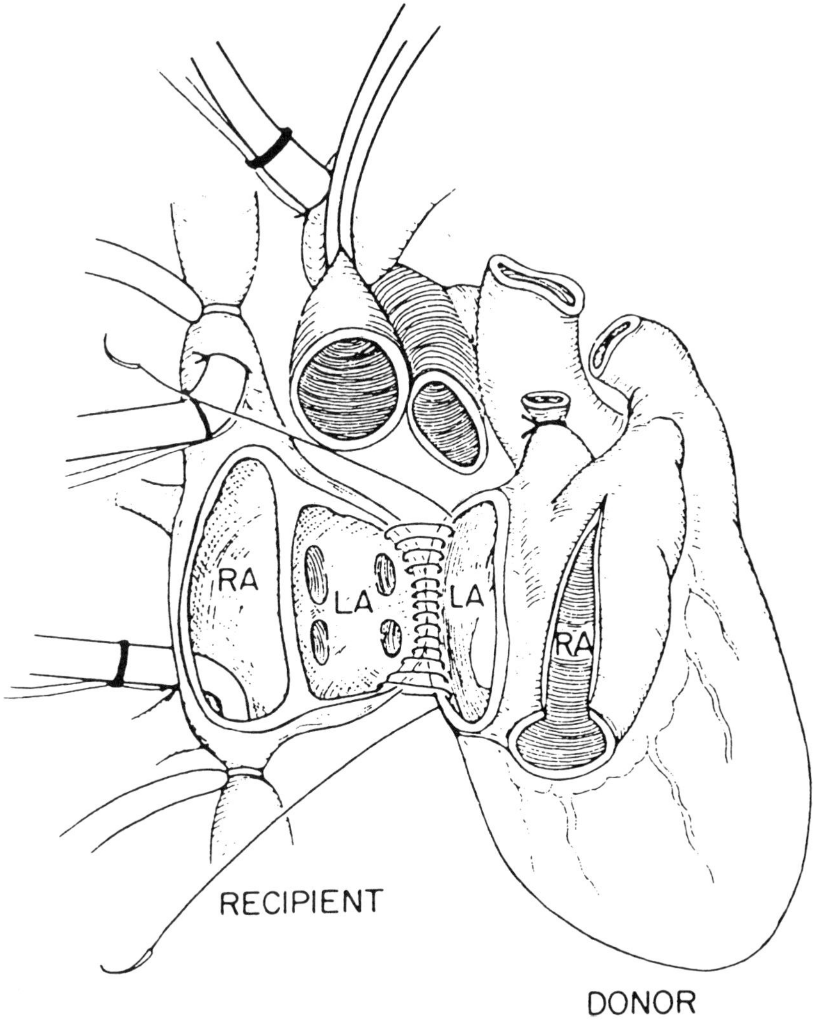

Figure 1. The anastomosis of the donor and recipient hearts. (Reproduced with permission from Bolman RM III. Cardiac transplantation: the operative technique. *Cardiovasc Clin* 20(2):133-145, 1990.)

heart, the aorta and pulmonary artery are separated carefully with electrocautery.

On arrival, the donor heart is kept in saline solution at 4 °C and prepared for implantation. First, the donor aorta and pulmonary artery are carefully separated, and the donor superior vena cava is ligated. At this point, an anastomotic site for the recipient left atrial cuff is created by removing that portion of the posterior donor left atrium that contains the pulmonary veins. An incision is then made from the inferior vena cava orifice toward the right atrial appendage to create an opening that will correspond to the recipient right atrial cuff. Care is taken to avoid harm to the donor sinoatrial node, which is in this region. The donor heart is also inspected at this time and any septal defects are oversewn if present.

The implantation of the donor heart is performed with continuous running sutures beginning at the left atria. The order of subsequent anastomoses is generally as follows: pulmonary arteries, segment of the right atria, aortas, and then the remainder of the right atria. During the anastamosis of the pulmonary arteries, the Swan-Ganz catheter is passed through the donor heart and placed into the recipient pulmonary artery. If the ischemic time of the donor heart is prolonged, the aortic anastomosis may be performed after the left atrial one. This maneuver, although more technically difficult, allows the aortic cross clamp to be removed and reperfusion of the donor heart to take place during the subsequent anastomoses.

Throughout the procedure, the donor heart is frequently bathed with iced saline at 4 °C. This may be done via pericardial lavage or through an additional line placed in the left atrial appendage. At the completion of the anastomosis, air is carefully removed from the new heart, and attention is directed to hemostasis. While systemic rewarming is being completed, the transplanted heart is usually given a significant period of reperfusion to ensure uniform warming, repletion of energy stores, and elimination of cardioplegia. Finally, temporary pacing wires are placed and separation from CPB proceeds as outlined previously.[45]

What are the Management Goals in the Immediate Postoperative Period?

First, rapid extubation is usually desirable on the first postoperative day to minimize the chance of pulmonary infection. Secondly, discontinuation of all invasive catheters is achieved as quickly as possible for the same reason. Weaning of pressor support is also begun; however, an isoproterenol infusion is usually continued for several days because junctional rhythms and bradycardias are quite common during this period. In fact, 5% to 15% of patients will go on to require permanent pacing.[7] Finally, immunosuppression is begun at this time if not done preoperatively. Most immunosuppression regimens utilize a combination of azathioprine, prednisone, and cyclosporine in order to provide an adequate level of immunosuppression while limiting the toxicities of each drug. With this triple drug approach, first tried at the University of Minnesota in 1981, survival has improved to 81.9% at 5 years, as reported by Heck et al. in the 1989 report of The Registry of the International Society for Heart Transplantation.[1]

What are the Most Common Complications of the Immediate Postsurgical Period?

Although infection and rejection are ever present concerns, their incidence is the highest during the first 3 months after surgery.[7] In the past, rejection of the donor heart was diagnosed by clinical findings such as fever, signs of congestive failure, friction rubs, arrhythmias, and reduced voltage on the electrocardiogram. A much more accurate method was provided by the technique of transvenous endomyocardial biopsy and the histologic grading system of rejection introduced by Caves and Billingham in the 1970s.[46,47] With these advances came the realization that many episodes of rejection under cyclosporine were clinically silent. For this reason, patients today undergo surveillance for rejection with periodic transvenous biopsies. If rejection is detected, it is classified as mild, moderate, or severe depending on the histological findings. The decision to treat a rejection episode is based on the histology and evidence of ventricular dysfunction. Augmentation of immunosuppression usually involves a short trial of high-dose steroids, while anti-T cell therapy with ATG/ALG or OKT_3 antibodies is usually reserved for severe episodes. At present, noninvasive methods to detect rejection, such as the use of Doppler echocardiography, are being investigated; none, however, has replaced the endomyocardial biopsy.[48]

In addition to rejection, infection is a major early complication following transplantation. In 1982, Pennock et al.[49] reported that infections were responsible for 58% of the deaths in transplant patients over a 13-year period. The lungs are the most commonly involved organ; and bacteria, notably the staphylococcus and gram-negative organisms, are the most common pathogens in the immediate postoperative period.[7] Many pulmonary infections may be asymptomatic until quite advanced; therefore, surveillance with frequent chest radiographs is an integral part of postoperative care. Opportunistic infections with viral, fungal, and protozoal organisms are seen to a lesser degree but are by no means rare. Typical opportunistic pathogens include herpes simplex virus (HSV), CMV, aspergillus, cryptococcus, pneumocystis, toxoplasma, and nocardia. With the introduction of cyclosporine and the widespread use of triple drug immunosuppression, the incidence of and the mortality from infection have been reduced.[50]

What are the Longer Term Complications?

Although many patients suffer from hypertension and progressive renal failure secondary to immunosuppressive therapy, perhaps the most interesting long-term complication is accelerated allograft atherosclerosis. This entity has been reported to have an incidence of 40% at 5 years after surgery.[2] The etiology of this process is not well understood; however, it is generally felt that traditional risk factors for coronary artery disease (CAD) are not primarily responsible, but rather that they are superimposed upon a process of immunologic endothelial injury resulting from ongoing rejection. The distribution of allograft coronary artery disease (CAD) distinguishes itself from traditional atherosclerosis in that it is a diffuse concentric process involving both the large epicardial arteries and the smaller intramyocardial arterioles without the benefit of collateral vessels.[51] For this reason, traditional therapies of percutaneous transluminal angioplasty (PTA) and coronary artery bypass grafting (CABG) are usually ineffective and only retransplantation remains a viable option with a 1-year survival rate of

55%.[52] As a result of the denervation of the donor heart, these patients do not present with anginal pain, but rather with sudden death or worsening heart failure. Efforts to combat the progression of this disease have included intensification of immunosuppression, modification of traditional risk factors for CAD, reduction in steroid doses, and anticoagulation. Attempts at earlier diagnosis have included periodic screening with tests of ventricular function and coronary angiography.[51]

REFERENCES

1. Heck CF, Shumway SJ, Kaye MP. The registry of the international society for heart transplantation: sixth official report—1989. *J Heart Transplant* 8(4):271-6, 1989.
2. Hunt SA, Schroeder JS. Managing patients after cardiac transplantation. *Hosp Prac* 24(10):83-7, 90-6, 99-100, 1989.
3. Lansman SL, Ergin MA, Griepp RB. The history of heart and heart-lung transplantation. *Cardiovasc Clin* 20(2):3-19, 1990.
4. McGregor, CG. Evolution of heart transplantation. *Cardiol Clin* 8(1):3-10, 1990.
5. Vagelos R, Fowler MB. Selection of patients for cardiac transplantation. *Cardiol Clin* 8(1):23-38, 1990.
6. Massie BM, Conway M. Survival of patients with congestive heart failure: past, present, and future prospects. *Circulation* 75(Suppl IV):IV-11-IV-19, 1987.
7. Shimon DV, Admon D, Zilberman S, et al. Heart transplantation-state of the art. *Isr J Med Sci* 25(10):575-82, 1989.
8. Jessup M, Brozena SC. Identification and management of potential heart transplant recipients. *Cardiol Clin* 8(1): 11-21, 1990.
9. Figulla HR, Rahlf G, Nieger M, et al. Spontaneous hemodynamic improvement or stabilization and associated biopsy findings in patients with congestive cardiomyopathy. *Circulation* 71(6):1095-1104, 1985.
10. Keogh AM, Freund J, Baron DW, et al. Timing of cardiac transplantation in idiopathic dilated cardiomyopathy. *Am J Cardiol* 61:418-22, 1988.
11. Hastillo A, Hess ML. Selection of patients for cardiac transplantation. *Cardiovasc Clin* 20(2):107-20, 1990.
12. Griepp RB, Stinson EB, Dong E Jr, et al. Determinants of operative risk in human heart transplantation. *Am J Surg* 122:192-7, 1971.
13. Ream AK, Fowles RE, Jamieson S. Cardiac Transplantation. In: Kaplan JA, ed. *Cardiac Anesthesia.* Orlando, FL: Grune and Stratton; 1987:881-891.
14. Greenberg A, Egel JW, Thompson ME, et al. Early and late forms of cyclosporine nephrotoxicity: Studies in cardiac transplant recipients. *Am J Kidney Dis* 9(1):12-22, 1987.

15. Olivari MT, Antolick A, Ring WS. Arterial hypertension in heart transplant recipients treated with triple-drug immunosuppressive therapy. *J Heart Transplant* 8(1):34-9, 1989.
16. Kaye MP. The Registry of the International Society for Heart Transplantation: Fourth Official Report—1987. *J Heart Transplant* 6(2):63-7, 1987.
17. Gradinac S, Frazier OH, VanBuren CT, et al. Heart transplants in diabetic patients (abstract). *Circulation* 78(Suppl II):A1003, 1988.
18. Rhenman MJ, Rhenman B, Icenogle T, et al. Diabetes and heart transplantation. *J Heart Transplant* 7(5):356-8, 1988.
19. Cooper DKC, Lanza RP, Barnard CN. Noncompliance in heart transplant recipients: the Cape Town experience. *Heart Transplant* 3:248-53, 1984.
20. Nieminen MS. Evaluation and selection of the heart transplantation patient. *Transplant Proc* 22(1): 186-7, 1990.
21. Pae WE, Miller CA, Pierce WS. Combined registry for the clinical use of mechanical ventricular assist pumps and the total artificial heart: third official report—1988. *J Heart Transplant* 8(4):277-80, 1989.
22. Macoviak JA, Dasse KA, Poirier VL. Mechanical cardiac assistance and replacement. *Cardiol Clin* 8(1):39-53, 1990.
23. Frist WH, Fanning WJ. Donor management and matching. *Cardiol Clin* 8(1):55-71, 1990.
24. Hensley FA, Martin DE, Larach DR, et al. Anesthetic management for cardiac transplantation in North America—1986 survey. *J Cardiothorac Anesth* 1:427-9, 1987.
25. Braunwald E. Pathophysiology of heart failure. In: Braunwald E, ed. *Heart Disease.* Philadelphia, PA: W.B. Saunders; 1987:447-50.
26. Weber KT, Janicki JS. The heart as a muscle-pump system and the concept of heart failure. *Am Heart J* 98:371-84, 1979.
27. Parmely WW. Pathophysiology of congestive heart failure. *Am J Cardiol* 56:7A-11A, 1985.
28. Braunwald E, Ross J. The ventricular end-diastolic pressure: appraisal of its value in the recognition of ventricular failure in man. *Am Med J* 34:147, 1963.
29. Fowler MB, Laser JA, Hopkins GL, et al. Assessment of the β-adrenergic receptor pathway in the intact failing human heart: progressive receptor down-regulation and subsensitivity to agonist response. *Circulation* 74:1290-1302, 1982.
30. Wyands JE, Wong P, Whaley DG, et al. Oxygen-fentanyl anesthesia in patients with poor ventricular function. *Anesth Analg* 62:476-82, 1983.
31. Tomicheck RC, Rosow CE, Keegan CR, et al. Diazepam-fentanyl interaction: hemodynamic and hormonal effects in coronary artery surgery. *Anesth Analg* 62:881-4, 1983.
32. Leier CV, Heban PT, Huss P. Comparative systemic and regional hemodynamic effects of dopamine and dobutamine in patients with cardiomyopathic heart failure. *Circulation* 58:466-75, 1978.

33. Borow KM, Neumann A, Arensman FW, et al. Left ventricular contractility and contractile reserve in humans after cardiac transplantation. *Circulation* 71:866-72, 1985.
34. Steen PA, Tinker JH, Pluth JR, et al. Efficacy of dopamine, dobutamine, and epinephrine during emergence from cardiopulmonary bypass in man. *Circulation* 57:378-84, 1978.
35. Uretsky BF. Physiology of the transplanted heart. *Cardiovasc Clin* 20(2): 23-56, 1990.
36. Pope SE, Stinson EB, Daughters GT II, et al. Exercise response of the denervated heart in long-term cardiac transplant recipients. *Am J Cardiol* 46:213-18, 1980.
37. Stinson EB, Griepp RB, Schroeder JS, et al. Hemodynamic observations one and two years after cardiac transplantation. *Circulation* 45:1183-91, 1972.
38. Cannon DS, Rider AK, Stinson EB, et al. Electrophysiologic studies in the denervated transplanted human heart. II. Response to norepinephrine, isoproterenol and propranolol. *Am J Cardiol* 36:859-66, 1975.
39. Firestone L. Autonomic influences on cardiac function: lessons from the transplanted (denervated) heart. *Int Anesth Clin* 27(4): 283-91, 1989.
40. Kanter SF, Samuels SI. Anesthesia for major operations on patients who have transplanted hearts, a review of 29 cases. *Anesthesiology* 46:65-8, 1977.
41. Cooper DKC, Becerra EA, Novitsky D, et al. Surgery in patients with heart transplants. *S Afr Med J* 70(3):137-42, 1986.
42. Bexton R, Nathan AW, Cory-Pearce R, et al. Electrophysiologic effects of nifedipine and verapamil in the transplanted human heart. *J Heart Transplant* 3:97-104, 1984.
43. Fonger JD, Borkon AM, Baumgartner WA, et al. Acute right ventricular failure following heart transplantation: improvement with prostaglandin E_1 and right ventricular assist. *J Heart Transplant* 5:317-21, 1986.
44. Ziskind, Z, Pohoryles L, Mohr R, et al. The effect of low-dose intravenous nitroglycerin on pulmonary hypertension immediately after replacement of a stenotic mitral valve. *Circulation* 72:164-9, 1985.
45. Bolman RM, III. Cardiac transplantation: the operative technique. *Cardiovasc Clin* 20(2):133-145, 1990.
46. Caves PK, Billingham ME, Schulz WP, et al. Transvenous biopsy from canine orthopic heart allografts. *Am Heart J* 85(4):525-30, 1973.
47. Caves PK, Billingham ME, Stinson EB, et al. Serial transvenous biopsy of the transplanted human heart: improved management of acute rejection episodes. *Lancet* 1:821-6, 1974.
48. O'Connell JB, Renlund DG. Diagnosis and treatment of cardiac allograft rejection. *Cardiovasc Clin* 20(2):147-62, 1990.
49. Pennock JL, Oyer PE, Reitz BA, et al. Cardiac transplantation in perspective for the future. *J Thoracic Cardiovasc Surg* 83:168-77, 1982.
50. Linder J. Infection as a complication of heart transplantation. *J Heart Transplant* 7(5):390-4, 1988.

51. Eich DM, Johnson DE, Hastillo A, et al. Accelerated coronary atherosclerosis in cardiac transplantation. *Cardiovasc Clin* 20(2):199-211, 1990.
52. Gao SZ, Schroeder JS, Hunt S, et al. Retransplantation for severe accelerated coronary artery disease in heart transplant recipients. *Am J Cardiol* 62:876-81, 1988.

Index